Ultrasonography of the Pancreas

Mirko D'Onofrio

Ultrasonography of the Pancreas

Imaging and Pathologic Correlations

Foreword by
Claudio Bassi
Paolo Pederzoli

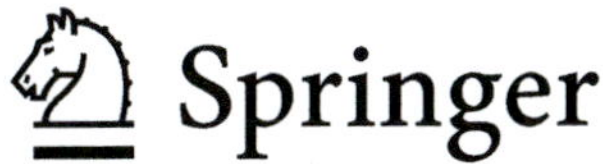
Springer

Editor
Mirko D'Onofrio
Department of Radiology
G.B. Rossi University Hospital
Verona, Italy

ISBN 978-88-470-2378-9
e-ISBN 978-88-470-2379-6

DOI 10.1007/978-88-470-2379-6

Springer Milan Dordrecht Heidelberg London New York

Library of Congress Control Number: 2011939492

9 8 7 6 5 4 3 2 1
2012 2013 2014

Cover design: Ikona S.r.l., Milan, Italy
Typesetting: Ikona S.r.l., Milan, Italy

Springer-Verlag Italia S.r.l. – Via Decembrio 28 – I-20137 Milan
Springer is a part of Springer Science+Business Media

To my Family
"…l'amor che move il sole e l'altre stelle."
Dante Alighieri. Divina Commedia, Paradiso, XXXIII Canto.

To my Friends
"If the doors of perception were cleansed everything
would appear to man as it is, infinite."
William Blake. The marriage of heaven and hell.

Foreword

It is with great enthusiasm and true pleasure that we commend this book to the attention of our colleagues.

In high-volume institutions, such as the Pancreas Center in Verona, ultrasonography plays an extremely important role in the study of pancreatic pathologies. This carefully assembled and up-to-date work on the topic will be very useful not only for radiologists but also for gastroenterologists, surgeons, oncologists and intensive care doctors!

In many applications, ultrasonography findings are now comparable to the results achieved with multidetector computed tomography (MCT); furthermore, in some specific applications, such as guidance of diagnostic interventional procedures, ultrasonography is preferable to both MCT and magnetic resonance imaging because it is faster, easier and cheaper to carry out.

Ultrasonography performed upon hospital admission or during consultation allows immediate confirmation of the presence of a pancreatic disease (in particular a tumour mass), assessment of surgical resectability and detection of liver involvement. Moreover, in non-resectable masses, ultrasound-guided percutaneous fine-needle aspiration with immediate cytological reading will give a definitive diagnosis within a few hours, and it is to be kept in mind that in experienced hands more than ten such procedures can be performed each half day.

Mirko D'Onofrio from the Radiological Department of our University Hospital is a skilled radiologist who focusses in particular on the use of ultrasonography. The work he carries out in this field is of extreme importance in planning our clinical pathways for the diagnosis and therapy of pancreatic diseases. On account of his enthusiasm and his continuous efforts to exploit the new technologies applicable in ultrasonography (in particular the use of ultrasound contrast media), the above-mentioned key features of ultrasonography are determinant factors in meeting our everyday needs, as surgeons, in staging patients suffering from pancreatic tumours.

This book presents the results that can now be achieved with ultrasonography of the pancreas in the hope that it will encourage wider use of this readily available and accurate imaging method for the study of pancreatic pathology.

Prof. Claudio Bassi
Prof. Paolo Pederzoli
Department of Surgery
G.B. Rossi University Hospital
Verona, Italy

Preface

Ultrasonography (US) of the pancreas is, in many cases, the initial imaging modality in most institutions to evaluate pancreatic pathologies and clinical symptoms which may be related to pancreatic diseases. However, the role of US of the pancreas is often questioned because the results of this examination are quite variable and not reproducible by different operators. The main reasons for this disagreement are variable operator experience, patient-related problems, e.g. meteorism and obesity, and/or low contrast and spatial resolution. However, many of these limitations have been overcome by technological advances in US which have had an extremely positive impact on the study of the pancreas, as in other organs.

Significant advances have been achieved in conventional, harmonic and Doppler imaging. Nowadays all portions of the normal pancreas can be visualized in the great majority of cases. Peri-pancreatic vessels are adequately visualized with conventional and Doppler imaging or with new advanced techniques. Therefore pancreatic pathologies can be adequately examined and pancreatic tumours, even if very small in diameter (e.g. insulinoma), can be detected with increased accuracy.

Contrast media have received growing attention in ultrasonography, with special emphasis on liver studies, where contrast-enhanced ultrasonography (CEUS) has become a well-established imaging modality. In the pancreas the contribution of contrast media in detecting and characterizing both solid and cystic exocrine or endocrine pancreatic neoplasms is increasing.

Furthermore, the applications of and indications for interventional, endoscopic and intraoperative US have increased significantly in recent years owing to technological advances.

All these new applications of US are extensively reviewed in this book in order to provide the reader with an up-to-date overview of modern imaging of the pancreas.

The book is organized into 14 chapters. Technical issues concerning modern US imaging, image-guided biopsy, endoscopic US, interventional US-guided procedures and intraoperative US are first addressed. An interesting chapter is then included on normal anatomy, including variants and pseudolesions of the pancreas. Thereafter a series of chapters are dedicated to pancreatic pathologies, namely pancreatitis, solid and cystic tumours, and rare pancreatic tumours, which are presented with emphasis on the imaging and pathologic correlation. Finally the role of US is discussed in the different flowcharts.

The book is supported by a large number of figures of excellent quality obtained with up-to-date US equipment and correlated with the findings of other imaging modalities, providing a complete overview of the present status and the real possibilities of modern US of the pancreas.

Prof. Roberto Pozzi Mucelli
Department of Radiology
G.B. Rossi University Hospital
Verona, Italy

Contents

1 Ultrasound Imaging 1
Anna Gallotti and Fabrizio Calliada

2 Transabdominal Ultrasonography of the Pancreas 17
Elisabetta Buscarini and Salvatore Greco

3 Endoscopic Ultrasonography of the Pancreas 31
Elisabetta Buscarini and Stefania De Lisi

**4 Percutaneous Ultrasound Guided Interventional Procedures
in Pancreatic Diseases** 47
Elisabetta Buscarini and Guido Manfredi

5 Intraoperative Ultrasonography of the Pancreas 55
Mirko D'Onofrio, Emilio Barbi, Riccardo De Robertis,
Francesco Principe, Anna Gallotti and Enrico Martone

6 Pancreatic Anatomy, Variants and Pseudolesions of the Pancreas 63
Emilio Barbi, Salvatore Sgroi, Paolo Tinazzi, Stefano Canestrini,
Anna Gallotti and Mirko D'Onofrio

7 Pancreatitis and Pseudocysts 83
Steffen Rickes and Holger Neye

8 Solid Pancreatic Tumors 93
Christoph F. Dietrich, Michael Hocke, Anna Gallotti and Mirko D'Onofrio

9 Cystic Pancreatic Tumors 111
Mirko D'Onofrio, Paolo Giorgio Arcidiacono and Massimo Falconi

10 Rare Pancreatic Tumors 135
Roberto Malagò, Ugolino Alfonsi, Camilla Barbiani, Andrea Pezzato
and Roberto Pozzi Mucelli

11 Imaging Correlation 147
Marie-Pierre Vullierme and Enrico Martone

12 Pancreatic Lesions: Pathologic Correlations 165
Paola Capelli and Alice Parisi

13 Clinical and Imaging Scenarios 187
Anna Gallotti and Riccardo Manfredi

14 Flowcharts in Pancreatic Diseases 191
Elisabetta Buscarini

Subject Index 199

Contributors

Ugolino Alfonsi Department of Radiology, G.B. Rossi University Hospital, Verona, Italy

Paolo Giorgio Arcidiacono Gastroenterology and Gastrointestinal Endoscopy Unit, Vita Salute San Raffaele University, San Raffaele Scientific Institute, Milan, Italy

Emilio Barbi Department of Radiology, Hospital "Casa di Cura Pederzoli", Peschiera del Garda (VR), Italy

Camilla Barbiani Department of Radiology, G.B. Rossi University Hospital, Verona, Italy

Elisabetta Buscarini Department of Gastroenterology, Maggiore Hospital, Crema, Italy

Fabrizio Calliada Department of Radiology, IRCCS Policlinico S. Matteo, Pavia, Italy

Stefano Canestrini Department of Radiology, G.B. Rossi University Hospital, Verona, Italy

Paola Capelli Department of Pathology, G.B. Rossi University Hospital, Verona, Italy

Stefania De Lisi Department of Endoscopy, European Institute of Oncology (IEO), Milan, Italy

Riccardo De Robertis Department of Radiology, G.B. Rossi University Hospital, Verona, Italy

Christoph F. Dietrich Department of Clinical Medicine, Caritas-Krankenhaus, Bad Mergentheim, Germany

Mirko D'Onofrio Department of Radiology, G.B. Rossi University Hospital, Verona, Italy

Massimo Falconi Department of Surgery, G.B. Rossi University Hospital, Verona, Italy

Anna Gallotti Department of Radiology, IRCCS Policlinico S. Matteo, Pavia, Italy

Salvatore Greco Department of Gastroenterology, Riuniti Hospital, Bergamo, Italy

Michael Hocke Department of Clinical Medicine, Caritas-Krankenhaus, Bad Mergentheim, Germany

Roberto Malagò Department of Radiology, G.B. Rossi University Hospital, Verona, Italy

Guido Manfredi Department of Gastroenterology, Maggiore Hospital, Crema, Italy

Riccardo Manfredi Department of Radiology, G.B. Rossi University Hospital, Verona, Italy

Enrico Martone Department of Radiology, G.B. Rossi University Hospital, Verona, Italy

Holger Neye Department of Internal Medicine, AMEOS Hospital St. Salvator, Halberstadt, Germany

Alice Parisi Department of Pathology, G.B. Rossi University Hospital, Verona, Italy

Andrea Pezzato Department of Radiology, G.B. Rossi University Hospital, Verona, Italy

Roberto Pozzi Mucelli Department of Radiology, G.B. Rossi University Hospital, Verona, Italy

Francesco Principe Department of Radiology, G.B. Rossi University Hospital, Verona, Italy

Steffen Rickes Department of Internal Medicine, AMEOS Hospital St. Salvator, Halberstadt, Germany

Salvatore Sgroi Department of Radiology, Hospital "Casa di Cura Pederzoli", Peschiera del Garda (VR), Italy

Paolo Tinazzi Department of Radiology, Hospital "Casa di Cura Pederzoli", Peschiera del Garda (VR), Italy

Marie-Pierre Vullierme Department of Radiology, Beaujon Hospital, Clichy, Paris, France

Ultrasound Imaging

Anna Gallotti and Fabrizio Calliada

1.1 Introduction

Ultrasonography (US) is usually the first imaging modality chosen for the primary evaluation of the pancreas. The pancreatic gland can almost always be visualized by US. Even though there are well-known and sometimes over-emphasized limitations, the pancreatic gland can be adequately visualized by using correct US techniques, imaging and settings. Conventional US is a noninvasive and relatively low cost imaging method which is widely available and easy to perform. Tissue harmonic imaging (THI) and Doppler imaging are well known technologies that provide significant complementary information to the conventional method, playing an important role in the diagnosis and staging of pancreatic diseases. In recent decades, new interesting US methods have been developed focused on the evaluation of mechanical strain properties of tissues, such as elastography and sonoelasticity. Acoustic radiation force impulse (ARFI) imaging is a promising new US method that allows the evaluation of mechanical strain properties of deep tissues with the potential to characterize tissue without the need for external compression. Contrast-enhanced ultrasonography (CEUS) advances the accuracy of this first line examination by characterizing focal solid and cystic lesions and providing an accurate real-time evaluation of macro- and microcirculation in and around a focal mass.

The aim of this chapter is to describe the US imaging methods and implementations now available for studying the pancreatic gland. Advantages and disadvantages of the US imaging methods are also mentioned. US approaches, such as transabdominal, endoscopic, laparoscopic and intraoperative procedures will be accurately illustrated in a dedicated chapter.

1.2 Conventional Imaging

Conventional US is a well-known, relatively low cost noninvasive imaging method which is widely available and easy to perform compared to computed tomography (CT) and magnetic resonance imaging (MRI), modalities which are usually used as second-line examinations. It is also free from side effects (i.e. lack of ionizing radiation) or contraindications, so is largely applicable also in young people. Two other important aspects are its real-time and multiplanar capabilities [1]. According to the literature, the pancreatic gland can almost always be visualized by US, even though in some cases this can be difficult due to the limited contrast between the pancreas and surrounding fat [2, 3]. In some overweight patients the visualization of the gland may also be difficult or unfeasible, despite several attempts. Examining the patient in different positions, such as erect or supine, with upleft or upright rotation, with suspended inspiration or expiration, may be suitable for achieving better pancreatic visualization. In the presence of abundant gas distension of the digestive tract, moving the transducer and applying compression can be useful to displace the bowel loops and visualize the pancreatic gland [2, 4]. Filling the stomach with degassed water (100-300 mL) or simethicone-water mixture may be used as a last option to improve US visualization of the pancreas since air bubble that cause artifacts will also be introduced into the stomach and a filled stomach is less compressible.

A. Gallotti (✉)
Department of Radiology
IRCCS Policlinico S. Matteo, Pavia, Italy
e-mail: annagallotti@virgilio.it

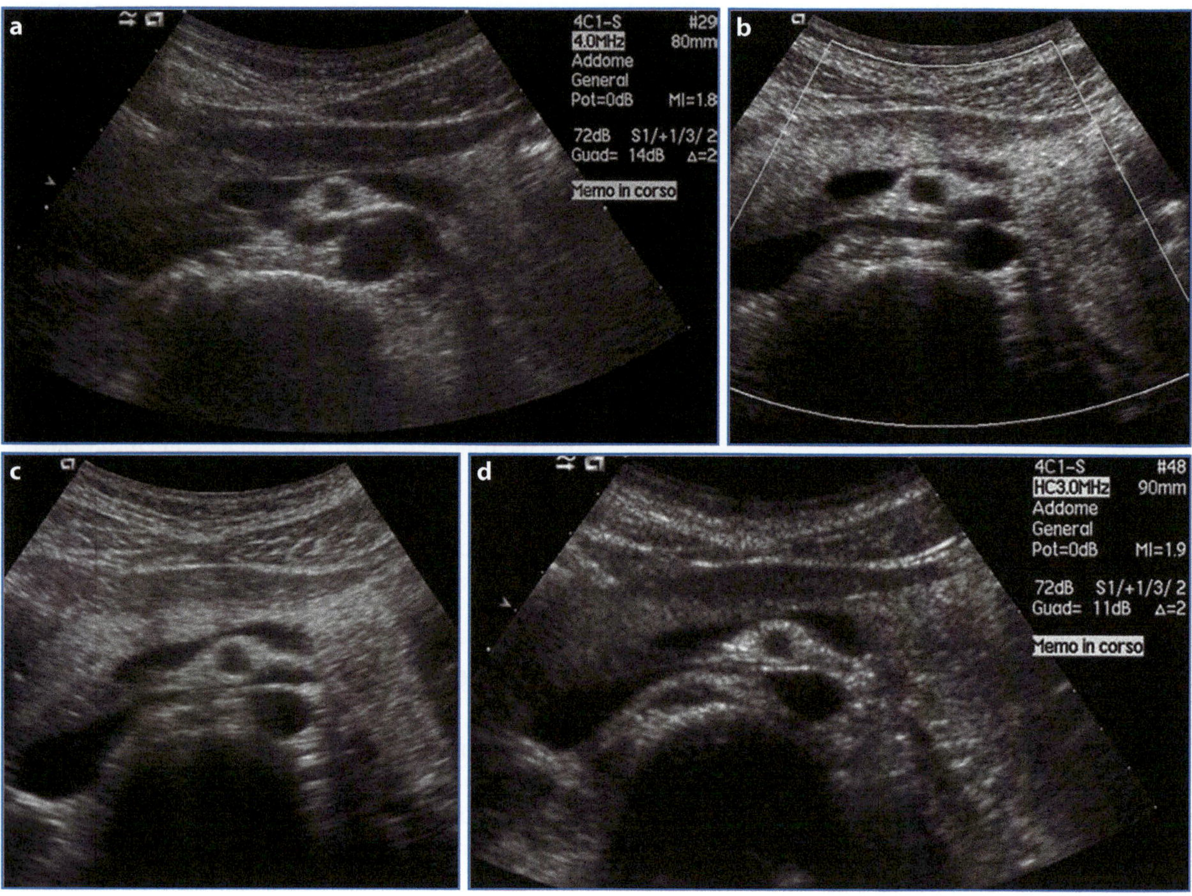

Fig. 1.1 a-d Pancreas. **a** B-mode image (4.0 Mhz). **b** Vascular enhancement image (4.0 Mhz). **c** Spatial compound image (4.0 Mhz). **d** Harmonic compound image (3.0 Mhz)

The US examination of the pancreas requires the use of multifrequency transducers (at least from 3 to 4 MHz) to study the entire gland with the proper frequencies for any depth (Fig. 1.1). The anatomic location, the body-size of the patient and the respiration phase may influence the depth of the pancreas, which is not a completely fixed retroperitoneal gland (see Chapter 6). Conventional US utilizes the same frequency bandwidth for both the transmitted and the received signal. The choice of frequency is mainly based on a compromise between the spatial resolution, which depends on the wavelength, and higher frequencies, which provide higher spatial resolution but which suffer greater tissue attenuation [5]. The basic US wave is a simple sinusoidal wave with a spectrum characterized by a *single line* and just one frequency of energy (f_0), also called the fundamental frequency or first harmonic. Furthermore, new technologies based on both the amplitude and the phase in-

formation of the return echo (e.g. coherent image formation, Acuson, Siemens) to create images are able to produce images with more information and detailed resolution [2].

The US study should be performed after a minimum fast of 6 hours to improve the visualization of the pancreas, creating the best situation for the evaluation of the gland. Through transverse, longitudinal and angled oblique scan planes (multiplanar view), the entire pancreatic gland should be recognizable. Beginning with the patient in the supine position, the probe should be slightly moved to the right of the midline to visualize the head and neck of the pancreas descending a little above the umbilical line for the uncinate process. To adequately study the body and tail of the pancreas the operator should move the transducer to the left of the midline with the end (right part) of the probe rotated slightly cranially. This positioning obviously reflects the most common location of the pancreatic gland, with the head at a more caudal plane than the tail [1]. The left lateral approach may also be useful for the evaluation of the pancreatic tail, which can be visualized between the spleen and the left kidney (see Chapter 6).

An accurate US study of the pancreas consists of the evaluation of the morphology, size, contour and echotexture of all the portions of the gland, the latter being comparable to the normal liver. The main pancreatic duct and the common bile duct, together with the main peri-pancreatic vascular structures, such as the celiac, superior mesenteric, hepatic and splenic arteries and the portal, superior mesenteric and splenic veins should be assessed. Lastly, the evaluation of the adjacent organs, in particular the liver, is always required for a complete study.

As reported in the literature, conventional B-mode US has a high sensitivity in detecting focal pancreatic disease due to differences in acoustic impedance between diseases and surrounding parenchyma. The *teardrop* sign, which is highly suggestive of vascular encasement in the presence of a neoplastic lesion, can only be detected in B-mode, which is also able to identify a dilation of the main pancreatic duct, parenchymal or ductal calcifications and potentially present peri-pancreatic fluid collections with great confidence [2].

Technical developments in recent years have led to image fusion, which is now currently available. This technology may help in diagnostic and interventional procedures by making the comparison between US and other imaging modalities more immediate. In interventional pancreatic procedures the advantages of US guidance, such as its dynamism and the possibility of innumerable manual scanning planes, would be maintained and it would also overcome the technical limitations of the technique, such as tympanites and obesity, through the simultaneous visualization of the previously acquired CT images matched and synchronized with the US images.

1.3   Harmonic Imaging

Tissue harmonic imaging (THI) is a well know technology that improves conventional US by providing images of higher quality [5-7]. While conventional US utilizes the same frequency bandwidth for both the transmitted and the received signal (f_0), THI uses low frequency for the transmitted signal and higher harmonic frequencies for the received signal. In other words, by using a Gaussian shaped transmit pulse the harmonic component can be separated from the returning echo without overlapping with fundamental reflections. In fact, nonlinear harmonic frequencies, generated by propagation of the US wave through the tissue, occur as whole-numbered multiples of the fundamental or transmitted sonographic frequency [5]. Therefore, the waveform changes compared to the basic US wave, resulting in a distorted wave with a complex form owing to the presence of both the fundamental and multiple harmonic frequencies [8].

THI takes advantages of nonlinear harmonic frequencies to correct the defocusing effects and to extensively reduce artifacts caused by low amplitude pulses [8]. As a consequence, THI produces images with improved lateral resolution by reducing side-lobe artifacts and improved signal-to-noise ratio compared with conventional US, thus resulting in an enhanced overall image quality [9]. The primary advantage is fewer artifacts in cavities, such as vascular structures, which can therefore be better evaluated. There are also advantages in fluid-solid differentiation, with the finely detailed depiction of anatomy such as the main pancreatic duct [7]. The physical basis depends on three main factors: (1) the contraction of the width of the harmonic wave; (2) the reduction of side-lobe artifacts; and (3) a received signal free of the original frequency transmitted.

Lateral resolution mostly depends on the width of the US wave. Since nonlinear harmonic waves are narrower than the fundamental, they also have lower side-lobe levels, thus improving lateral resolution which is most evident in fluid-filled structures (Fig. 1.2). The signal-to-noise ratio is consequently enhanced, with higher contrast resolution, resulting in images characterized by brighter tissues and darker cavities (e.g. main pancreatic duct, vascular structures, cystic lesions). Therefore, a narrow-bandwidth low-frequency pulse is transmitted, a filter automatically processes the received signal, and only the returning echo, characterized by high-frequency harmonic signal is used to generate the image.

THI has been incorporated in all state-of-the-art systems. By pushing the specific button on the US scanner, the receiver automatically is regulated on a frequency higher than the fundamental, with little or no overlap between them, and all the components that are in the transmitted pulses are rejected. Harmonic band filtering and phase inversion are the two main methods used for

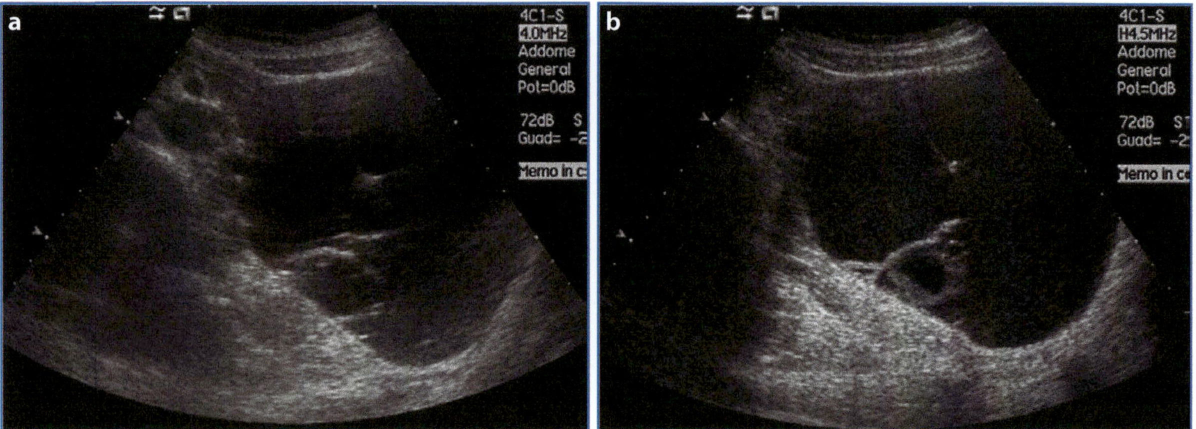

Fig. 1.2 a,b Pancreatic mucinous cystic neoplasm. Better definition of the cystic wall and intralesional septa moving from conventional US (a) to harmonic US (b) imaging

the generation of harmonic images [8]. In harmonic band filtering, there is little or no overlap between the transmitted and received pulses, but through a high-pass filter to the received signal, just the higher harmonic frequencies should be used. However, to separate them a fine bandwidth of the fundamental transmitted frequency must be selected and, as a consequence, decreased spatial resolution is the result. The same processes are also applied to the receiver, with a consequent decrease in contrast resolution [10]. These shortcomings can be overcome with the phase inversion method. This uses two sequential pulses, the second of which is phase reversed, and is able to remove the fundamental frequency by electronically storing the reflected signal following the first pulse and adding it to the second one, leaving only the harmonic waves [8]. The disadvantages are that the frame rate is halved and motion artifacts can occur.

The pancreatic examination requires the use of the same multifrequency curved array transducers (at least from 3 to 4 MHz) used for conventional US. Typically, the frequency setting consists of a transmitted frequency of 2.0 MHz and a received frequency of 4.0 MHz (second harmonic). The examination protocol is similar to that reported above for conventional US.

As reported in the literature, an accurate pancreatic THI examination is characterized by a higher sensitivity than conventional B-mode US regarding the detection of focal solid and cystic pancreatic lesions [8, 11]. THI is able to more clearly delineate lesion margins as well as internal solid components of a mass with more confidence [7]. Compared to conventional US, THI provides a higher soft tissue differentiation, allowing both the detection of even small lesions with little changes in echogenicity with respect to the surrounding parenchyma and the identification of calcifications [11, 12]. Moreover, other important advantages consist of the ability to clearly study deep structures and overweight patients, due to the rejection of low-amplitude pulses which generate artifacts in the conventional examination [8]. In a nutshell, in the study of the pancreas and compared to conventional B-mode US, THI can increase both spatial and contrast resolution, providing an enhanced overall image quality, better lesion conspicuity, and advantages in fluid-solid differentiation, thus achieving a better detection of pancreatic cancer.

1.4 Compound and Volumetric Imaging

State-of-the-art systems provide images with high detail resolution owing to both amplitude and phase information of the return echo and compound technology. Compounding is able to improve contrast and spatial resolution in the B-mode image (Fig. 1.1), reducing the intrinsic acoustic noise of US imaging (*speckle*) by generating several independent frames of data and then averaging them [2]. There are different types of compounding technology available, such as frequency compounding and spatial compounding (Fig. 1.1).

The introduction of *volumetric image acquisition*,

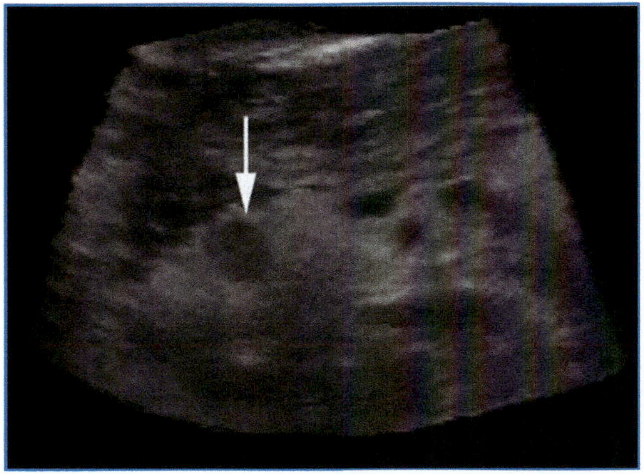

Fig. 1.3 Solid focal pancreatic lesion. Volumetric imaging of a solid focal hypoechoic (*arrow*) pancreatic head lesion

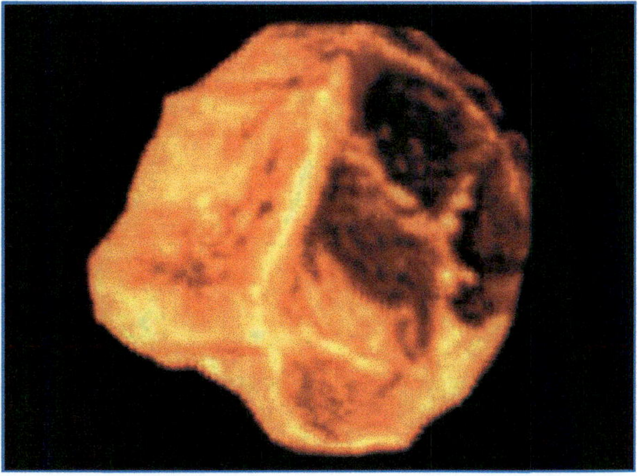

Fig. 1.4 Pancreatic mucinous cystic neoplasm. Volumetric imaging of a cystic pancreatic mass completely included in the automated acquisition scan

which maintains the real-time and multiplanar capabilities of conventional US, opens up new clinical opportunities for a more complete evaluation of the pancreatic gland [1]. Volumetric US imaging is a relatively new technique based on the acquisition of a volume dataset of anatomic structures (Fig. 1.3). Automated volumetric imaging is able to overcome the low reproducibility of the previous volume freehand sweep acquisition, owing to the possibility of a standardized and objective acquisition during the study. The whole volume of a region of interest is automatically acquired during a breath hold of a few seconds without moving the probe (Fig. 1.4). With the volumetric electromechanical transducers, such as 4D3C (GE Healthcare, Waukesha, WI, USA), the acquisition is related to the internal movement of the piezoelectric elements inside the probe with an angle of acquisition from 40° to 60°. Therefore the entire volume is uniformly and automatically acquired, and then reviewed and studied by means of different applications: volume review for reviewing the whole volume acquired to obtain a virtual scan of the pancreas; tomographic imaging for allowing the multiplanar vision of the region of interest; volume rendering for allowing the volumetric visualization of a pancreatic lesion. Moreover, when studying a pancreatic mass the evaluation of the involvement of the peri-pancreatic vessels can be improved by using multiplanar reconstruction (Fig. 1.5). In general, the correct application of these new technologies in the US study of the pancreas results in a conventional imaging of the gland with very high spatial and contrast resolution.

1.5 Doppler Imaging

Doppler imaging is a well-known technology that advances and completes the conventional US examination, providing significant complementary information about the vascular structures. Since its high sensitivity in evaluating flow in all the main peri-pancreatic arterial (i.e. celiac, superior mesenteric, hepatic and splenic arteries) and venous (i.e. portal, superior mesenteric and splenic veins) structures, together with its increased sensitivity in recognizing smaller intrapancreatic and intratumoral vessels, this technology plays an important role in diagnosing and staging pancreatic diseases [6, 13].

While conventional US is based on short pulses of US, Doppler signals derive from both continuous and pulsed waves and are mostly due to scattering from red blood cells. Some special methods have been developed for Doppler study. Continuous-wave technique, which is very sensitive to small vessels, enables measurements of a wide velocity range, but is unable to obtain information about the source of the Doppler signal because any moving object produces a signal. To overcome this shortcoming, the pulsed-wave technique, which is based on the pulse length and the duty cycle, enables the selective measurement of the wave speed at precise locations in the beam, even though the exact source of the Doppler signal remains difficult to determine because an image of the subsurface anatomy is not reported and is prone to false velocity indications (i.e. aliasing). The real advance in the application of Doppler technology is

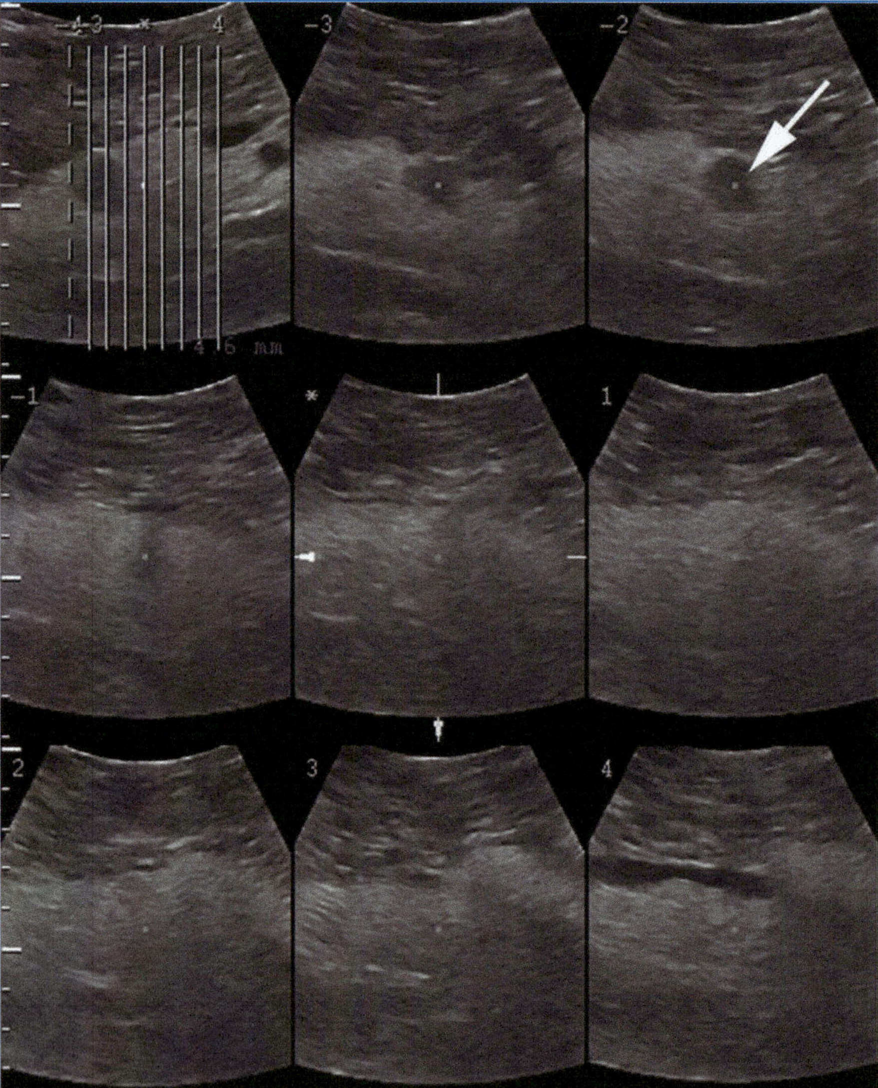

Fig. 1.5 Solid focal pancreatic lesion. Sagittal views of a solid focal hypoechoic (*arrow*) pancreatic head lesion after automated volumetric acquisition scan

duplex Doppler imaging. This is more complex and expensive as it combines both previous techniques, but it does enable the precise location of the signal; image and both peak velocity and velocity distribution are provided in real-time together with indications of the sample size. Lastly, color-flow Doppler imaging, which combines both anatomic and velocity data, provides qualitative and quantitative information adding velocity information to the conventional images as color data: red represents blood moving toward the transducer, whereas blue represents blood moving away. Variation of the velocity is also reproduced as a different color intensity. Typically, the lighter the color is, the higher the velocity (i.e. aliasing in the presence of improper velocity range) [14].

Doppler technology has been incorporated in all state-of-the-art systems. The pancreatic examination requires the use of the same multifrequency curved array transducers (at least from 3 to 4 MHz) used for conventional US and is based on an adequate visualization of the gland and of the targeted vascular structures at B-mode US. Color gain and velocity settings are tuned to provide good color filling of the vascular structures avoiding the generation of artifacts [15]. Typically, the frequency setting varies from 1 to 4 MHz, mostly depending on two factors: first, the targeted vascular structures, since lower frequencies allow an adequate evaluation of the peri-pancreatic main vessels owing to their higher penetration, while higher frequencies allow the evaluation of smaller vessels characterized by slower flows or vascular structures in thin patients whose pancreas is less deep; second, the patient's habitus. An accurate velocity measurement requires: (1) a correct angle between the vessel, the Doppler angle and the axis of the US beam, which should be as small as possible to generate signals with high signal-to-noise ratios; (2) the gate has to be located in the vessel center, with a size as small as possible; and (3) a correct angle for the velocity measurement has to be chosen, usually less than 60°. High-pass filters are used to reduce the influence of vessel wall and other non-vascular movements [14]. The examination protocol is similar to that reported above for conventional US.

Doppler technology implements conventional US in studying vascular structures, providing useful anatomic information and an accurate evaluation of patency (color-power study) and blood flow (color-Doppler study). At color-power imaging, a patent vessel of course appears colored. The color study offers an adequate evaluation of large vessels, providing information about the direction of flow, but it is dependent on the angle and is potentially affected by aliasing due to the difficulty in separating background noise from true flow in slow-flow states. Smaller vascular structures are better identified by the power study, which along with being relatively angle independent and unaffected by aliasing is characterized by higher signal persistence with better definition of vessel margins. However, it also suffers from increased movement artifacts and is unable to demonstrate flow direction or to estimate flow velocity [16]. Moreover, both technologies may provide useful information about the vascular network of focal lesions which may be present. Therefore, spectral waveform changes in peri-pancreatic vessels may depend on the effect of pancreatic diseases on the vascular structures [13].

As reported in the literature, an accurate pancreatic Doppler examination is based on the evaluation of all peripancreatic, intrapancreatic and intratumoral vessels. The most important applications are the identification of the vascular nature of an anechoic lesion (Fig. 1.6) detected at conventional US (i.e. pseudoaneurysm) and the differentiation between resectable (Fig. 1.7) and non-resectable (Fig. 1.7) pancreatic tumor (i.e. localized aliasing with reverse flow, mosaic pattern and accelerated flow velocity are detected at the site of stenosis, while *parvus et tardus* flow is observed downstream from an infiltrated tract) [17-19] with a reported accuracy of 85-90.5% [19]. As well described in the literature, a locally advanced pancreatic mass is defined by the extended invasion of a main arterial or venous vessel, by the encasement of a main arterial structure and/or by the occlusion of a main venous structure [19, 20]. Splenic arterial or venous encasement is not a contraindication for surgical resection [6]. If both a dilation of small peripancreatic veins and a tumor surrounding three quarters of a main vessel lumen allow the diagnosis of a vascular infiltration, while the *teardrop* sign, due to a tumor surrounding more than a half but less than three quarters of a main vessel lumen is highly suggestive of vascular encasement, a simple contiguity (less than a half of the vessel circumference) between tumor and vessel does not necessary correspond to vascular invasion [20].

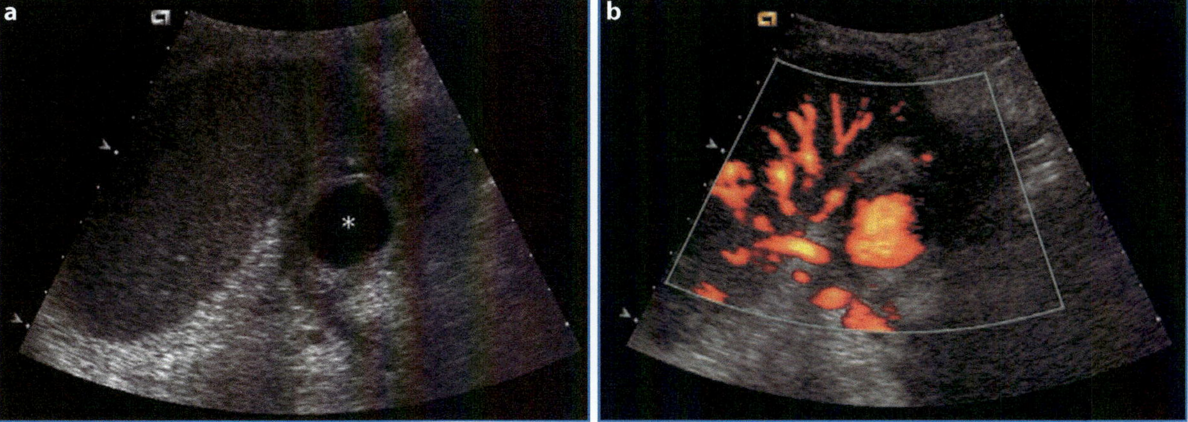

Fig. 1.6 a,b Pseudoaneurysm. Cystic lesion (*asterisk*) in the pancreatic tail at conventional imaging (**a**) in patient with chronic pancreatitis with final diagnosis of pseudoaneurysm at Doppler study (**b**)

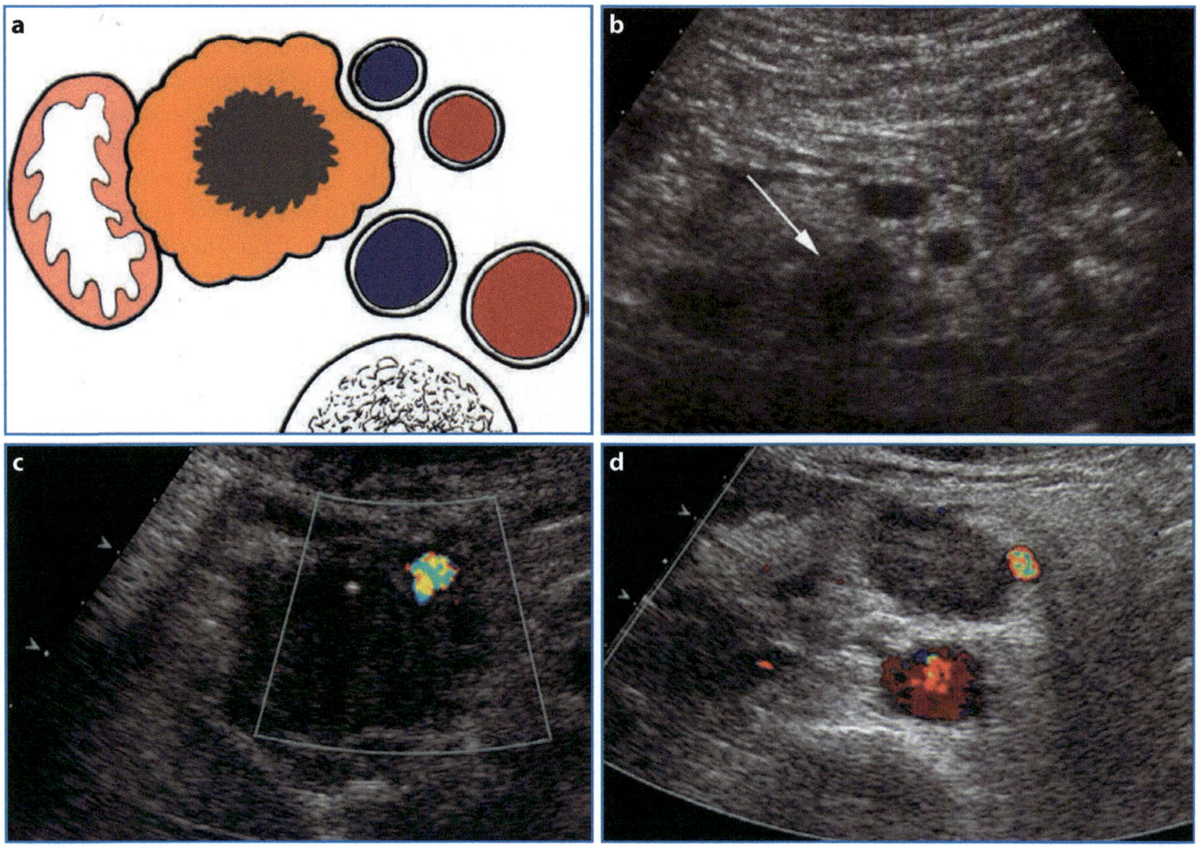

Fig. 1.7 a-d Pancreatic mass resectability. **a** Schematic representation of a resectable pancreatic head mass. **b** US detection of a resectable hypoechoic mass (*arrow*) of the pancreatic head. **c** Pancreatic head solid mass infiltrating the superior mesenteric vein at conventional imaging and confirmed at Doppler study. **d** Pancreatic head solid mass infiltrating the superior mesenteric artery at conventional imaging and confirmed at Doppler study

Some new technologies have been developed: wideband Doppler, which improves both spatial and temporal resolution of the color-Doppler signal with decreased artifacts [13]; power-like flow systems such as B-flow (General Electric) and e-flow (Aloka) imaging which are able to suppress tissue clutter and improve sensitivity to directly visualize blood reflectors and consequently provide images characterized by better spatial resolution [13]; color flow imaging (CFI), mostly used to image the blood movement through arteries and veins, but also to represent the motion of solid tissues [21]. The weak signals from blood echoes are enhanced and correlated with the corresponding signals of the adjacent frames to suppress non-moving tissues. The remaining aspects of the data processing are essentially the same as in conventional grey-scale imaging. In comparison with Doppler techniques these new

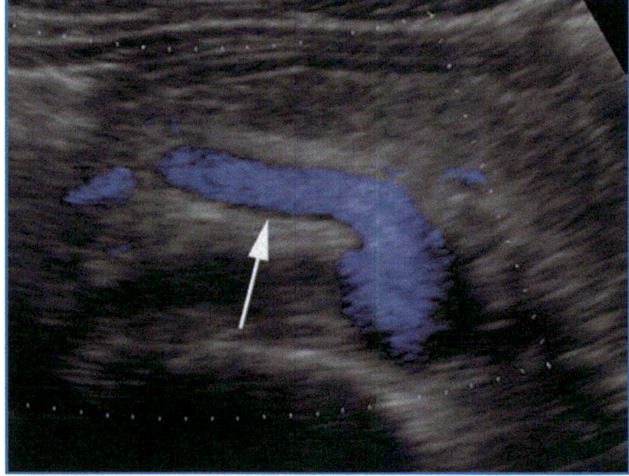

Fig. 1.8 Superior mesenteric artery. Doppler based US imaging of superior mesenteric artery shows flow only inside the lumen of the artery with a perfect detection of the arterial wall (*arrow*)

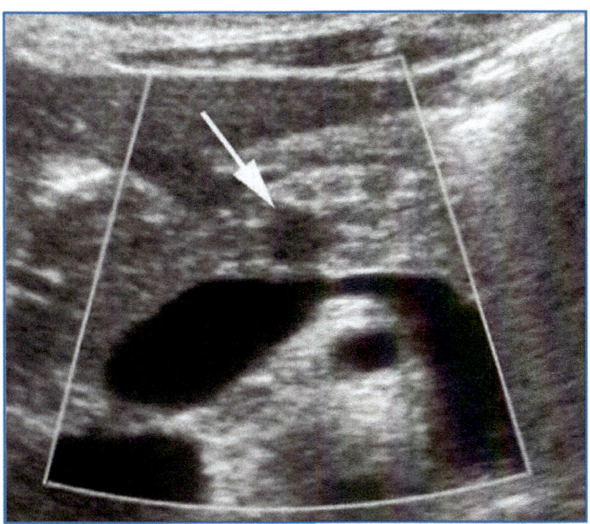

Fig. 1.9 Small solid focal pancreatic lesion. Doppler based US imaging of a very small solid focal hypoechoic (*arrow*) pancreatic lesion in the pancreatic body

US flow imaging modalities are not affected by aliasing and have the advantages of a significantly lower angle dependency and better spatial resolution with reduced overwriting. As a consequence, evaluation of vessel profiles is markedly improved (Fig. 1.8).

Other new Doppler-based technologies are able to improve image quality, owing to the immediate identification of the vascular structures in B-mode. For example, Clarify Vascular Enhancement (Acuson, Siemens) enables image optimization by enhancing the B-Mode display with information derived from power-Doppler, clearly differentiating vascular anatomy from acoustic artifacts and surrounding tissue (Fig. 1.9). In studying the pancreas, the resulting images can immediately appear diagnostic or more informative.

1.6 Elastography Imaging

In recent decades, new and interesting US techniques have been developed focused on the evaluation of mechanical strain properties of tissues. The noninvasive analysis of tissue stiffness immediately received major interest, owing to a revolutionary approach in the study of focal and diffuse diseases able to provide a new diagnostic tool. Tissue stiffness has long been an asset in physical palpation for clinicians and surgeons. Since the introduction of these new technologies, it has become a new and useful technique for radiologists able to complement other traditional data when making a diagnosis.

The first imaging techniques developed to image tissue elasticity consisted of elastography, the static US approach [22], and sonoelasticity, the dynamic US approach [23]. In elastography, the longitudinal stress and strain of superficial tissues can be estimated by tracking tissue motion mainly derived from external mechanical compression applied by the US probe [24]. In sonoelasticity, externally applied vibrations at low amplitude (less than 0.1 mm displacement) and low frequencies (10-1000 Hz) are used to induce oscillations within tissues and this motion is detected by Doppler US [25]. Through a color or grey scale map, a qualitative evaluation of the elastic properties of tissues is provided. As a consequence, isoechoic lesions which are undetectable at conventional US often might be identified at elastography and sonoelasticity imaging, owing to their altered vibration response. US elastography and sonoelasticity have been implemented as simple add-ons alongside conventional US scanners or as dedicated units. Transient US elastography utilizes a displacement wave generated by a piston or acoustic force which provides the stress to the tissue, without producing an image, but only numeric data of the tissue stiffness. This has mainly been used in the evaluation of diffuse liver diseases [26].

As widely reported in the literature, several clinical applications have been studied: for diagnostic purposes and biopsy targeting in breast and prostate; to differentiate benign from malignant nodules in the thyroid gland; to differentiate benign from malignant lymph nodes [27-30]; and in the evaluation of liver fibrosis [31].

Elastography has the same problems as B-mode sonography. The stress propagating into a tissue is in fact attenuated by tissues, causing it to spread into other directions from the primary incidental direction and to interact with a boundary between two media of different elastic properties, with potential distraction.

A more recent elastographic technique called acoustic radiation force impulse (ARFI) imaging has been developed [32, 33]. This new promising US method enables the evaluation of mechanical strain properties of deep tissues without the need for external compression. It produces a high intensity push pulse to displace the tissue and lower intensity pulses for imaging. The physical basis depends on the evaluation of the transverse wave spread away from the target tissue. There are two basic types of wave motion for mechanical waves, most widely used in US testing: longitudinal or compression waves and transverse or shear waves. Whereas the particle displacement is parallel to the direction of wave propagation in a longitudinal wave, in a transverse wave the particle displacement is perpendicular to the direction of wave propagation. In other words, if compression waves can be generated in liquids as well as solids, shear waves are not effectively propagated in gas or fluids owing to the absence of a mechanism for driving motion perpendicular to the sound beam. Transverse waves are also relatively weak when compared to longitudinal waves, since they are usually generated using some of the energy from longitudinal waves. As is well known, sound travels at different speeds in different materials, mostly because elastic constants are different for different media. Young's modulus deals with the velocity of a longitudinal wave, while the shear modulus deals with the velocity of a shear wave.

ARFI imaging has been incorporated in only a few US systems, and all papers present in the literature at this moment describe the application of the Siemens ACUSON S2000 scanner (Siemens, Erlanger, Germany). The pancreatic examination requires the use of the same multifrequency curved array transducers (at least from 3 to 4 MHz) used for conventional US. A single transducer is used both to generate radiation force and to track the resulting displacements. Pushing the specific button on the US scanner, the transducer is automatically regulated on the THI imaging, with a received frequency of 4.0 MHz. On a traditional harmonic US image, the target region of interest (ROI) is selected utilizing a box with fixed dimensions of 1 x 0.5 cm, able to descend at a maximum depth of 5.5 cm (8 cm in the most recent scanner). The box has to be completely included in the target tissue (i.e. organ in cases of diffuse diseases or lesion in cases of focal diseases), taking care not to comprise any fluid structures, such as vessels or ducts. Once the target ROI has been correctly located, the patient should maintain a proper suspended inspiration or expiration, to minimize motion artifacts. Pushing a specific button on the US scanner, acoustic push pulses are then transmitted. The push pulse is characterized by short duration (less than 1 msec) and runs immediately on the right side of the target ROI. Owing to its very high speed, it is minimally and not significantly influenced by the structures encountered through the path away from the transducer up to the box. The acoustic beam is able to generate localized, micron-scale displacements in the selected ROI proportional to the tissue elasticity. As a consequence, detection waves of lower intensity (1:100) are generated. The shear waves produced, which run

away perpendicular to the acoustic beam, are measured. The speed of the shear waves reflects the tissue elasticity, being dependent on the elasticity modulus that is mainly related to the resistance offered by the tissue to the wave propagation, and is proportional to the tissue stiffness: the stiffer a tissue is, the higher the shear wave speed it generates [34]. As a result, according to the interaction between waves and transducer previously selected by the operator, the response may be reported as qualitative or quantitative information (Fig. 1.10). The qualitative response consists of a grey scale map of the previously selected ROI, characterized by a lack of anatomic details, but with high contrast resolution, in which a bright shade corresponds to soft tissue, while a dark shade represents stiff tissue. The implementation of ARFI imaging able to provide this kind of response is called Virtual Touch tissue imaging. Obviously, this new advance could play an important role in the presence of focal disease. The quantitative response consists of a numeric wave velocity value, expressed in m/s, which derives from multiple measurements automatically made by the system for the previously selected ROI. It provides objective and reproducible data regarding the shear wave speed: the stiffer a tissue is, the higher the shear wave speed. The implementation of ARFI imaging able to provide this numerical response is called Virtual Touch tissue quantification and can be applied both in the presence of focal and diffuse disease [35].

The most significant advantages of ARFI technology over previous elastographic techniques are: (1) its in-

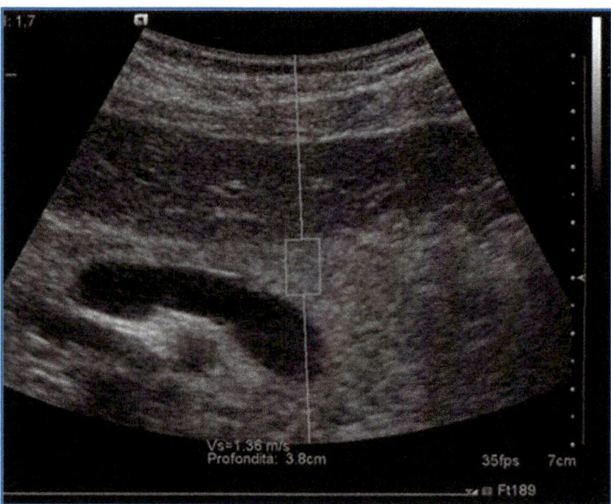

Fig. 1.10 Pancreas. Acoustic radiation force impulse (ARFI) US imaging with virtual touch quantification shows normal shear wave velocity in the normal pancreas of a healthy volunteer

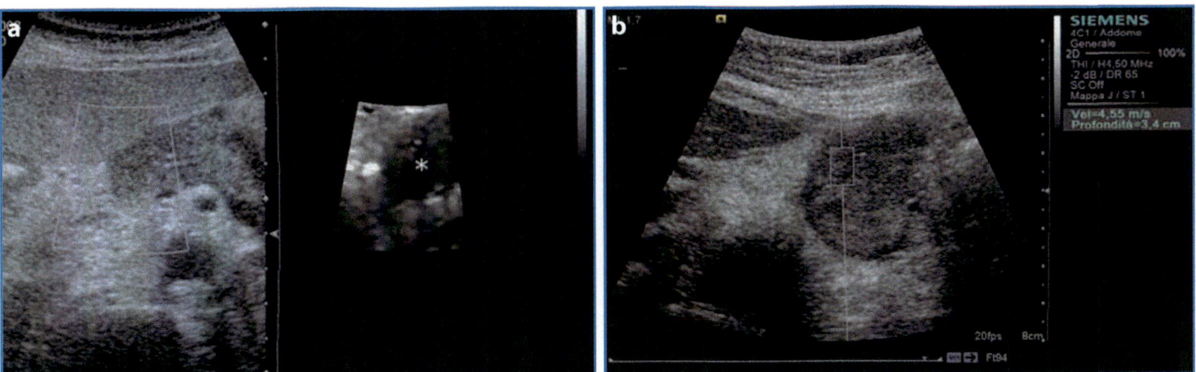

Fig. 1.11 a,b Pancreatic ductal adenocarcinoma. **a** Acoustic radiation force impulse (ARFI) US imaging shows a solid mass in the pancreatic body appearing black (*asterisk*) and therefore stiff at virtual touch imaging. **b** Acoustic radiation force impulse (ARFI) US imaging shows a solid mass in the pancreatic body with very high value of shear wave velocity at virtual touch quantification and therefore stiff

tegration into a conventional US system, thus allowing the visualization of B-mode, color-Doppler mode and ARFI images with the same equipment; (2) the consequent selection of an ROI in the target tissue on a conventional US image; (3) the subsequent possibility of precisely studying target lesions during a real-time visualization at conventional US; (4) the opportunity to also study deep tissues, since there is no need for external compression; and (5) the objective quantification of the tissue stiffness expressed as a numeric value, by Virtual Touch tissue quantification. There are nonetheless some important limitations: (1) the fixed box dimensions of the target ROI, while less important in cases of diffuse disease, could be significantly limiting in cases of focal lesions; and (2) a high sensitivity to movement artifacts, such as lack of suspended respiration or heart motion.

The US examination should be performed after a minimum fast of 6 hours to improve the visualization of the pancreas, creating the best situation for the evaluation of the gland. The good visualization of the target tissue at conventional US is a mandatory condition for performing the ARFI examination.

As reported in the literature, the mean wave velocity value obtained in the healthy pancreas (Fig. 1.10) is about 1.40 m/s [6, 35]. An accurate pancreatic US examination consists of the application of both qualitative and quantitative implementations of ARFI technology, whenever possible, to assess the concordance of the results. Different focal and diffuse diseases that alter the tissue stiffness should be characterized by different shades and wave velocity values. For example, since

pancreatic ductal adenocarcinoma is a firm mass which is stiffer than the adjacent parenchyma (see also Chapter 8) owing to the presence of fibrosis and marked desmoplasia, it should appear as a dark shade with higher values (Fig. 1.11).

According to the physical principles of the shear waves, ARFI imaging has been tested in the study of solid tissues. However, fluids in vivo, and as a consequence pancreatic cystic lesions, can be markedly different and different responses at ARFI technology might be expected. The qualitative evaluation should give a bright shade, while as recently reported in the literature, it seems that the quantitative study usually gives non numeric values in serous cystadenoma (see also Chapter 9), which contains a simple fluid, and mainly numeric values in mucinous tumors (Fig. 1.12), which contain a more complex content [36, 37].

Since its recent introduction, few data regarding the usefulness of ARFI technology in the study of pancreatic diseases are available in the literature. However, it seems to be potentially able to allow tissue characterization by imaging and may constitute a feasible alternative to invasive needle-biopsy in the future.

1.7 Contrast-enhanced Ultrasound

Contrast-enhanced ultrasonography (CEUS) is a relatively recent implementation of conventional US which significantly advances the accuracy of this first line examination in characterizing focal solid and cystic diseases. The administration of microbubbles allows an

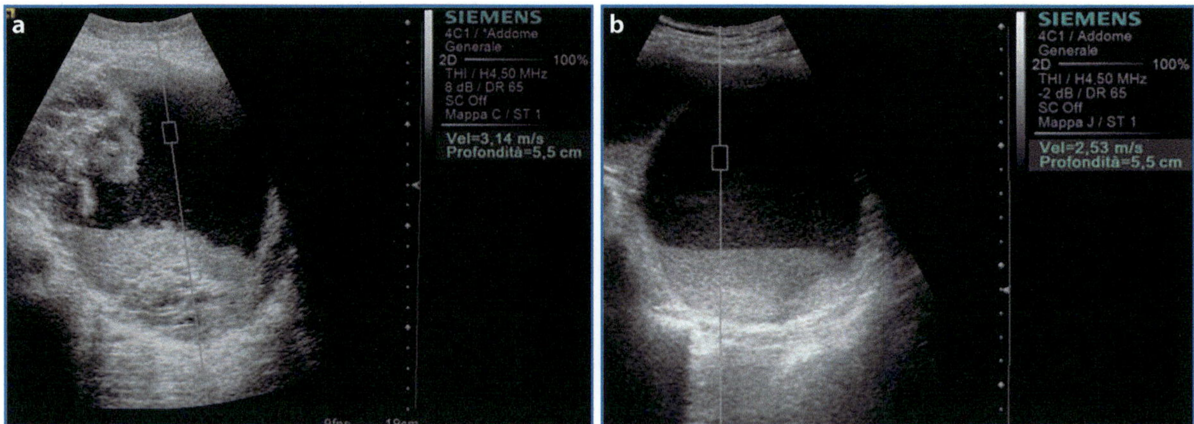

Fig. 1.12 a,b Pancreatic mucinous cystic neoplasm. Acoustic radiation force impulse (ARFI) US imaging of a cystic mass with numerical value of shear wave velocity at virtual touch quantification of the fluid content

accurate evaluation of macro- and microcirculation, in and around a focal mass, giving more detailed and advanced results than the color-Doppler study thanks to its high spatial, contrast and temporal resolution. This new technology has been widely used to study hepatic diseases and also more recently applied in the study of the pancreas, giving promising results in diagnosis and staging of pancreatic diseases already detected at conventional US [6, 38].

The introduction of US contrast agents goes back some decades and their effects during cardiac catheterization were first described at the end of the 1960s. Today their use has been approved in Europe, Asia and Canada, but the Food and Drug Administration in the United States has not yet approved their application for non-cardiac use. Only the administration in pregnancy and pediatrics is off label. Some recommendations exist, especially for second generation contrast agents filled with sulfur-hexafluoride: they are not recommended in patients with recent acute coronary syndrome, unstable angina, recent acute heart attack, recent coronary artery intervention, acute or class III or IV chronic heart failure or severe arrhythmias. No interactions with other drugs have been reported and only rarely some subtle and usually transient adverse reactions have been described, such as tissue irritation and cutaneous eruptions, dyspnea, chest pain, hypo- or hypertension, nausea and vomiting. No severe effects have been described in humans to date [39, 40].

US contrast agents consist of microbubbles, characterized by a diameter that ranges from 2 to 6 microns, a shell of biocompatible materials, such as proteins, lipids or biopolymers and a filling gas, such as air or gas with high molecular weight and low solubility (e.g. perfluorocarbon or sulfur hexafluoride). Their small diameter allows their passage through the pulmonary district, thus microbubbles are exhaled during respiration 10-15 minutes after injection, while the components of the shell are metabolized or filtered by the kidney and eliminated by the liver. Shell and gas influence the time of circulation and acoustic behavior of microbubbles. The thin shell ranges from 10 to 200 nm and allows the passage through the pulmonary district with a consequent systemic effect and a more prolonged contrast effect. The filling gas produces a vapor concentration inside the microbubbles higher than the surrounding blood, increasing their stability in the peripheral circulation [38, 41].

Both the shell and the filling gases have been changed over the years, passing from first generation contrast media to second generation agents. The first generation contrast media were characterized by a stiff shell (denatured albumin) and air as filling gas. The stiff shell allows more stability in the peripheral blood, with a reduction in non-linear behavior. Therefore, as the microbubbles have a short half-life because they are easily destroyed, their US response depends on the echogenicity and the concentration. The second generation contrast media are both more stable and resistant. They are characterized by a flexible shell (phospholipids), which allows the prevalence of nonlinear behavior, and filling gas other than air. Their US response consists of the generation of nonlinear harmonic frequencies, since at low acoustic power of insonation

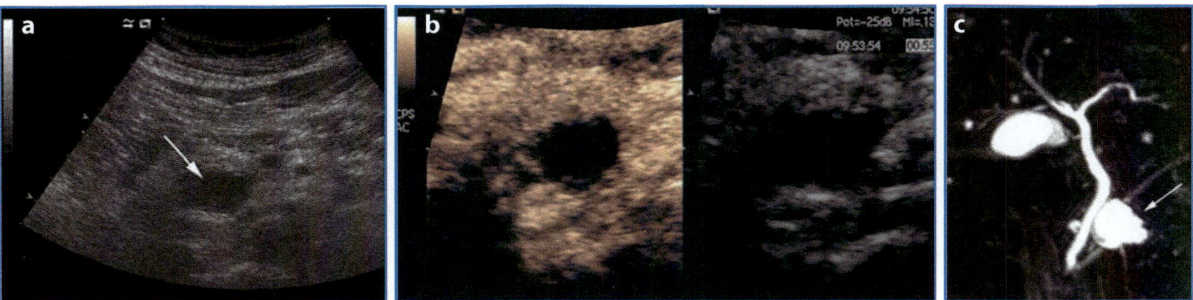

Fig. 1.13 a-c Pancreatic intraductal papillary mucinous neoplasm. **a** Pseudosolid appearance of the pancreatic head lesion at conventional US resulting hypoechoic (*arrow*) but avascular with cystic appearance at CEUS (**b**). The cystic nature (*arrow*) of the lesion is confirmed at MRI (**c**)

(about 30-70 kPa), the degree of microbubble expansion is greater than its compression [41].

Several contrast-specific software applications have been developed for CEUS examination, even though the most promising techniques are phase and amplitude modulation. Pulse inversion is the most common phase modulation technique [42], while power modulation is a well-known amplitude modulation software application [41]. Cadence contrast pulse sequencing (CPS) is a more advanced combined phase and amplitude modulation technique [38, 43].

The CEUS examination should be performed after an accurate conventional US of the pancreas with the evidence of a focal or diffuse pancreatic disease [44]. The pancreatic examination requires the use of the same multifrequency curved array transducers (at least from 3 to 4 MHz) used for conventional US. Nowadays, second generation contrast agents are used. Harmonic microbubble-specific software applications are required to filter all the background tissue signals so only vascularized structures related to the harmonic responses of the microbubbles are visualized after injection. The dual screen should be used to adequately and continuously compare B-mode and contrast images. Focus and depth should be regulated simultaneously in both images and low acoustic US pressures should be selected (mechanical index less than 0.2). The examination protocol and technique are similar to those reported above for conventional US.

The dynamic evaluation begins immediately after the intravenous administration of a 2.4-mL bolus of microbubble contrast agent. Since the pancreatic blood supply is exclusively arterial, the enhancement of the gland begins almost together with the arteries. Enhancement of the pancreatic gland begins almost at the same time as aortic enhancement. After this early phase (arterial/pan-

creatic; from 10 s to 30 s), as with other dynamic imaging modalities there is a second phase, the venous phase (from 30 to approximately 120 s) defined by hyperechogenicity within the spleno-mesenteric-portal venous axis. The late phase (about 120 s after injection) is defined by hyperechogenicity of the hepatic veins.

US specific contrast agents have a purely intravascular distribution without any interstitial phase, so they differ from all contrast media used during CT and MRI examinations [45]. Moreover, CEUS with second generation contrast media enables real-time evaluation of target tissues, with high spatial, temporal and contrast resolution. Unlike other imaging modalities, as reported above, only vascularized structures are visible after the administration of microbubbles (see Chapter 11). Therefore, compared to conventional US and other imaging modalities, pancreatic CEUS is better able to differentiate between solid and cystic lesions (Fig. 1.13), characterize focal masses and provide a clear differentiation between remnant tissue, fibrosis and necrosis [44]. Moreover, the CEUS examination covers an important role in evaluating the resectability or non-resectability of a focal mass [46], together with Doppler imaging for the assessment of the relationship between the tumor and the adjacent main vessels, and during the late phase to exclude the presence of liver metastases.

Some new applications of CEUS have been developed: the use of CEUS enhancement as a prognostic factor, both in the diagnostic workup and in the follow-up of patients. In fact, as reported in the literature, in the presence of focal pancreatic lesions, the accurate description of the enhancement pattern at CEUS is mandatory for a prompt prognostic evaluation. The association between intratumoral microvessel density (MVD) and tumor aggressiveness has already been proven [46]. The use of

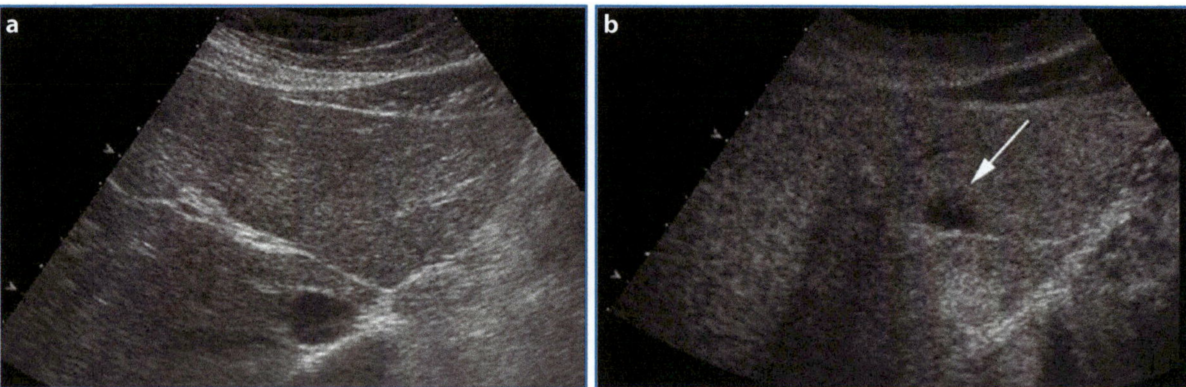

Fig. 1.14 a,b Liver metastatic pancreatic adenocarcinoma. **a** At US no focal liver lesion was detected. **b** At late phase of contrast-enhanced US a hypoechoic solid metastatic lesion (*arrow*) was detected in the left lobe of the liver

microbubbles as a vehicle for targeted therapies is an interesting future possibility [47]. Moreover, the development of new software applications for the perfusion study has been recently improved. Some papers have reported the qualitative, subjective evaluation of the enhancement pattern of different pancreatic tumors studied at CEUS [48], while other studies have described the potential quantitative evaluation of the CEUS enhancement, derived from the offline evaluations of different pancreatic tumors [46, 49]. More recently, a few US systems have been developed to quantitatively evaluate the enhancement at CEUS, based on either the video intensity analysis or the raw data analysis, which are able to immediately achieve repeatable results comparable to those derived from perfusion CT examinations [50].

An accurate pancreatic CEUS examination should be performed only after an adequate conventional US and consists of a real-time continuous observation of the target tissue (pancreatic gland in cases of diffuse disease or focal lesion already detected at conventional US in cases of focal disease [51]) during all the dynamic phases after the administration of microbubbles. At the end, in all cases a liver study during the late phase should be performed (Fig. 1.14).

References

1. Wilson SR, Gupta C, Eliasziw M et al (2009) Volume imaging in the abdomen with ultrasound: how we do it. Am J Roentgenol 193:79-85
2. Martínez-Noguera A, D'Onofrio M (2007) Ultrasonography of the pancreas. 1. Conventional imaging. Abdom Imaging 32:136-149
3. Martínez-Noguera A, Montserrat E, Torrubia S et al (2001) Ultrasound of the pancreas: update and controversies. Eur Radiol 11:1594-1606
4. Abu-Yousef MM, El-Zein Y (2000) Improved US visualization of the pancreatic tail with simethicone, water, and patient rotation. Radiology 217:780-785
5. Shapiro RS, Wagreich J, Parsons RB et al (1998) Tissue harmonic imaging sonography: evaluation of image quality compared with conventional sonography. Am J Roentgenol 171:1203-1206
6. D'Onofrio M, Gallotti A, Pozzi Mucelli R (2010) Imaging techniques in pancreatic tumors. Expert Rev Med Devices 7:257-273. Review
7. Desser TS, Jeffrey RB (2001) Tissue harmonic imaging techniques: physical principles and clinical applications. Semin Ultrasound CT MR 22:1-10
8. Hohl C, Schmidt T, Honnef D et al (2007) Ultrasonography of the pancreas. 2. Harmonic Imaging. Abdom Imaging 32::150-160. Review
9. Ward B, Baker AC, Humphrey VF (1997) Nonlinear propagation applied to the improvement of resolution in diagnostic medical ultrasound. J Acoust Soc Am 101:143-154
10. Duck FA (2002) Nonlinear acoustics in diagnostic ultrasound. Ultrasound Med Biol 28:1-18
11. Hohl C, Schmidt T, Haage P et al (2004) Phase-inversion tissue harmonic imaging compared with conventional B-mode ultrasound in the evaluation of pancreatic lesions. Eur Radiol 14:1109-1117
12. Sparchez Z (2003) Tissue harmonic imaging: Is it useful in hepatobiliary and pancreatic ultrasonography? Rom J Gastroenterol 12:239-246
13. Bertolotto M, D'Onofrio M, Martone E et al (2007) Ultrasonography of the pancreas. 3. Doppler imaging. Abdom Imaging 32:161-170
14. Nelson TR, Pretorius TH (1998) The Doppler signal: Where does it come from and what does it mean? Am J Roentgenol 151:439-447
15. Angeli E, Venturini M, Vanzulli A et al (1997) Color-Doppler imaging in the assessment of vascular involvement by pancreatic carcinoma. Am J Roentgenol 168:193-197. Review
16. Hamper UM, DeJong MR, Caskey CI et al (1997) Power

Doppler Imaging: clinical experience and correlation with color Doppler US and other imaging modalities. Radiographics 1:499-513

17. Yassa NA, Yang J, Stein S et al (1997) Gray-scale and color flow sonography of pancreatic ductal adenocarcinoma. J Clin Ultrasound 25:473-480

18. Ueno N, Tomiyama T, Tano S et al (1997) Color-Doppler ultrasonography in the diagnosis of portal vein invasion in patients with pancreatic cancer. J Ultrasound Med 16:825-830

19. Minniti S, Bruno C, Biasiutti C et al (2003) Sonography versus helical CT in identification and staging of pancreatic ductal adenocarcinoma. J Clin Ultrasound 31:175-182

20. Lu DSK, Reber HA, Krasny RM et al (1997) Local staging of pancreatic cancer: criteria for unresectability of major vessels as revealed by pancreatic-phase, thin-section helical CT. Am J Roentgenol 168:1439-1443

21. Evans DH (2010) Colour flow and motion imaging. Proc Inst Mech Eng H 224:241-253

22. Ophir J, Céspedes I, Ponnekanti H et al (1991) Elastography: a quantitative method for imaging the elasticity of biological tissues. Ultrason Imaging 13:111-134

23. Lerner RM, Huang SR, Parker KJ (1990) "Sonoelasticity" images derived from ultrasound signals in mechanically vibrated tissues. Ultrasound Med Biol 16:231-239

24. Garra BS (2007) Imaging and estimation of tissue elasticity by ultrasound. Ultrasound Q 23:255-268. Review

25. McLaughlin J, Renzi D, Parker K et al (2007) Shear wave speed recovery using moving interference patterns obtained in sonoelastography experiments. J Acoust Soc Am 121:2438-2446

26. Sandrin L, Catheline S, Tanter M et al (1999) Time-resolved pulsed elastography with ultrafast ultrasonic imaging. Ultrason Imaging 21:259-272

27. Itoh A, Ueno E, Tohno E et al (2006) Breast disease: clinical application of US elastography for diagnosis. Radiology 239:341-350

28. Cochlin DL, Ganatra RH, Griffiths DF (2002) Elastography in the detection of prostatic cancer. Clin Radiol 57:1014-1020

29. Lyshchik A, Higashi T, Asato R et al (2005) Thyroid gland tumor diagnosis at US elastography. Radiology 237:202-211

30. Lyshchik A, Higashi T, Asato R et al (2007) Cervical lymph node metastases: diagnosis at sonoelastography - initial experience. Radiology 243:258-267

31. Lamproye A, Belaiche J, Delwaide J (2007) The FibroScan: a new non invasive method of liver fibrosis evaluation. Rev Med Liege 62:68-72

32. Fahey BJ, Nelson RC, Bradway DP et al (2008) In vivo visualization of abdominal malignancies with acoustic radiation force elastography. Phys Med Biol 53:279-293

33. Nightingale K, Soo MS, Nightingale R et al (2002) Acoustic radiation force impulse imaging: in vivo demonstration of clinical feasibility. Ultrasound Med Biol 28:227-235

34. Fahey BJ, Nightingale KR, Nelson RC et al (2005) Acoustic radiation force impulse imaging of the abdomen: demonstration of feasibility and utility. Ultrasound Med Biol 31:1185-1198

35. Gallotti A, D'Onofrio M, Pozzi Mucelli R (2010) Acoustic Radiation Force Impulse (ARFI) technique in ultrasound with Virtual Touch tissue quantification of the upper abdomen. Radiol Med 115:889-897

36. D'Onofrio M, Gallotti A, Salvia R et al (2010) Acoustic Radiation Force Impulse (ARFI) ultrasound imaging of pancreatic cystic lesions. Eur J Radiol 2010. doi:10.1016/j.ejrad. 2010.06.015

37. D'Onofrio M, Gallotti A, Pozzi Mucelli R (2010) Pancreatic mucinous cystadenoma at ultrasound Acoustic Radiation Force Impulse (ARFI) imaging. Pancreas 39:684-685

38. D'Onofrio M, Zamboni G, Faccioli N et al 82007) Ultrasonography of the pancreas. 4. Contrast-enhanced imaging. Abdom imaging 32:171-181

39. Correas JM, Bridal L, Lesavre A et al (2001) Ultrasound contrast agents: properties, principles of action, tolerance, and artifacts. Eur Radiol 11:1316-1328

40. Torzilli G (2005) Adverse effects associated with SonoVue use. Expert Opin Drug Saf 4:399-401

41. Quaia E (2007) Microbubble ultrasound contrast agents: an update. Eur Radiol 17:1995-2008

42. Burns PN, Wilson SR, Hope Simpson D (2000) Pulse inversion imaging of liver blood flow: an improved method for characterization of focal masses with microbubble contrast. Invest Radiol 35:58-71

43. Whittingham T (2005) Contrast-specific imaging techniques: technical perspective. In: Quaia E (ed) Contrast media in ultrasonography: Basic principles and clinical applications. Springer, Berlin Heidelberg New York, pp 43-70

44. D'Onofrio, Martone E, Malagò R et al (2007) Contrast-enhanced ultrasonography of the pancreas. JOP J Pancreas. 8[1 Suppl]:71-76

45. D'Onofrio M, Malagò R, Zamboni G et al (2005) Contrast-enhanced ultrasonography better identifies pancreatic tumor vascularization than helical CT. Pancreatology 5:398-402

46. D'Onofrio M, Zamboni GA, Malagò R et al (2009) Resectable pancreatic adenocarcinoma: is the enhancement pattern at contrast-enhanced ultrasonography a pre-operative prognostic factor? Ultrasound Med Biol 35:1929-1937

47. van Wamel A, Bouakaz A, Bernard B et al (2005) Controlled drug delivery with ultrasound and gas microbubbles. J Control Release 101:389-391

48. Tawada K, Yamaguchi T, Kobayashi A et al (2009) Changes in tumor vascularity depicted by contrast-enhanced ultrasonography as a predictor of chemotherapeutic effect in patients with unresectable pancreatic cancers. Pancreas 38:30-35

49. Kersting S, Konopke R, Kersting F et al (2009) Quantitative perfusion analysis of transabdominal contrast-enhanced ultrasonography of pancreatic masses and carcinomas. Gastroenterology 137:1903-1911

50. Xu J, Liang Z, Hao S et al (2009) Pancreatic adenocarcinoma: dynamic-64 slices helical CT with perfusion imaging. Abdom Imaging 34:759-766

51. EFSUMB Study Group (2008) Guidelines and good clinical practice recommendations for contrast enhanced ultrasound (CEUS) – update 2008. Ultraschall Med 29:28-44

Transabdominal Ultrasonography of the Pancreas

Elisabetta Buscarini and Salvatore Greco

2.1 Introduction

Transabdominal conventional ultrasonography (US) is a widely performed, relatively low-cost and readily available examination for the study of the pancreas, and is very often the first diagnostic imaging modality in the study of pancreatic diseases.

2.2 Examination Technique

2.2.1 Equipment

In adults the transducer frequency may vary from 3 MHz to 5 MHz, whereas in children a 5-MHz or 7.5-MHz transducer can be used routinely. The focal zone of the transducer should be matched to the depth of the pancreas. The transducer gain control must be adjusted to optimize visualization of the entire pancreas.

2.2.2 Preparation

The US examination of the pancreas is best performed on patients who have fasted overnight. To improve the evaluation of the pancreas, only if it is poorly seen, the water technique can be used: the patient drinks 250–500 ml of water, which may provide a sonic window into the pancreas.

2.2.3 Position of the Patient

The examination is generally begun with the patient in the supine position. Changing patient position is then very often required (see also Chapters 6 and 8) to gain the best visualization of the pancreas.

2.2.4 Scans and Normal Findings

The goal of every pancreatic US examination is to visualize the gland in its entirety. To do this, the examiner should find or produce a suitable acoustic window through which the pancreas can be visualized (Fig. 2.1). For transverse scans, the left lobe of the liver can be used to start the examination as a first window into the pancreatic bed. Then if access is impaired by the superimposed stomach or small bowel, graded compression with the probe or deep inspiration may displace the viscera (see also Chapters 6 and 8) leading to the expected direct visualization of the pancreas. Visualization of the abdominal aorta and inferior vena cava ensures that adequate deep penetration has been attained to image the pancreas. Sagittal scanning begins in the midline, with identification of the great vessels, and proceeds to the right until the right kidney is seen and then left to the splenic hilum (or until the pancreas is obscured by gastric or colonic gas).

Anatomic landmarks should be identified in scans of the pancreas, in the following order: (1) aorta, (2) inferior vena cava, (3) superior mesenteric artery, (4) superior mesenteric vein, (5) splenic vein, (6) gastric wall and (7) common bile duct (Fig. 2.1).

The pancreas can be localized with US by identifying its parenchymal architecture and the surrounding anatomic landmarks (see also Chapter 6). The level of the pancreas changes slightly with the phase of respi-

E. Buscarini (✉)
Department of Gastroenterology
Maggiore Hospital, Crema, Italy
e-mail: ebuscarini@rim.it

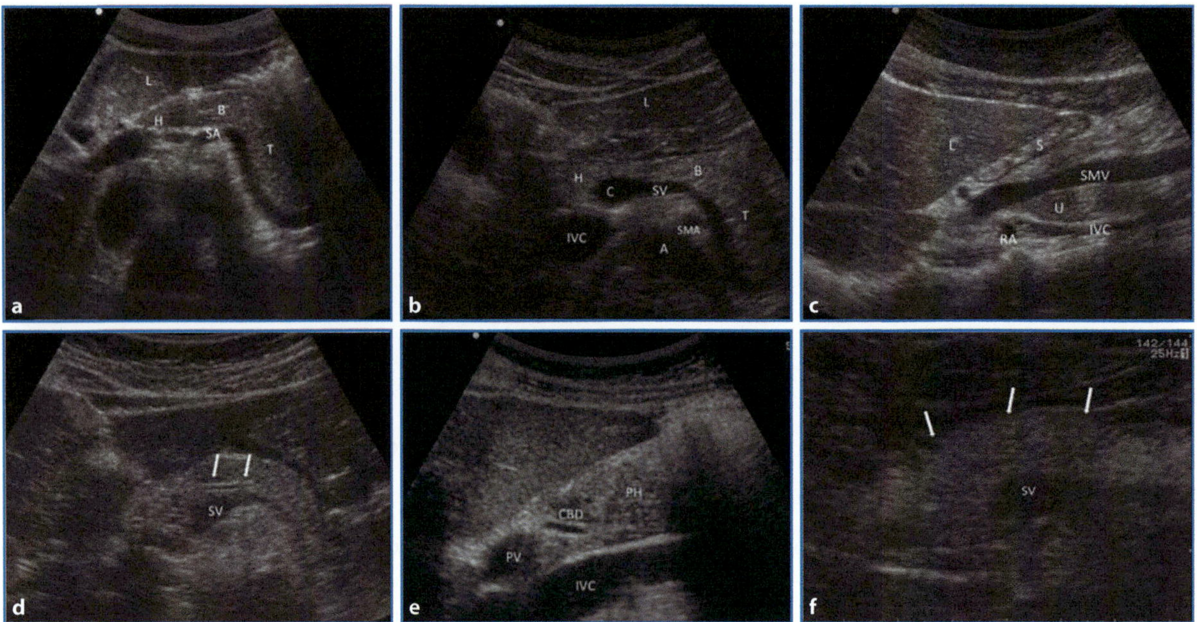

Fig. 2.1 a-f Pancreas, normal US anatomy. **a** Transverse scan in the supine position shows the head (*H*), body (*B*) and tail (*T*) of the pancreas (*SA*, splenic artery; *L*, liver). **b** Transverse scan shows the head (*H*), body (*B*) and tail (*T*) of the pancreas (*C*, spleno-mesenteric confluence; *SV*, splenic vein; *IVC*, inferior vena cava; *SMA*; superior mesenteric artery; *A*, aorta; *L*, liver). **c** Sagittal scan in the supine position shows the pancreas head wrapped around the confluence of the splenic and the superior mesenteric (*SMV*) veins, the uncinate process (*U*) lying posterior to the vein, and the inferior vena cava (*IVC*) on which the head of the pancreas lies (*RA*, right renal artery; *S*, stomach). **d** Normal pancreatic duct on transverse scan (*arrows*) appears as double-line pancreatic duct (*SV*, splenic vein). **e** Longitudinal scan of the pancreatic head showing the intrapancreatic common bile duct (*CBD*) (*PH*, pancreatic head; *PV*, portal vein; *IVC* , inferior vena cava). **f** Transverse scan of the pancreas shows the diffusely increased echogenicity of the pancreas (*arrows*) in an elderly patient (*SV*, splenic vein)

ration: at maximal inspiration and expiration, the organ can shift 2–8 cm along the craniocaudal axis. These respiratory excursions should be considered when imaging the pancreas and especially during US-guided biopsy. The pancreas is a nonencapsulated, retroperitoneal structure that lies in the anterior pararenal space between the duodenal loop and the splenic hilum over a length of 12.5–15 cm. Standard views are the transverse and longitudinal planes in the upper abdomen (see also Chapter 6).

2.2.4.1 Transverse Scan

The head, uncinate process, neck, body and tail constitute the different parts of the pancreas. The superior mesenteric artery is surrounded by brightly echogenic fat at the root of the mesentery. Anterior to the superior mesenteric artery and in its transverse course is the splenic vein, which forms the dorsal border of the pancreas from the splenic hilum to its junction with the superior mesenteric vein at the neck of the pancreas. At

this point, the head and the uncinate process actually wrap around the venous junction, which forms the portal vein, and pancreatic tissue is observed both anterior and posterior to the vein. The uncinate process forms the medial extension of the head and lies behind the superior mesenteric vessels. The superior mesenteric vessels run posterior to the neck of the pancreas, separating the head from the body. No anatomic landmark separates the body from the tail, but the left lateral border of the vertebral column is considered to be the arbitrary plane that demarcates these two segments. Two other important landmarks are the common bile duct and the gastroduodenal artery. In transverse scans, the gastroduodenal artery is visible anterior to the neck of the pancreas and the common bile duct at the posterior part of the head of the pancreas (Fig. 2.1). The right margin of the pancreas is formed by the second portion of the duodenum. Anterior to the pancreas lies the lesser sac, which under normal circumstances is only a potential space and is thus not visible, and the stomach, which are identified by the alternating hyper- and hypoechoic layers of its submucosa and muscularis propria, respectively.

2.2.4.2 Sagittal Scan

On the right, and lateral to the head, a sagittal right paramedian scan shows the inferior vena cava, on which the head of the pancreas lies (Fig. 2.1). At the level of the neck, the superior mesenteric vein is observed posterior to the pancreas. The uncinate process of the head is located posterior to the superior mesenteric vein. The third portion of the duodenum projects inferiorly. The stomach lies anteriorly at the levels of the body and the tail (Fig. 2.1). A cross-section of the splenic vein is observed posteriorly, whereas a cross-section of the splenic artery appears cranially. The pancreatic duct may be seen as a single echogenic line within the gland (Fig. 2.1). This is considered normal as long as the internal diameter of the duct does not exceed 2–2.5 mm [1, 2]. In the normal subject, however, the diameter of the duct of Wirsung may be more than 2 mm in physiologic conditions, such as postprandially [3]. Visualization of the duct has been reported in up to 86% of normal people. The echotexture of the normal pancreas is usually homogeneous, but a mottled appearance may sometimes be observed. The texture of the pancreas varies with age. In infants and young children, the gland may be more hypoechoic than the normal liver. With aging and obesity, the pancreas becomes more echogenic (see also Chapter 6) as a result of the presence of fatty infiltration (Fig. 2.1); in up to 35% of cases, it may be as echogenic as the adjacent retroperitoneal fat. Other causes of fatty infiltration of the pancreas include chronic pancreatitis, dietary deficiency, viral infection, corticosteroid therapy, cystic fibrosis, diabetes mellitus, hereditary pancreatitis and obstruction caused by a stone or a pancreatic carcinoma. The normal size of the pancreas is a matter of some debate. Most authors consider the normal anteroposterior measurements to be approximately 3.5 cm for the head, 2.0 cm for the neck, 2.5 cm for the body and 2.5 cm for the tail. The size of the pancreas diminishes with age. In practice, focal enlargement or localized changes in texture are more significant than an abnormal measurement. The normal pancreas is the result of the fusion of two embryonic buds: the ventral bud arises from the common bile duct (CBD), forming the uncinate process and part of the head, and the dorsal bud arises from the posterior wall of the duodenum (see Chapter 6). Developmental anomalies of the pancreas occur as a result of a failure of the dorsal and ventral pancreatic ducts to fuse, i.e. pancreas divisum (see Chapter 6).

2.3 Indications

2.3.1 Acute Pancreatitis

Acute inflammation of the pancreas has a number of possible causes but is most commonly associated with gallstones or alcoholism. Clinically, it presents with severe epigastric pain, abdominal distension and nausea or vomiting. Biochemically, increased levels of amylase and lipase are present in the blood and urine. Acute inflammation causes the pancreatic tissue to become necrosed, releasing the pancreatic enzymes, which can further destroy the pancreatic tissue and the capillary walls.

Acute pancreatitis (see also Chapter 7) is classified as mild (interstitial edema) or severe (necrosis, fluid collections).

The role of US in acute pancreatitis consists of:

1. etiological determination and mainly the detection of gallbladder or CBD stones; US should also exclude a pancreatic lesion;
2. survey of possible complications, such as peripancreatic fluid;
3. follow-up of complications arising from acute pancreatitis;
4. guidance for interventional procedures.

2.3.1.1 Sonographic Criteria of Acute Pancreatitis

The sensitivity of sonography is limited because in 30% of patients with purely edematous pancreatitis, no abnormality is discernible. If the pancreas is easily identified, sonographic findings have a high specificity and a strong positive predictive value.

Edematous pancreatitis

- Swelling of part of or the entire pancreas is indicated by an increased volume with concomitant hypoechoic texture (Fig. 2.2). The extent of hypoechogenicity depends on the pancreatic texture and is less pronounced in preexisting chronic pancreatitis, old age, or pancreatic lipomatosis.
- Acute focal pancreatitis is often localized in the head of the pancreas [4, 5].
- Acute-on-chronic pancreatitis is characterized by focal hypoechogenicity or adjacent hyper-and hypoechoic zones.
- Fluid-filled lesser sac.
- As it is compressed by edema, the pancreatic duct

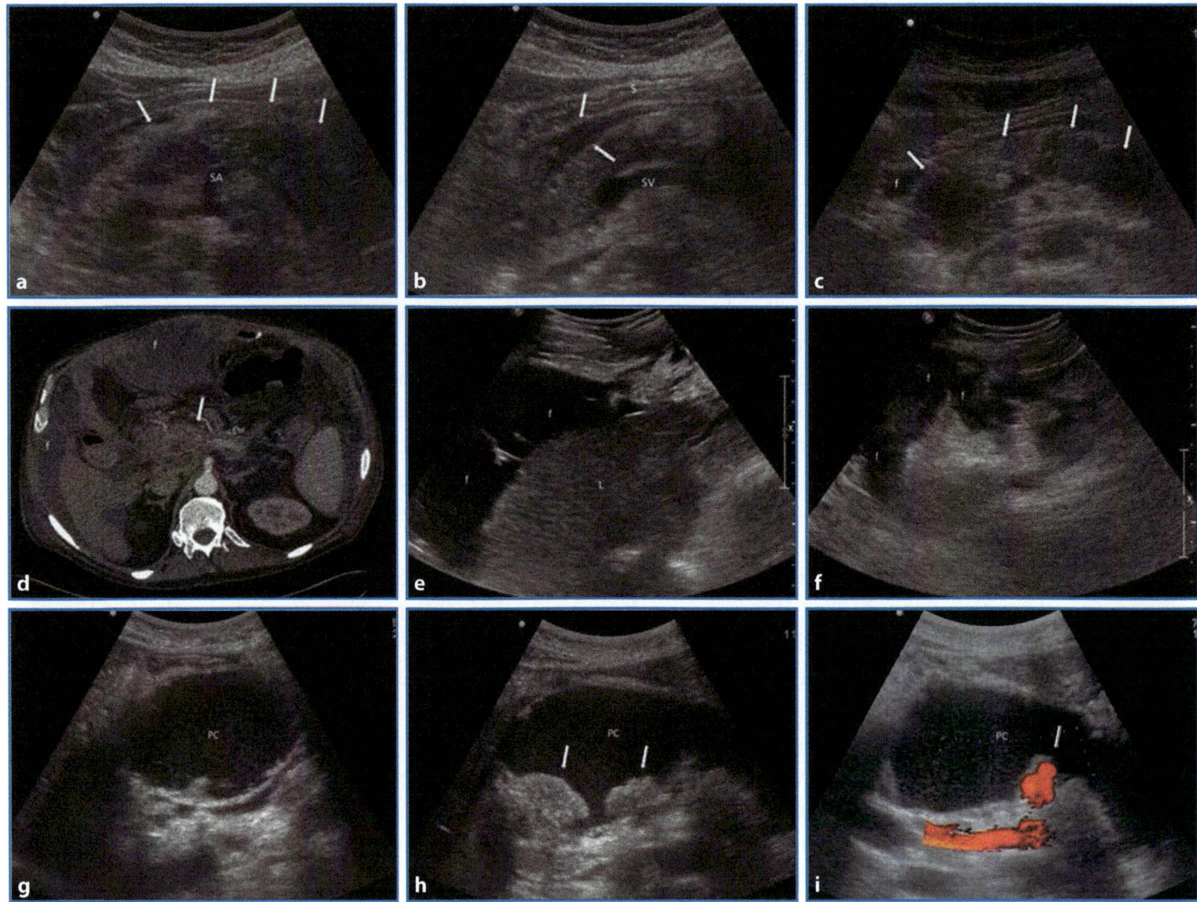

Fig. 2.2 a-i Acute pancreatitis. **a** Transverse scan shows a diffusely enlarged pancreas (*arrows*) with inhomogeneous hypoechogenicity (*SA*, splenic artery). **b** Transverse scan demonstrates a diffusely enlarged pancreas with fluid (*arrows*) posterior to the stomach (*S*) (*SV*, splenic vein). **c** Transverse scan shows inhomogeneously echo-poor pancreas with frayed contours (*arrows*) and a small amount of fluid (*f*) anterior to the pancreatic head. **d** CT scan in a case of severe acute pancreatitis showing an enlarged pancreatic head (*arrow*) with hypodense areas, with substantial peritoneal effusion around the liver and between GI loops (*f*). **e** In the same patient, US shows the fluid (*f*) collection around the liver (*L*), and (**f**) the fluid (*f*) between GI loops. **g** Transverse scan shows a pancreatic pseudocyst (*PC*) with well-defined echorich wall, and echogenic content. **h** This large pseudocyst (*PC*) content is markedly heterogeneous because of gross debris (*arrows*). **i** Transverse scan shows splenic artery (*arrow*) included in the pseudocyst (*PC*) wall

usually cannot be discerned, with the exception of prevailing pancreatic duct dilatation in chronic pancreatitis or pancreatic duct obstruction.

Necrotizing pancreatitis
US findings as in edematous pancreatitis, plus:
- Liquefaction of pancreatic parenchyma, i.e. areas of rather hypoechoic to almost anechoic sonotexture.
- Frayed contour of the pancreas (Fig. 2.2).
- Band of fat necrosis visualized as hypo- to anechoic structures bilaterally in the anterior perirenal space, as well as in the mesocolon, mesentery, and greater and lesser omentum.

- Bowel wall edema secondary to chemical peritonitis and/or impaired perfusion (systemic capillary damage, involvement of the mesentery).

Complications
The complications of acute pancreatitis that may be demonstrated sonographically are:
- Fluid collections (Fig. 2.2): abdominal collections, more often around the pancreas, in the anterior pararenal space and lesser sac [6-8]; pleural effusion (more often on the left).
- Pancreatic pseudocysts are fluid collections that have developed well-defined, non-epithelized walls in re-

sponse to extravasated enzymes [7]. These are generally spherical and distinct from other structures. Fluid must collect over 4–6 weeks for the fluid collection to enclose itself by forming a wall consisting of collagen and vascular granulation tissue. Classically, a pseudocyst is seen on sonographic examination as a well-defined, smooth-walled anechoic structure with acoustic enhancement (Fig. 2.2); its content is generally heterogeneous because of the presence of debris. Pseudocysts occur in 30% of cases of acute pancreatitis, can extend into adjacent organs, and can cause either duodenal or biliary obstruction or stomach compression. Pseudocysts can also be infected. They tend to spontaneously resolve in half of the cases and remain stable in 20% of cases.

- Pancreatic abscesses consist of an encapsulated collection of purulent material within or near the pancreas. They develop several weeks after the onset of pancreatitis. On US, they appear as anechoic or heterogeneous masses containing bright echoes from pus, debris, or gas bubbles [9]. A pancreatic abscess should be suspected based on the clinical evidence and when changes in the echogenicity of the content of pseudocysts are documented on US examination [9]. Pancreatic abscesses require percutaneous drainage or surgical debridement [10, 11]. Pancreatic phlegmons are a combination of fat necrosis, tissue necrosis, extravasated pancreatic fluid, and occasionally, hemorrhage. Differentiating pancreatic phlegmons from pancreatic abscesses is essential for appropriate clinical treatment.
- Vascular complications: venous thrombosis most often occurs in the splenic vein and/or superior mesenteric vein; Doppler US is useful in assessing associated vascular complications. Prolonged and repeated attacks of acute pancreatitis may cause the splenic vein to become encased and compressed, leading to splenic and/or portal vein thrombosis; pseudoaneurysms of adjacent vessels may be found on US examination. Pseudoaneurysms may be related to pancreatitis or may occur secondary to pseudocyst formation. Strong suspicion is crucial for the diagnosis of a pseudoaneurysm because it can be mistaken for a pseudocyst, which is a much more common complication of this condition. Hemorrhage can also occur as a result of vascular injury. US examination can also reveal delayed gastric emptying in paralytic ileus or stenosis of the duodenum, resulting from pancreas swelling or pseudocyst formation in the head; the enlargement of the pancreas in acute pancreatitis may also obstruct the CBD, causing biliary dilatation.

2.3.2 Chronic Pancreatitis

Chronic pancreatitis (see also Chapter 7) is an inflammatory disease that is characterized by progressive replacement of the normal pancreas by fibrous tissue, which may encase the nerves in the celiac plexus, causing abdominal pain, particularly postprandially. Due to decreased capacity to produce digestive enzymes, the patient develops steatorrhea. Common etiologies of chronic pancreatitis include alcohol, hyperlipidemia, hyperthyroidism, cystic fibrosis, and hereditary and idiopathic causes [12]. The diagnosis of chronic pancreatitis is based on clinical findings, laboratory evaluation of endocrine and exocrine pancreatic function, and imaging findings. Although early morphologic changes in chronic pancreatitis are difficult to recognize on various imaging techniques, the findings of advanced disease are readily detected.

Sonographic findings in chronic pancreatitis consist of changes in:
- the size of the pancreas
- the echotexture of the pancreas
- focal mass lesions
- calcifications
- pancreatic duct dilatation
- pseudocyst formation

Alterations in the size of the pancreas may be observed in fewer than half of the patients with chronic pancreatitis [13, 14]. This percentage decreases dramatically in the early stages of the disease. However, the finding of a gland of normal size does not exclude a diagnosis of chronic pancreatitis [13]. Atrophy and focal alterations in the size of the pancreas are the most easily identified alterations (Fig. 2.3). However, these changes in pancreatic volume are an expression of advanced stages of the disease in which the glandular contours appear to be irregular, sharp, and sometimes lumpy (Fig. 2.3).

Echogenicity of the pancreas is usually increased in chronic pancreatitis due to adipose infiltration and fibrosis [15]. Hyperechogenicity is not a specific parameter, however, as it is also present in elderly and obese subjects.

Alteration of parenchymal echo structure is a more specific sign of chronic pancreatitis. The pancreatic echotexture is inhomogeneous and coarse due to the coexistence of hyperechoic and hypoechoic foci (Fig. 2.3), which are foci of fibrosis and inflammation, re-

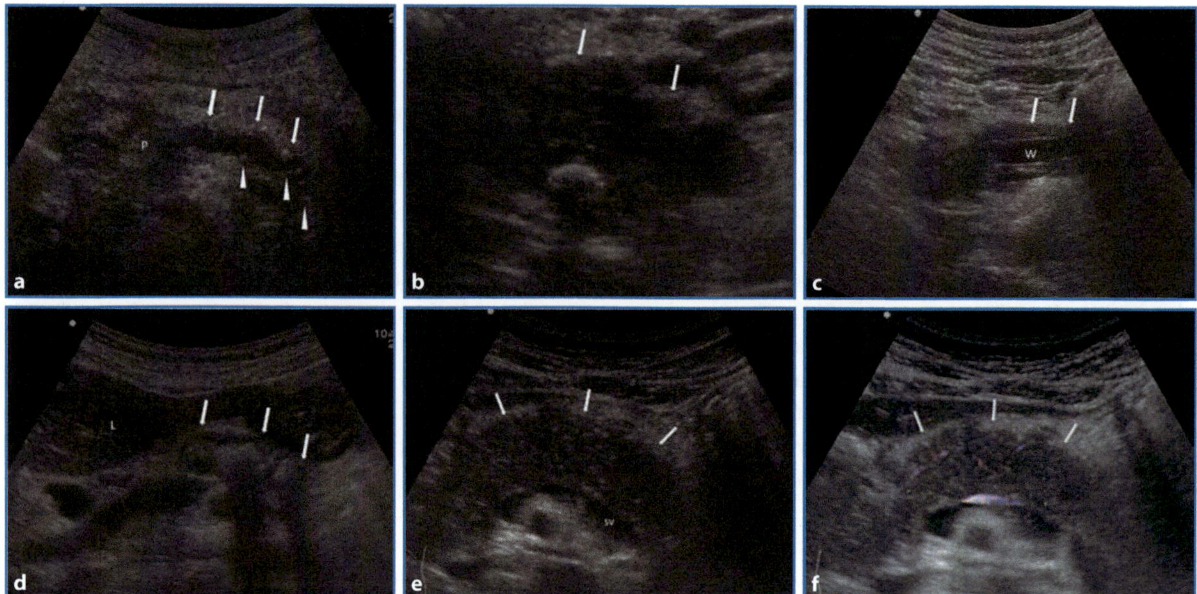

Fig. 2.3 a-f Chronic pancreatitis. **a** Transverse image of the pancreas (*P*) shows diffusely inhomogeneous echotexture and a dilated and irregular duct (*arrows*). Note multiple pancreatic calcifications (*arrowheads*) scattered throughout the pancreas. **b** Transverse scan shows a stone (*between calipers*) with posterior shadowing within the duct (pancreatic head, *arrows*). **c** In the same case the duct (*w*) upstream to the stone is markedly dilated with atrophy of pancreatic body and tail (*arrows*). **d** Transverse scan shows multiple calcifications (*arrows*) with posterior shadowing in the pancreatic body and tail (*L*, liver). **e** Transverse scan shows a substantially and diffusely enlarged pancreatic gland (*arrows*) with echopoor echotexture and normal sized main pancreatic duct, in a case of autoimmune pancreatitis; note the compressed splenic vein (*SV*). **f** In the same case, power Doppler shows increased vascular signals within the gland (*arrows*) which reflect the inflammatory condition

spectively [15]. These findings are described in 50%–70% of cases [13, 14]. In patients affected by severe exocrine pancreatic insufficiency, this percentage increases to approximately 80%, showing a fairly good sensitivity of this finding.

According to the Japan Pancreas Society [16], the most important diagnostic criterion for chronic pancreatitis is the presence of pancreatic calcifications (Fig. 2.3), the identification of which is pathognomonic. Pancreatic calcifications are calcium carbonate deposits, usually on a protein matrix (plug) or on interstitial necrotic areas [13]. On US, these appear as hyperechoic spots with posterior shading, which may, however, be difficult to detect if the calcification is small. The demonstration of pancreatic calcifications may be improved with the use of harmonic imaging and high-resolution US using a high US beam frequency and thus increasing US diagnostic accuracy. Plugs with few or no calcium carbonate deposits, usually located in ducts, appear at US as echoic spots almost without posterior shading.

In chronic pancreatitis, the main pancreatic duct can show a dilation greater than 3 mm [15]. In chronic pan-

creatitis, duct dilation is the most easily identified US sign (Fig. 2.3). Duct of Wirsung alterations have a sensitivity of approximately 60%–70% [14], but most importantly they have a high specificity of approximately 80%–90% [14, 17, 18] for the diagnosis. The limits of the reported sensitivity reflect the minor frequency of duct dilation in initial and/or mild cases of chronic pancreatitis. In the early phases of chronic pancreatitis, the duct of Wirsung may have a normal diameter. Chronic pancreatitis may also manifest as a marked reduction in duct of Wirsung diameter, as in autoimmune pancreatitis [19].

Intraductal calculi (Fig. 2.3) are protein aggregates with calcium carbonate deposits, which appear at US as round echoic particles that are usually mobile. Intraductal protein matrix (plug) echogenicity increases with their calcium content, until they become real intraductal calcifications (calculi). The mobility of intraductal calculi depends on the relationship between the ductal dilation and the diameter of the calculus itself. When possible, high-resolution US with a high US beam frequency may be useful to demonstrate the intraductal calculi inclusions. Intraductal calculi must be considered to be pathognomonic of chronic pancreatitis [16].

Focal pancreatitis reportedly occurs in 20% of cases and typically involves the pancreatic head [20]. Differentiation between pseudotumors in cases of chronic pancreatitis and pancreatic carcinoma may be difficult due to their similar patterns. Autoimmune pancreatitis is a particular type of chronic pancreatitis [19] that is caused by an autoimmune mechanism [21, 22]. It is characterized by periductal inflammation that is mainly sustained by lymphoplasmacytic infiltration, with evolution to fibrosis [19]. Unlike the other forms of chronic pancreatitis, the pancreas is usually diffusely enlarged with the typical *sausage* appearance, and the duct of Wirsung is compressed or string-like [19]. US features include focal or diffuse pancreatic enlargement (Fig. 2.3); US findings are characteristic in the diffuse form when the entire gland is involved. Echogenicity is markedly reduced, gland volume is increased, and the duct of Wirsung is compressed by parenchyma, in which vessels are easily demonstrated at color power Doppler US. The differential diagnosis of focal forms of autoimmune chronic pancreatitis with ductal adenocarcinoma is very challenging. The overall sensitivity of US in the diagnosis of chronic pancreatitis is variable, with an average range in most series of 60%–70% [12].

2.3.3 Malignant Pancreatic Lesions

Adenocarcinoma of the pancreas (see also Chapter 8) is a major cause of cancer-related death. It carries a very poor prognosis, with a 5-year survival rate of less than 5% due to its late presentation [23-27]. The presenting symptoms depend on the size of the lesion, its location within the pancreas and the extent of metastatic deposits. Most pancreatic carcinomas (60%) are detected in the head of the pancreas, and patients present with the associated symptoms of jaundice due to obstruction of the CBD. The majority of pancreatic cancers are ductal adenocarcinomas, most of which are located in the head of pancreas.

Endocrine tumors (see also Chapter 8), which originate in the islet cells of the pancreas, tend to be either insulinomas (generally benign) or gastrinomas (malignant). These present with hormonal abnormalities while the tumor is still small. Most of them are insulinomas (60%) or gastrinomas (18%); less common endocrine tumors include glucagonomas, VIPomas, somatostatinomas, and nonsecreting islet cell tumors. Approximately

99% of all insulinomas are intrapancreatic, and approximately 90% are solitary; only 30% of gastrinomas are intrapancreatic and are primarily located in the head of the pancreas [28].

2.3.3.1 Sonographic Criteria of Pancreatic Cancer

Pancreatic cancer may alter the size, shape and texture of the pancreas. Adenocarcinoma originating from the ductal epithelium is the most common tumor of the pancreas, with approximately 75% arising in the head of the pancreas. The role of sonography in suspected pancreatic cancer is based on the detection of pancreatic masses and on the differentiation between chronic pancreatitis and malignant masses. When pancreatic malignancy is strongly suspected, US can assess the anatomic relationships and possible inoperability.

The most common sonographic finding in pancreatic carcinoma is a poorly defined, homogeneous or inhomogeneous hypoechoic mass in the pancreas (Fig. 2.4). Dilatation of the pancreatic duct proximal to a pancreatic mass is also a common finding (Fig. 2.4). Other sonographic findings include bile duct dilatation (Fig. 2.4), atrophic changes of the gland proximal to an obstructing mass and encasement of adjacent major vessels. Dilatation of the common bile duct associated with the pancreatic duct is known as the *double-duct sign*. Necrosis, which is observed as a cystic area within the mass, is a rare manifestation of pancreatic carcinoma.

US criteria of inoperability include the following:
- peritoneal carcinomatosis
- distant spread (most commonly to the liver)
- tumor growth beyond the pancreatic head with invasion of neighboring organs (except for the duodenum)
- extensive invasion of the portal vein/superior mesenteric vein or superior mesenteric artery

Apart from direct tumor demonstration, indirect signs of pancreatic head cancer may be dilatation of bile and pancreatic ducts, liver metastases, ascites, lymphadenopathy and delayed gastric emptying. In a series of 62 pancreatic cancers, biliary dilatation occurred in 69%, pancreatic duct dilatation in 37% and the double duct sign (pancreatic and biliary duct dilatation) in 34% of patients [29]. The sensitivity of US tumor detection ranges from 72% to 98%, and the specificity exceeds 90%. However, even though some small pancreatic tumors are better resolved with US than with CT, con-

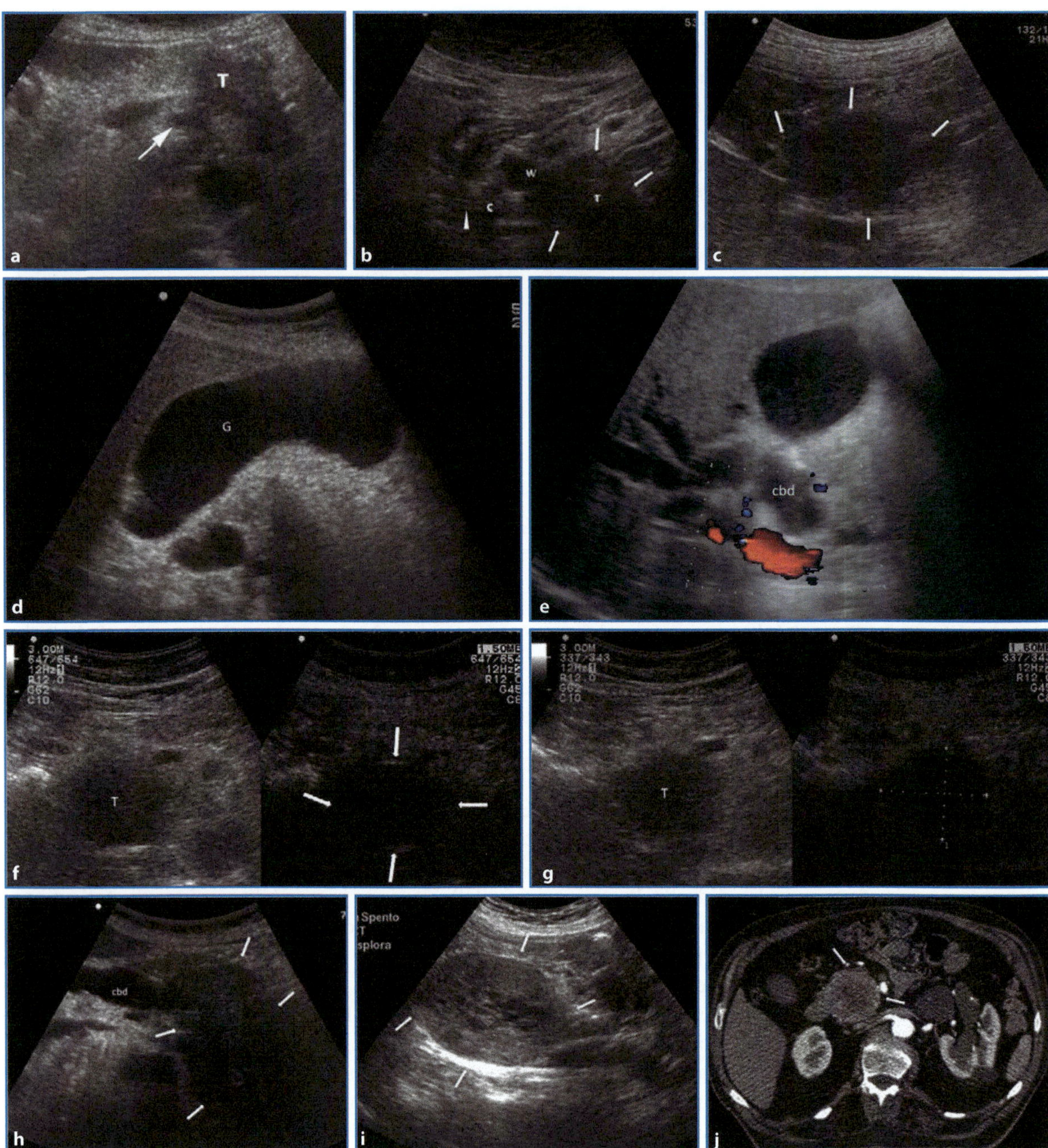

Fig. 2.4 a-j Solid pancreatic tumors. **a** Transverse sonogram shows an ill-defined heterogeneous hypoechoic mass (*T*) at the pancreatic body involving the splenic vein and the superior mesenteric artery (*arrow*). **b** Transverse scan shows a markedly dilated Wirsung duct (*W*) and bile duct (*C*) with a biliary stent (*arrowhead*) inside, upstream to a solid hypoechoic mass (*T, arrows*) in the pancreatic head. **c** Transverse scan demonstrates a hypoechoic mass (*arrows*) in the pancreatic head. **d** In the same case, US shows the signs of the biliary obstruction caused by the pancreatic head tumor: gallbladder (*G*) distension (Courvoisier-Terrier sign), together with (**e**) dilatation of the common bile duct (*cbd*) and intrahepatic bile ducts. **f** CEUS of a pancreatic head tumor (*T*) shows absence of contrast enhancement in arterial phase (*arrows*), and (**g**) also in late phase the tumor (*T, between calipers*) shows no enhancement. **h** A transverse sonograms shows the pancreas is diffusely infiltrated by a gross echopoor mass, extending beyond the gland (*arrows*) and causing biliary obstruction (*cbd*): a pancreatic lymphoma was diagnosed at percutaneous biopsy. **i** Neuroendocrine carcinoma. Transverse view demonstrates a large well-defined echogenic mass (*arrows*) in the pancreatic head, with small central echopoor areas. **j** The corresponding CT findings (*arrows*)

trast-enhanced CT has a higher sensitivity than US [27]. The integration of different imaging methods may be necessary for tumor detection.

Endocrine tumors or islet cell tumors arise from the neuroendocrine cells of the pancreas. These tumors are classified as functioning or nonfunctioning based on the presence or absence of symptoms related to hormone production.

Insulinomas and gastrinomas are the most common functioning islet cell tumors and are usually small at the time of detection. Nonfunctioning tumors are frequently large at diagnosis and are often malignant (Fig. 2.4) [28]. The diagnosis is usually based on clinical and biochemical findings. The tasks of imaging are to localize the tumor and study its relationship to vital structures for surgical resection. Insulinomas are usually benign, solitary pancreatic lesions, whereas gastrinomas tend to be malignant and consist of multiple lesions. Insulinomas are the most common functioning neuroendocrine tumors of the pancreas (approximately 60% of all neuroendocrine tumors) and, in the majority of cases, are benign (85%–99%) and solitary (93%–98%) [28, 30]. Preoperative US detection of insulinomas is generally difficult but is possible in 25%–60% of cases [30]. The majority of insulinomas appear as hypoechoic pancreatic nodules, which are usually capsulated (Fig. 2.4). In some cases, very small calcifications may be present, especially in larger lesions [31]. At the time of clinical presentation, 50% of the tumors are smaller than 1.5 cm [32]. When malignant, their diameter is generally >3 cm, and approximately a third of these have metastases at the time of diagnosis [28]. Gastrinomas are the second most common functioning neuroendocrine tumors of the pancreas (approximately 20% of all neuroendocrine tumors) [31, 32]. These tumors differ from insulinomas in localization, size, and vasculature [31, 33]. They occur within the gastrinoma triangle (junction of the cystic duct and common bile duct – junction of the second and third parts of the duodenum – junction of the head and neck of the pancreas), of which only the pancreatic side can be adequately explored by US. Liver metastases are present in 60% of cases at the time of diagnosis [32].

Other functioning neuroendocrine tumors (VIPoma, glucagonoma, and somatostatinoma) are rarer; altogether, they account for about 20% of functioning neuroendocrine tumors of the pancreas [31, 32].

Nonfunctioning islet cell tumors account for up to 33% of neuroendocrine tumors of the pancreas; they range from 1 to 20 cm in diameter and show a high malignancy rate, up to 90% [34]. They are, however, less aggressive than adenocarcinomas (Fig. 2.4). The clinical presentation of nonfunctioning islet cell tumors is nonspecific. These tumors, characterized by predominantly expansive growth, are not clinically apparent until adjacent viscera and structures have become involved. At US they appear to have clear borders and are usually easy to detect, thanks to their size (Fig. 2.4). Due to their dimensions, these tumors tend towards necrosis and hemorrhage, developing a typical nonhomogeneous appearance that is sometimes accompanied by very small intralesional calcifications. Larger nonfunctioning islet cell tumors show cystic degeneration or cystic change [31]. Characterization of these tumors depends on the demonstration of their hypervascularity [31, 34].

Pancreatic lymphoma (see also Chapter 10) is mainly represented by the non-Hodgkin B-cell histotype, and in the majority of cases, it is associated with lymph nodes or lesions in other organs. US shows focal or diffuse pancreatic enlargement that is hypoechoic to normal pancreatic parenchyma (Fig. 2.5). Diffuse pancreatic enlargement may be due to a diffuse pancreatic tumor or pancreatitis associated with tumor. Primary tumors that most frequently metastasize to the pancreas are from the lung, breast, kidney, or melanoma [23, 35]. Pancreatic metastases (see also Chapter 10) can appear as focal or multifocal lesions or diffuse enlargements of the pancreas in a patient with a known primary neoplasm.

2.3.4 Cystic Pancreatic Lesions

Benign cysts in the pancreas are rare and tend to be associated with other conditions, such as polycystic disease, cystic fibrosis or von Hippel-Lindau disease (an autosomal dominant disease characterized by pancreatic and renal cysts, renal carcinoma, pheochromocytoma and/or hemangioblastomas in the cerebellum and spine) (Fig. 2.5) [36]. The presence of a cystic mass in the absence of these conditions should raise suspicion for one of the rarer types of cystic neoplasm or a pseudocyst associated with previous history of acute pancreatitis.

Cystic neoplasms (see also Chapter 9) account for approximately 10–15% of pancreatic cysts and only approximately 1% of pancreatic malignancies [37]. Two distinct forms of cystic neoplasm of the pancreas are recognized; both are generally easily distinguished from the much more common carcinoma.

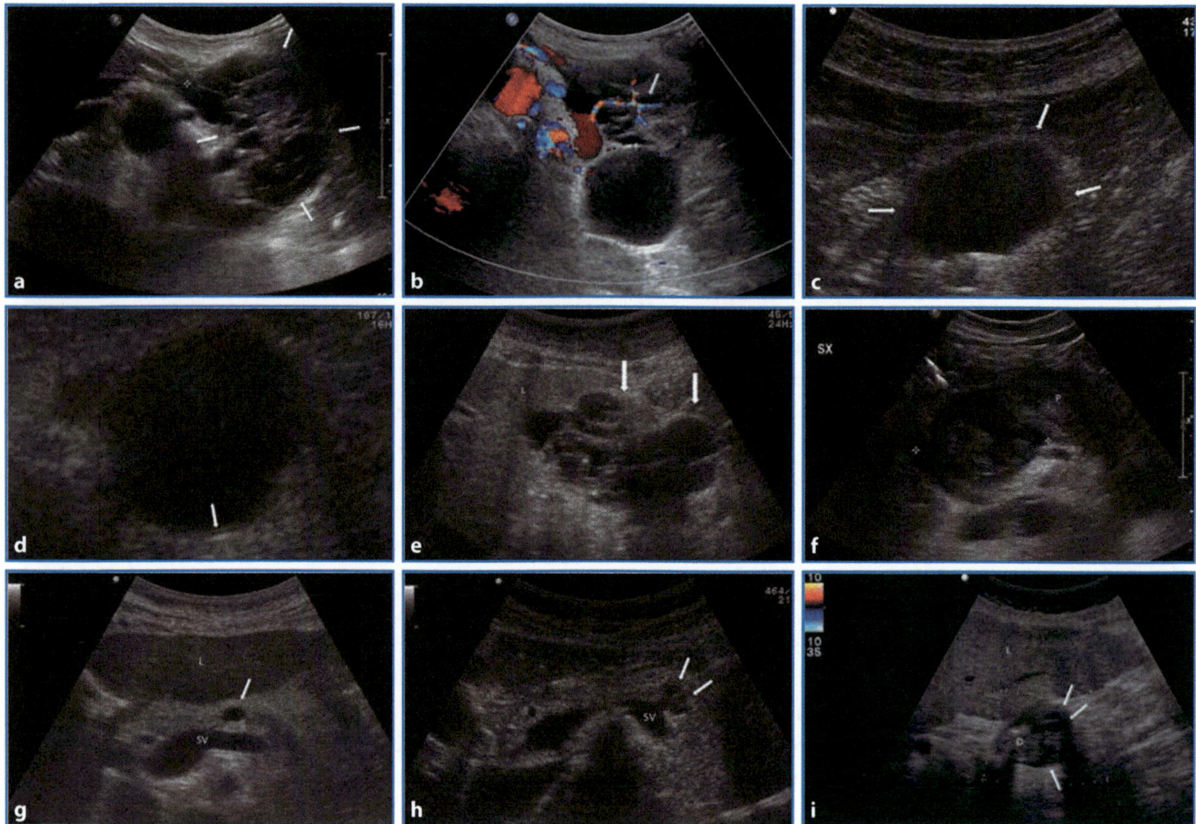

Fig. 2.5 a-i Cystic neoplasms of the pancreas. **a** Serous cystadenoma. Transverse sonogram demonstrates a heterogeneously echogenic, solid-appearing mass (*arrows*) with small-medium cystic components in the body and tail of the pancreas. Note posterior acoustic enhancement behind the mass. **b** In the same patient color Doppler analysis shows the central vessel (*arrow*) of the serous cystadenoma; the largest cyst of this cystadenoma (*between calipers*) is 3.5 cm large. **c** Mucinous cystadenoma. Transverse scan shows a unilocular cystic lesion (*arrows*) of approximately 5 cm at the junction of the pancreatic body and tail. **d** A detail of the previous image shows the thick wall (*arrow*) typical of the mucinous cystadenoma. **e** Multiloculated cystic lesions of pancreas (*arrows*) in Von Hippel Lindau disease (*L*, liver). **f** Intraductal papillary mucinous tumor of pancreas head – main duct type. Transverse scan reveals a cystic lesion (*between calipers*) with solid echogenic components (*P*, pancreatic body). **g** Intraductal papillary mucinous tumor of pancreas body – side branch type. Transverse scan shows a small unilocular cystic lesion of the pancreatic body (*arrow*), with a normal Wirsung duct (*SV*, splenic vein; *L*, liver). **h** Intraductal papillary mucinous tumor of pancreas body-tail – side branch type. Transverse scan shows a small grape-like multilocular cystic lesion of the pancreatic body-tail (*arrows*), with a normal Wirsung duct (*SV*, splenic vein). **i** Cystic dystrophy on aberrant pancreas of duodenal wall: transverse scan shows the presence of multiple cystic lesions (*arrows*) within the thickened duodenum (*D*) wall

Microcystic cystadenoma (serous cystadenoma) is always histologically benign and frequently found in elderly women. It is composed of cysts that are small (1–2 mm), generating an appearance of a hyperechoic mass, frequently with lobular outlines (Fig. 2.5). A central echogenic stellate scar is an inconstant feature of this tumor. Oligocystic serous cystadenoma, which has fewer but much larger cysts, is a variant of serous cystadenoma and accounts for 10–25% of serous cystadenomas of the pancreas. Sonographic findings in oligo-

cystic serous cystadenoma are similar to those of mucinous cystadenoma; however, lobulated outer margins and more frequent pancreatic duct dilatation proximal to the lesion can allow its differentiation from oligocystic serous cystadenoma. Serous cystadenomas do not communicate with the main pancreatic duct. The demonstration of this is fundamental, especially when the lesion is large, because it might compress the main pancreatic duct that is dilated proximally. Demonstration of the absence of communication, however, is impossible with US and is a specific issue for magnetic resonance imaging and endoscopic retrograde cholangiopancreatography. Differential diagnosis between serous and mucinous cystic tumors is a fundamental issue of imaging, considering the different management required for these two lesions, so that aggressive surgical intervention for serous cystadenomas can be avoided [37]. Serous cystadenoma, being a benign lesion, can be conservatively managed.

Mucinous cystic neoplasms are malignant or potentially malignant lesions. They are more common in women in their fourth to sixth decade and are most often located in the body or tail of the pancreas. The mucinous cystic tumor is peripherally located in the pancreatic parenchyma and shows cysts which are less numerous and larger in size than are typically seen with serous cystadenoma. The content of the cyst is mucin. At US, a mucinous cystic neoplasm appears as round to ovoid, with unilocular or multilocular cystic lesions, each >20 mm. Mucinous cystic tumors are characterized by the presence of thick walls and, occasionally, peripheral calcifications (Fig. 2.5). The mucinous content is viscous, may generate fine echoes in the internal part of the lesion covering the internal wall of the cystic tumor, and may mask the inclusions, such as internal septa and/or solid papillary projections. Demonstration of these inclusions, and if possible, demonstration of their vasculature, is fundamental for the diagnosis. The number and thickness of intralesional septa and nodules are not always related to the grade of malignancy. Mucinous tumors may spread, involve lymph nodes, and produce liver metastases [38, 39].

Intraductal papillary mucinous tumors (IPMTs) originate from the main pancreatic duct or its branches. Their histology ranges from benign to frankly malignant. The lesion is identifiable as a dilatation of the main pancreatic duct and/or its branches or cyst formation, with proliferation of pancreatic ductal epithelium and excessive production of mucin. IPMTs are classified in main duct type, branch duct type, or a combination of the two [39-41]. The main duct type can be localized or diffuse. The main pancreatic duct type presents as a segmental, diffuse dilatation of the main duct with or without side-branch dilatation. The main duct type of mucin-secreting tumors appears predominantly cystic on US, tends to be located in the body or tail of the pancreas and metastasizes late, which represents a much less aggressive course than adeno-

carcinomas. These tumors have a much higher curative rate with surgery [39]. The localized main duct type of IPMT is characterized by highly inhomogeneous masses, which are related to neoplastic intraductal proliferation, with upstream dilation of the main pancreatic duct (Fig. 2.5). The diffuse main type may be difficult to distinguish from chronic pancreatitis. At US examination, the mucin of IPMT may not be easily differentiated from the solid portions of the tumor, which can therefore be mistakenly reported as solid. Harmonic imaging, with its better contrast resolution [42, 43], may lead to the identification of the part of the IPMT that is not solid. With US, a final diagnosis of IPMT by demonstration of the communication between the tumor and the pancreatic duct is difficult. The combination of other imaging techniques, mainly magnetic resonance and endoscopic US, may better show the cystic dilatation of branch ducts as well as nodules and septa inside the cystic lesion [39]. The IPMT branch duct type manifests as a single or multiple cysts (Fig. 2.5) which are generally incidentally discovered during US examination. As they are mostly benign, imaging follow-up has been suggested, depending on their characteristics. Based on limited published data, it appears that asymptomatic cystic lesions without main duct dilation, those without mural nodules, and those smaller than 30 mm in size have a low risk of prevalent cancer and a low risk of progressing to invasive cancer in near-term follow-up (12 to 36 months). Ideally, the imaging modality at baseline and follow-up should provide adequate information regarding the size of the lesion, size of the main pancreatic duct, and presence of intramural nodules, which can be barely evaluated with US but can be assessed satisfactorily by using multidetector high-resolution computed tomography or magnetic resonance cholangiopancreatography or with endoscopic US. Transabdominal US is useful for the initial evaluation and for follow-up in thin patients with clearly visualized cysts. The interval between follow-up examinations has been suggested as follows: yearly follow-up if the lesion is <10 mm in size, 6–12-monthly follow-up for lesions between 10 and 20 mm, and 3–6-monthly follow-up for lesions >20 mm. On follow-up studies, the appearance of symptoms attributable to the cyst (e.g. pancreatitis), the presence of intramural nodules, cyst size >30 mm, and dilation of the main pancreatic duct (>6 mm) would be indications for resection. The follow-up interval can be lengthened after 2 years of no change [39].

Cystic dystrophy of the duodenal wall and groove pancreatitis occur in a border site (groove region) between the pancreas and the duodenum, which is difficult to access for a correct US evaluation. Identification of small cystic formations in the thickened duodenal wall on the pancreatic side is a specific finding [44] for cystic dystrophy of the duodenal wall (Fig. 2.5).

2.4 Comments

Pancreatic lesions are commonly detected during US examination, as this modality is used very often as the first line of diagnostic imaging [45]. Basically the differential diagnosis of pancreatic masses must always be considered. For this task, more recent technologic improvements in US (elastography, contrast-enhanced US) should be integrated, if possible in the same examination session, to achieve the best US definition (see related chapters).

References

1. Lawson TL, Berland LL, Foley WD et al (1982) Ultrasonic visualization of the pancreatic duct. Radiology 144:865-871
2. Niederau C, Grendell JH (1985) Diagnosis of chronic pancreatitis. Gastroenterology 88:1973-1995
3. Brogna A, Bucceri AM, Catalano F et al (1991) Ultrasonographic study of the Wirsung duct caliber after meal. Ital J Gastroenterol 23:208-210
4. Loren I, Lasson A, Fork T et al (1999) New sonographic imaging observations in focal pancreatitis. Eur Radiol 9:862-867
5. Jacobs JE, Coleman BG, Arger PH, Langer JE (1994) Pancreatic sparing of focal fatty infiltration. Radiology 190:437-439
6. Baron HT, Morgan ED (1997) The diagnosis and management of fluid collections associated with pancreatitis. Am J Med 102:555-563
7. Procacci C (2001) Pancreatic neoplasms and tumor-like conditions. Eur Radiol 11[Suppl 2]:S167-S192
8. Kourtesis G, Wilson S, Williams R (1990) The clinical significance of fluid collections in acute pancreatitis. Am Surg 56:796-799
9. Procacci C, Mansueto G, D'Onofrio M et al (2002) Non-traumatic abdominal emergencies: imaging and intervention in acute pancreatic conditions. Eur Radiol 12:2407-2434
10. Balthazar EJ, Freeny PC, Van Sonnenberg E (1994) Imaging and intervention in acute pancreatitis. Radiology 193:297-306
11. Ranson J, Rifkind R, Roses D (1975) Prognostic signs and role of operative management in acute pancreatitis. Surg Gynecol Obstet 139:69-80
12. Freeny P, Lawson T (1982) Radiology of the pancreas. New York, Springer-Verlag, p. 449
13. Alpern MB, Sandler MA, Kellman GM, Madrazo BL (1985) Chronic pancreatitis: ultrasonic features. Radiology 155:215-219
14. Bolondi L, Priori P, Gullo L et al. (1987) Relationship between morphological changes detected by ultrasonography and pancreatic esocrine function in chronic pancreatitis. Pancreas 2:222-229
15. Remer EM, Baker MB (2002) Imaging of chronic pancreatitis. Radiol Clin N Am 40:1229-1242
16. Homma T, Harada H, Koizumi M (1997) Diagnostic criteria for chronic pancreatitis by the Japan Pancreas Society. Pancreas 15:14-15
17. Glasbrenner B, Kahl S, Malfertheiner P (2002) Modern diagnostics of chronic pancreatitis. Eur J Gastroenterol Hepatol 14:935-941
18. Hessel ST, Siegelman SS, McNeil BJ et al (1982) A prospective evaluation of computer tomography and US of the pancreas. Radiology 143:129-133
19. Furukawa N, Muranaka T, Yasumori K et al (1998) Autoimmune pancreatitis: radiologic findings in three histologically proven cases. J Comput Assist Tomogr 22:880-883
20. Neff CC, Simeone JF, Witenberg J et al (1984) Inflammatory pancreatic masses. Problems in differentiating focal pancreatitis from carcinoma. Radiology 150:35-38
21. Irie H, Honda H, Baba S et al (1998) Autoimmune pancreatitis: CT and MR characteristics. Am J Roentgenol 170:1323-1327
22. Buscarini E, Frulloni L, De Lisi S et al (2010) Autoimmune pancreatitis: A challenging diagnostic puzzle for clinicians. Digest Liver Dis 42:92-98
23. Martinez-Noguera A, D'Onofrio M (2007) Ultrasonography of the pancreas.1. Conventional imaging. Abdom Imaging 32:137-149
24. Rosewicz S, Wiedenman B (1997) Pancreatic carcinoma. Lancet 349:485-489
25. Ichikawa T, Haradome H, Hachiya J et al (1997) Pancreatic ductal adenocarcinoma: preoperative assessment with helical CT versus dynamic MR imaging. Radiology 202:655-662
26. Minniti S, Bruno C, Biasiutti C et al (2003) Sonography versus helical CT in identification and staging of pancreatic ductal adenocarcinoma. J Clin US 31:175-182
27. Karlson BM, Ekbom A, Lindgren PG et al (1999) Abdominal US for diagnosis of pancreatic tumor: prospective cohort analysis. Radiology 213:107-111
28. Buetow PC, Miller DL, Parrino TV (1997) Islet cell tumors of the pancreas: clinical, radiologic, and pathologic correlation in diagnosis and localization. Radiographics 17:453-472
29. Yassa N, Yang J, Stein S et al (1997) Gray-scale and colour flow sonography of pancreatic ductal adenocarcinoma. J Clin US 25:473-480
30. Angeli E, Vanzulli A, Castrucci M et al (1997) Value of abdominal sonography and MR imaging at 0.5 T in preoperative detection of pancreatic insulinoma: a comparison with dynamic CT and angiography. Abdom Imaging 22:295-303
31. D'Onofrio M, Mansueto GC, Falconi M, Procacci C (2004) Neuroendocrine pancreatic tumor: value of contrast enhanced ultrasonography. Abdom Imaging 29:246-258
32. Ros PR, Mortele KJ (2001) Imaging features of pancreatic neoplasms. JBRBT-R 84:239-249
33. Pereira PL, Wiskirchen J (2003) Morphological and functional investigations of neuroendocrine tumors of the pancreas. Eur Radiol 13:2133-2146

34. Procacci C, Carbognin G, Accordini S et al (2001) Non-functioning endocrine tumors of the pancreas: possibilities of spiral CT characterization. Eur Radiol 11:1175-1183
35. Merkle EM, Braz T, Kolkythas O et al (1998) Metastases to the pancreas. Br J Radiol 71:1208-1214
36. Elli L, Buscarini E, Portugalli V et al (2006) Pancreatic involvement in von Hippel-Lindau disease: report of two cases and review of the literature. Am J Gastroenterol 101:2655-2658
37. Yeo CJ, Sarr MG (1994) Cystic and pseudocystic diseases of the pancreas. Curr Probl Surg 31:165-243
38. Hammond N, Miller F, Silca G, Gore R (2002) Imaging of cystic disease of the pancreas. Radiol Clin N Am 40:1243-1262
39. Tanaka M, Chari S, Adsay V et al (2006) International consensus guidelines for management of intraductal papillary mucinous neoplasms and mucinous cystic neoplasms of the pancreas. Pancreatology 6:17-32
40. Kalra MK, Maher MM, Sahani DV et al (2002) Current status of imaging in pancreatic diseases. J Comput Assist Tomogr 26:661-675
41. Procacci C, Megibow AJ, Carbognin G et al (1999) Intraductal papillary mucinous tumor of the pancreas: a pictorial essay. Radiographics 19:1447-1463
42. Shapiro RS, Wagreich J, Parsons RB et al (1998) Tissue harmonic imaging sonography: evaluation of image quality compared with conventional sonography. Am J Roentgenol 171:1203-1206
43. Bennett GL, Hann LE (2001) Pancreatic ultrasonography. Surg Clin North Am 81:259-281
44. Procacci C, Graziani R, Zamboni G et al (1997) Cystic dystrophy of the duodenal wall: radiologic findings. Radiology 205:741-747
45. D'Onofrio M, Gallotti A, Pozzi Mucelli R (2010) Imaging techniques in pancreatic tumors. Expert Rev Med Devices 7:257-273

Endoscopic Ultrasonography of the Pancreas

3

Elisabetta Buscarini and Stefania De Lisi

3.1 Introduction

Endoscopic ultrasonography (EUS) joins a high frequency (5–20 MHz) US transducer to a flexible endoscope. In contrast to transabdominal US, EUS provides a high-resolution view of the pancreatic parenchyma because of the close proximity of the probe to the gland without interference from bowel gas or fat tissue, and it is one of the most accurate methods for diagnosing and staging pancreatic diseases. Indeed, EUS is the most sensitive technique for the detection of lesions to screen subjects who are at high risk of developing pancreatic cancer, showing a sensitivity of 93% compared to magnetic resonance imaging (MRI) (81%) and computed tomography (CT) (27%) [1].

3.2 Technical Equipment

The instruments that are currently available for the examination of the pancreas are radial scanning echoendoscopes, linear scanning echoendoscopes and more recently developed electronic radial scopes. The radial scanning instruments display a 360° or 270° cross-sectional image that is perpendicular to the long axis of the scope, whereas the image of linear echoendoscopes is parallel to the long axis of the scope, and sampling of pancreatic and nodal lesions is possible using EUS-guided fine-needle aspiration (EUS-FNA) (Fig. 3.1).

E. Buscarini (✉)
Department of Gastroenterology
Maggiore Hospital, Crema, Italy
e-mail: ebuscarini@rim.it

As with linear scopes, electronic radial instruments have high resolution and Doppler capability.

FNA needles are available in 19-, 21-, 22- and 25-gauge sizes. A recent randomized trial showed that EUS-FNA of solid pancreatic lesions reached higher diagnostic accuracy and fewer blood contaminations with 25-gauge needles than with 22-gauge ones [2]. Tru-cut biopsy needles are used for histologic diagnosis, but they have technical limitations, especially for biopsy from the duodenum. Miniature high-frequency US probes (12–30 MHz) can be introduced in the operative channel of a standard duodenoscope, allowing for intraductal ultrasonography (IDUS) of the main pancreatic duct. Mechanical rotation of the transducer provides a 360° cross-sectional image of the structures near the probe (2 cm). EUS color Doppler is useful for discriminating between a venous vessel and an arterial vessel; it adds information about vascular involvement by pancreatic tumors, and it is essential for avoiding vessel puncture during interventional procedures. EUS power Doppler has been employed with contrast-enhanced EUS (CE-EUS), which is performed after the administration of intravenous contrast agents, improving the characterization of the vascular patterns of pancreatic masses. However, contrast-enhanced power Doppler presents artifacts, such as blooming and variability with Doppler gain. Contrast-enhanced harmonic has been recently developed to overcome these artifacts, allowing for a more detailed evaluation of tissue vasculature. As with transabdominal CEUS, arterial, portal venous, and parenchymal contrast enhancement is possible. During the arterial phase, which lasts approximately 10 to 20 seconds, the celiac axis, common hepatic artery, and splenic artery can be characterized; in the venous phase (30–120 seconds), enhancement of the splenic vein, portal vein and superior mesenteric vein can be observed.

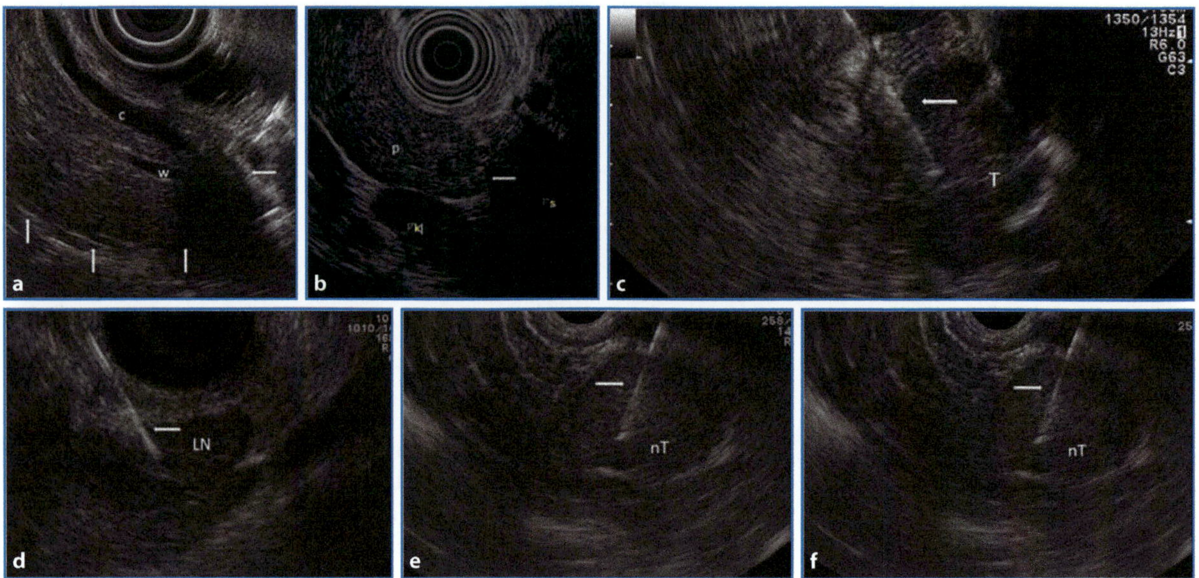

Fig. 3.1 a-f Normal EUS anatomy of pancreas. **a** EUS scan from the second part of the duodenum shows the pancreas head (*arrows*), the common bile duct (*c*) and the duct of Wirsung (*w*). **b** EUS scanning from the stomach shows the pancreatic body and tail (*p*); the *arrow* indicates the tail tip (*k*, kidney; *s*, spleen). **c** EUS-FNA of a pancreatic tumor (*T*). **d** EUS-FNA of a peripancreatic lymphnode (*LN*). **e** EUS-FNA of a pancreatic neuroendocrine tumor (*nT*). **f** EUS-FNA of a pancreatic cystic lesion (*c*)

3.3 EUS Examination

Prior to upper GI tract endoscopy, the patient should fast for six hours, and the examination is performed with the patient lying in the left lateral decubitus position. Usually, conscious sedation is achieved with the administration of midazolam. In particular cases, opioid drugs (e.g. pethidine) or deep anesthesia can be used.

Particular attention should be paid during the esophageal intubation and the maneuvers of transit into the descending duodenum because of the rigid and prominent tip of the echoendoscope. Cervical esophageal perforation is a rare event; an incidence of 0.06% has been reported in elderly women undergoing EUS with a linear echoendoscope by a skilled operator [3]. To scan the pancreas, good acoustic coupling can be achieved by inflating the balloon and filling the gastrointestinal lumen with water. The administration of spasmolytic agents (e.g. butylscopolamine) is still controversial.

Radial scanning with the echoendoscope placed in the descending duodenum displays the pancreatic head, the uncinate process and the region of major papilla, and the pancreatic neck and common bile duct can be visualized from the duodenal bulb. The body and the tail of the pancreas can be imaged by scanning from the stomach.

Linear scanning from the stomach may display the whole gland; from the descending duodenum, the pancreatic head and the region of major papilla can be imaged.

Pancreatic EUS examination is limited in cases of surgically altered anatomy; the head of the pancreas cannot be imaged after Roux-en-Y surgery, whereas a complete examination including FNA may be possible after Billroth II surgery if the afferent loop is intubated [4]. Because EUS-FNA is a procedure with a high risk of bleeding, a pre-examination check of coagulation parameters and platelet count is mandatory when the procedure is scheduled. Similarly, antithrombotic drugs should be discontinued before the procedure [5]. Intravenous antibiotics should be administered before aspiration of a pancreatic cyst.

3.4 Normal EUS Pancreatic Findings

The normal pancreatic parenchyma has a fine granular pattern with echogenicity that is equal to or slightly higher than that of the liver (Fig. 3.1). Hyperechoic pancreas is a common condition; risk factors are fatty liver, age older than 60 years, male gender and hypertension [6].

A physiologic difference between the ventral and the dorsal portion of the pancreatic head can be observed in half of normal pancreases: the former appears hypoechoic, and the latter appears hyperechoic. The border of the gland is smooth.

The main pancreatic duct appears as a tubular anechoic structure with hyperechoic walls. Its normal caliber ranges from 3 mm in the head to 1 mm in the pancreatic tail.

On IDUS, the wall of a normal main pancreatic duct is visualized as a single hyperechoic layer, and the surrounding pancreatic parenchyma is demonstrated as a homogeneous pattern in normal cases. The course of the normal pancreatic duct is tortuous, and the lumen caliber is not sufficient for performing IDUS in the body and tail.

3.5 Pathologic EUS Features of the Pancreas

3.5.1 Pancreatic Cancer

On EUS, pancreatic adenocarcinoma appears essentially as a hypoechoic, inhomogeneous lesion with irregular margins (Fig. 3.2). Small cancers can show a homogeneous echopattern with smooth margins; when the tu-

mor grows, hypoechoic and hyperechoic areas can occur, indicating intralesional necrosis and calcifications, respectively. A post-stenotic dilatation of the main pancreatic duct can be observed, which is joined to the common bile duct dilatation if the mass involves the pancreatic head (Fig. 3.2).

Multiple, patchy, hypoechoic areas adjacent to the dilated main pancreatic duct can be observed in patients with pancreatic cancer, as reported in a retrospective analysis of EUS images performed in 84 patients with main pancreatic duct dilatation. This was observed more frequently in patients with malignancy than in patients with benign disease (73.8% versus 14.3%) [7].

EUS allows for detailed evaluation of peri-pancreatic vessels that are invaded by tumors. The splenic vein and artery are easily depicted, whereas it is more difficult to image the superior mesenteric vessels [8]. EUS criteria for vascular involvement by pancreatic tumors have been published (Fig. 3.2) [9, 10].

The following EUS findings appear to be reliable signs for the identification of venous tumor invasion:
1. Clear separation between tumor and vessel, with interposed hyperechoic tissue;

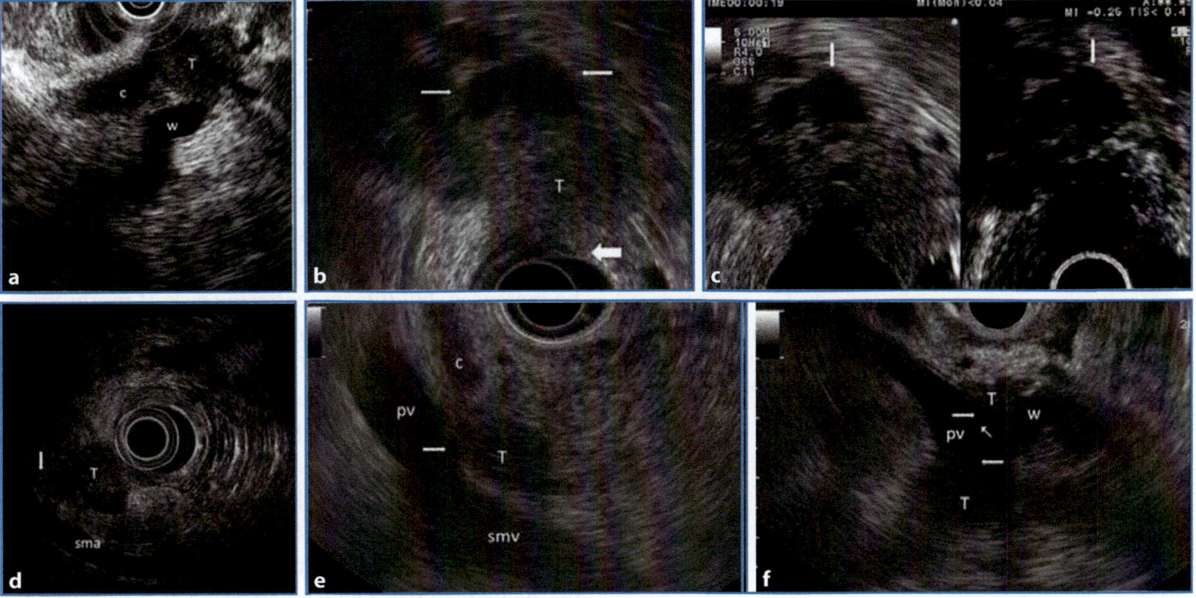

Fig. 3.2 a–f Pancreatic cancer. **a** EUS scan of pancreatic head shows a small tumor (*T*) obstructing both common bile duct (*c*) and duct of Wirsung (*w*). **b** EUS shows a cystadenocarcinoma (*T*) of the pancreatic head, invading the duodenal wall (*thick arrow*), with two cystic areas (*arrows*). **c** CE-EUS shows that the lesion enhances during the arterial phase irregularly and only to the boundaries. **d** EUS staging of a pancreatic tumor (*T*) shows a clear interface (*arrow*) with the superior mesenteric artery (*sma*). **e** EUS staging of a pancreatic tumor (*T*) shows the contact (*arrow*) with the superior mesenteric artery (*smv*) and portal vein (*pv*) wall (*c*, common bile duct). **f** EUS staging of a pancreatic tumor (*T*) shows the loss of interface (*arrows*) with the portal vein (*pv*) which is surrounded by the tumor; the duct of Wirsung (*w*) is obstructed by the tumor

2. Tumor border at the vessel, without interruption of the vessel wall;
3. Abnormal vessel contour with loss of the vessel–parenchymal sonographic interface;
4. Tumor border at the vessel, echo-rich vessel wall interrupted or not visible;
5. Partial or complete vascular lumen obstruction by the tumor;
6. Peri-pancreatic venous collateral vessels.

To diagnose arterial invasion, criteria 1 and 2 as well as tumor encasement are used.

Staging of pancreatic cancer is currently based on the tumor–node–metastasis (TNM) classification revised by the American Joint Committee for Cancer in 2003 [11] (Table 3.1). According to this classification, pancreatic cancer is considered non-resectable when (a) the tumor involves the celiac or superior mesenteric artery or other major arteries of the upper abdomen, or (b) there is nodal involvement beyond the peripancreatic tissue and/or (c) there is distant metastasis. The resectability of neoplasms involving the superior mesenteric vein or portal vein and its confluence is still controversial. Survival after resection was comparable to that of patients without vascular invasion in one study [12], whereas another surgical series did not confirm a survival benefit [13].

Table 3.1 TNM staging classification of pancreatic adenocarcinoma [11]

Tumor
T-x: Primary tumor cannot be assessed
T-0: No evidence of primary tumor
T-is: Carcinoma in situ
T-1: Tumor limited to the pancreas, ≤ 2 cm
T-2: Tumor limited to the pancreas, > 2 cm
T-3: Tumor extension beyond the pancreas (without involvement of the celiac axis or the superior mesenteric artery)
T-4: Tumor involving the celiac axis and superior mesenteric artery (unresectable tumor)
Regional lymph nodes
N-x: Regional lymph nodes cannot be assessed
N-0: No regional lymph node metastasis
N-1: Regional lymph node metastasis
Distant metastasis
M-x: Distant metastasis cannot be assessed
M-0: No distant metastasis
Stage 0 – Tis, N0, M0
Stage IA – T1, N0, M0
Stage IB – T2, N0, M0
Stage IIA – T3, N0, M0
Stage IIB – T1, N1, M0 or T2, N1, M0 or T3, N1, M0
Stage III – T4, any N, M0
Stage IV – any T, any N, M1

To correctly interpret EUS images and avoid artifacts, the scanning should be performed by multiple stations and angles.

EUS can detect enlarged perigastric, periduodenal and celiac lymph nodes. EUS criteria that are highly predictive of nodal metastasis by esophageal cancer have been defined [14]. They include size (>1 cm in diameter in the short axis), hypoechoic appearance, round shape, and clear borders.

When all four criteria are present, the accuracy of predicting malignant invasion is approximately 80%, but all four criteria are present in only 25% of cases [15]. For this reason, EUS criteria alone are not able to define the nature of lymph nodes, and EUS-FNA is required for nodal staging of pancreatic cancer.

EUS-FNA is essential for a histologic diagnosis of adenocarcinoma and to rule out other causes of pancreatic masses which may require different treatment. The sensitivity of EUS-FNA for pancreatic cancer ranges between 60% and 90% [16, 17].

The risk of complications due to EUS-FNA is low, as revealed by a recent multicenter study of 808 patients (of which 541 were pancreatic biopsies) undergoing EUS-FNA, with a 0.9% rate of complications, represented by acute pancreatitis (0.02%) and bleeding (0.07%) [18]. The risk of seeding is generally low, and to minimize it, sampling of pancreatic head lesions is usually performed through the duodenal wall, which is then resected during surgery.

Although EUS-FNA provides cytologic diagnosis with high accuracy, false-negative results can still be a problem, especially in the setting of chronic pancreatitis. To overcome this limitation, the number of passes should be increased, but this increases the risk of morbidity.

In recent years, two noninvasive methods of standard US have been applied to EUS to improve the differential diagnosis between pancreatic cancer and chronic pancreatitis: CE-EUS aids in the delineation of the margins of pancreatic lesions and in the evaluation of their relationships with perilesional vessels. Initial studies used CE-EUS with Levovist, showing tumor hypovascularity in 92% of the patients with ductal adenocarcinoma of the pancreas [19]. Other relevant findings involve the irregular vascular network of malignant lesions after contrast enhancement with only arterial vessels, whereas in benign masses both venous and arterial vessels can be imaged [20].

In a recent study, CE-EUS was performed with a new prototype echoendoscope and using SonoVue (Fig. 3.2).

The microvascular pattern was compared to the final pathologic diagnosis based on surgery or EUS-FNA. The results revealed that 16 of 18 hypovascular lesions (88.8%) were pancreatic carcinomas. The sensitivity, specificity and accuracy of hypovascularity for diagnosing pancreatic adenocarcinoma were 89%, 88%, and 88.5 %, compared with corresponding values of 72%, 100%, and 86%, respectively, for EUS-FNA [21]. Hyperenhancement of pancreatic cancer on CE-EUS has been reported for poorly differentiated adenocarcinoma [22].

EUS elastography provides a real-time evaluation of tissue stiffness to discriminate between malignant and benign lesions. A score for the classification of pancreatic mass sonoelastography has been proposed [23]:

Score 1 indicates a homogenous, low elastograph area (soft, green) and corresponds to the normal pancreas tissue.

Score 2 indicates a heterogeneous pattern in the soft tissue range (green, yellow and red) and corresponds to fibrosis.

Score 3 indicates an elastograph image that is largely blue (hard), with minimal heterogeneity, and corresponds to a small (less than 25 mm), early pancreatic adenocarcinoma.

Score 4 indicates lesions with a hypoechoic central region, which is small and appears green surrounded by blue or harder tissue, and corresponds to a hypervascular lesion, such as a neuroendocrine tumor or small pancreatic metastasis.

Score 5 is assigned to lesions that are largely blue on the elastograph, but with heterogeneity of softer tissue colors (green, red), which represents necrosis, and is seen in advanced pancreatic adenocarcinoma.

This scoring system was validated in a multicenter study of 121 patients undergoing EUS for pancreatic lesions; scores 1 and 2 were considered benign and scores 3–5 were considered malignant. The sensibility, specificity, positive predictive value (PPV) and negative predictive value (NPV) of EUS elastography to differentiate benign from malignant pancreatic masses were, respectively, 80.6%, 92.3%, 93.3% and 78.1%, with a global accuracy of this new technology of 89.2%. The NPV for malignancy of scores 1 and 2 was 77.4%, and the PPV for malignancy of scores 3–5 was 92.8% [24]. A recent study attempted to overcome the main limitation of EUS elastography, which is the subjectivity of the evaluation; the accuracy of quantitative, second-generation EUS elastography in the differential diagnosis of solid pancreatic masses was assessed using a *strain ratio* between the region of interest and a reference area. A significant difference between the strain ratio values was reported in pancreatic cancer compared to chronic pancreatitis with an inflammatory mass [25].

3.5.1.1 EUS Performance in Staging of Pancreatic Cancer

Poor prognosis of pancreatic cancer is due mainly to late-stage diagnosis. In this setting, a sensitive tool is essential for early diagnosis and assessment of resectability. EUS is a technique with particularly high sensitivity for the detection of masses smaller than 3 cm.

In early studies comparing EUS with conventional CT, EUS sensitivity for tumor detection ranged from 91% to 98%, which is higher than that of CT (63–85%) [26-29] (Table 3.2). Even more recent studies that compared EUS to helical CT confirmed the superior sensitivity of EUS to that of CT [17, 30-33] (Table 3.2).

A systematic review analyzed 11 studies comparing helical CT with EUS for the diagnosis of pancreatic cancer. In all of these studies, EUS sensitivity was higher than that of helical CT, especially for pancreatic tumors smaller than 3 cm [34]. Moreover, a retrospective series

Table 3.2 Sensitivity (%) of EUS and other imaging techniques for diagnosis of pancreatic lesions

Reference	Patients included	EUS	CT	MRI	US	PET
Rosch (1992) [26]	60	98	85		78	
Palazzo (1993) [27]	49	91	66		64	
Muller (1994) [28]	33	94	69	83		
Marty (1995) [29]	37	92	63			
Mertz (2000) [30]	31	93	53			87
Rivadeneira (2003) [31]	44	100	68			
Agarwal (2004) [17]	71	100	86			
Dewitt (2004) [32]	80	98	86			
Mansfield (2008) [33]	84	95	97			

showed that EUS, performed by skilled operators, is a valuable tool to rule out the presence of a pancreatic tumor, with a negative predictive value of 100% [35].

A recent meta-analysis evaluated the accuracy of EUS for vascular invasion in pancreatic and periampullary cancers [8]. Because EUS technology and EUS criteria for diagnosing vascular invasion have changed over time, the 29 studies included in the analysis were grouped into three time periods. Although this allowed for a comparison among studies using similar methods, the heterogeneity in the number and type of EUS vascular criteria of the included studies affected the findings of the meta-analysis. Indeed, its results show that the pooled specificity of EUS is high (90.2%), whereas the pooled sensitivity is 73%, which is lower than previously reported.

The role of EUS in the assessment of vascular invasion should be re-evaluated because of the use of helical CT and MRI. Currently available studies report equivalent results for the three modalities, so their use depends on local expertise and availability [36, 37].

3.5.2 Cystic Lesions

In recent years, the relatively rare cystic neoplasms have become increasingly identified because of the advancement of imaging studies. Cystic tumors can range from benign adenoma to premalignant and malignant lesions.

Serous cystadenomas (Fig. 3.3) are frequently located in the body or tail of the pancreas. The typical EUS findings of these benign lesions are several microcysts with a honeycomb, sponge-like structure, and possibly with central calcification. Large serous cystadenomas can show a hyperechoic central stellate scar, and microcysts can combine into a single macrocyst. The presence of debris in the fluid of the cysts is not usual, and it suggests a mucinous cystadenoma.

Mucinous cystadenomas (Fig. 3.3) are characteristically well-demarcated, unilocular, single cysts with thin walls that can show peripheral calcification. Multilocular cysts divided by thin septa can be observed. Thickening of the cystic wall (≥3 mm) or the appearance of a solid hypoechoic component should be carefully examined because these features are suggestive of malignant evolution of a mucinous cyst. No communication with the main pancreatic duct is seen. The cystic fluid can contain floating mucinous debris.

Intraductal papillary mucinous tumors (IPMT) (Fig. 3.3) include three forms: the main type, in which the tumors arise from the main pancreatic duct; the branch-duct type, which involves a side branch; and the mixed type, which involves both ductal systems. The EUS features of the main type IPMT are segmental or diffuse main duct dilatation, whereas a cystic dilatation of a side branch of the pancreatic duct communicating to a normal main duct is diagnostic of a branch-duct type IPMT. In this setting, IDUS may be a complementary tool for evaluating the involvement of the main pancreatic duct. IDUS can show the spread of branch-duct type IPMT into the main pancreatic duct as an irregular thickening of the main pancreatic duct wall, as reported in a recent study, which showed a diagnostic accuracy of 92% and indicated an important role for the determination of the resection line in surgical candidates [38]. Although EUS morphology alone cannot distinguish benign from malignant pancreatic cysts, EUS findings that are suggestive of IPMT malignancy have been proposed: main pancreatic duct dilatation >10 mm, branch type tumors >40 mm with irregular septa, and mural nodules (>10 mm) [39]. IPMT have a malignant potential, which is higher for main duct IPMT than for branch-duct tumors. Their natural history has been evaluated in a study on 103 patients with branch-duct type IPMT: 5.8% of the patients developed cancer during the long-term follow up (median 59 months), an IPM carcinoma was diagnosed in four patients, and a ductal carcinoma was found in the remaining two patients [40]. These findings underscore the value of regular follow-up imaging with accurate examination of the whole gland. Papillary cystic tumors are rare lesions with low malignant potential and frequent localizations to the pancreatic body or tail. On EUS, they appear as large, well-demarcated mixed masses, each with a solid and a cystic component.

Pseudocysts, which have to be differentiated from cystic neoplasm, can develop in both acute and chronic pancreatitis. On EUS, they usually appear as unilocular cysts with thin walls and floating debris in the cystic fluid. Chronic pseudocysts may display septa and a thick wall that is adherent to the stomach or duodenum; a final diagnosis is often reached, taking into account features of the surrounding parenchyma and the clinical history of the patients.

EUS-FNA is a useful tool for differentiating between serous and mucinous cysts. In this setting, FNA may be targeted to the cystic fluid, cystic wall, septa or nodule. Aspirated cystic fluid may be examined for tumor markers and for chemical and molecular analysis. CEA is considered the most predictive marker for diagnosing mucinous cysts. A cutoff of 192 ng/mL has an accuracy of 79% [41]. Low levels of CEA can be observed in

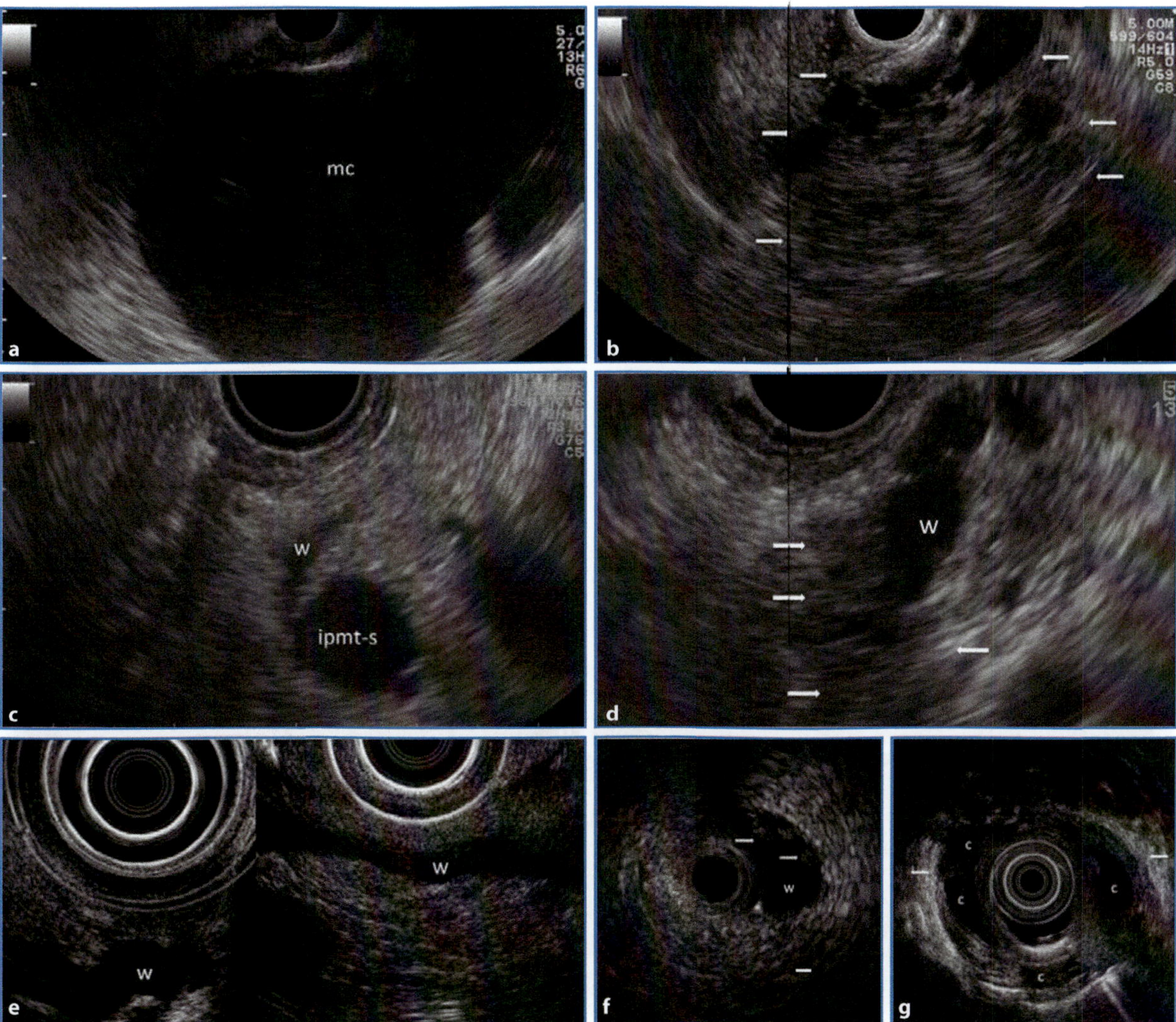

Fig. 3.3 a–g Cystic lesions of pancreas. **a** Mucinous cystadenoma: EUS shows a large roundish cystic lesion (*mc*) of the pancreatic tail, with thick wall and anechoic content. **b** Serous cystadenoma: EUS shows the multiple microcysts composing this cystic tumor (*arrows*) of the pancreatic body. **c** IPMT-side branch type: EUS reveals a small cystic lesion (*ipmt-s*) of the pancreatic isthmus, with a normal sized duct of Wirsung (*w*). **d** IPMT-main duct type: EUS shows the dilated duct of Wirsung (*w*) upstream to an ill-defined lesion (*arrows*) arising from the duct and which infiltrates the surrounding parenchyma. **e** In this patient EUS shows the duct of Wirsung (*w*) dilated in all pancreatic sections, but without lesions detected. **f** In the same patient the intraductal US (IDUS) of the duct of Wirsung (*w*) shows some small nodules (*arrows*) of the duct wall: IPMT. **g** Cystic dystrophy of aberrant pancreas of duodenal wall: EUS shows multiple cystic lesions (*c*) within the edematous and thickened duodenal wall (*arrows*)

serous cystadenomas and pseudocysts. Amylase levels are high in cystic lesions with a direct communication to the pancreatic ducts (IPMT and pseudocysts).

The performance of cytology based on EUS-FNA for the diagnosis of mucinous lesions has been assessed by a meta-analysis of 11 studies, with histopathology as the criterion standard. The pooled sensitivity and specificity in diagnosing mucinous cystic lesions were 63% and 88%, respectively [42].

EUS-FNA–based cytology has a low overall sensitivity, which could be improved by cystic brushing, which is an emerging technique in which a through-the-needle cytology brush of the cystic wall or mural nodule may be performed. A prospective study has recently compared the diagnostic yield of brushing and FNA in suspected mucinous cysts. Cytology brushing has a significantly higher detection rate of mucinous epithelium specimens than standard FNA [43].

3.5.3 Ampullary Tumors

Tumors of the major papilla can range from benign adenomas to adenocarcinomas; early detection affects treatment and prognosis.

Ampullary adenomas appear on EUS as hypoechoic, homogeneous thickening of the duodenal wall in the region of the major papilla, without involvement of the duodenal wall. As the tumor grows, it can acquire an inhomogeneous pattern and invade the duodenal wall and the pancreas. A post-stenotic dilatation of the main pancreatic duct and common bile duct can be observed.

A recent study compared the accuracy of EUS, CT and MRI in the diagnosis and staging of ampullary tumors. EUS was superior to CT and equivalent to MRI for tumor detection and locoregional staging. EUS accuracy was not affected by biliary stents or tumor size [44].

3.5.4 Endocrine Tumors

A careful examination of the pancreas, the peripancreatic area and the gastroduodenal wall is required for a

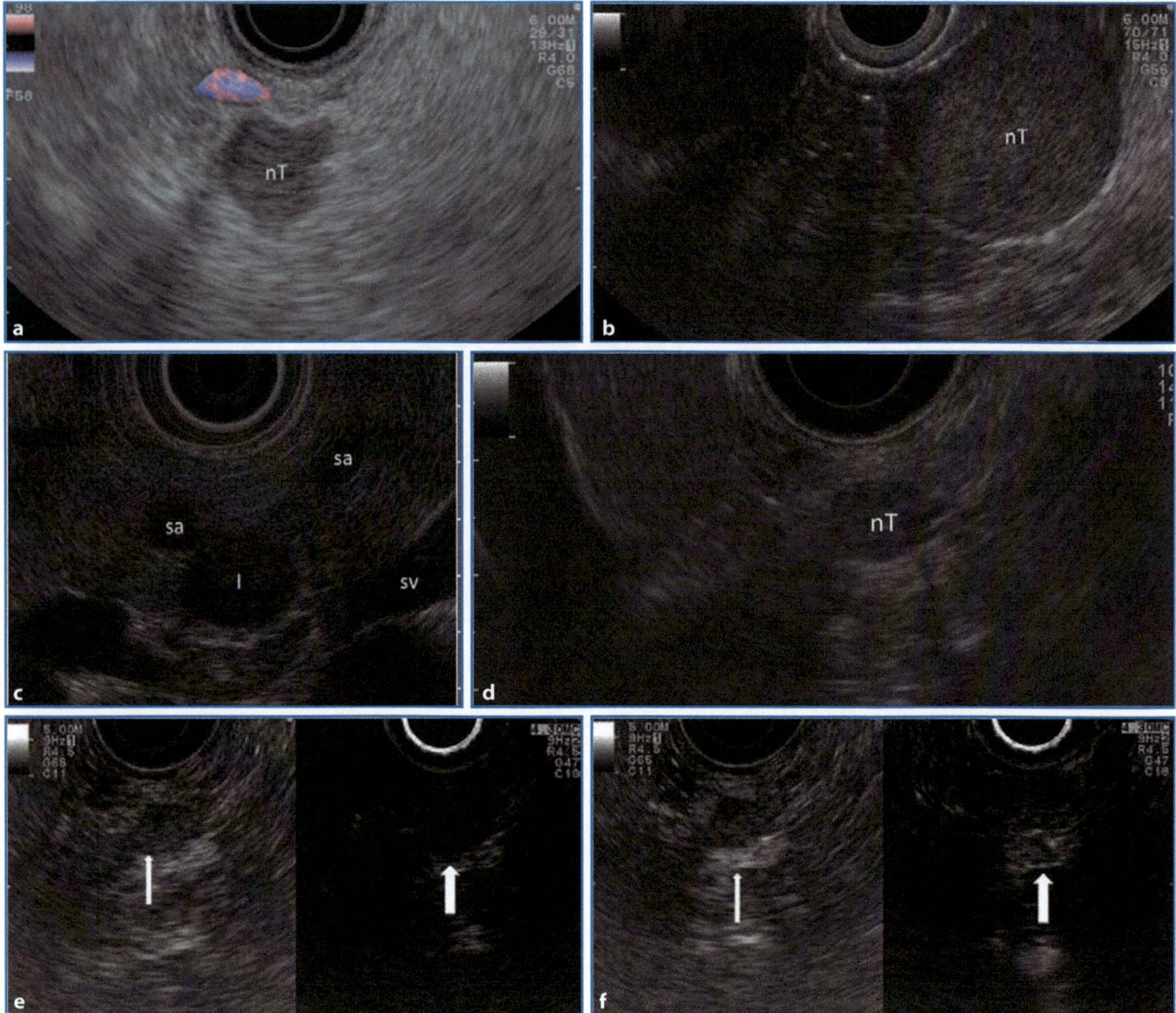

Fig. 3.4 a-f Endocrine tumors. **a** EUS shows this small neuroendocrine tumor (*nT*), well-defined from surrounding parenchyma, with internal vascular signals. **b** EUS shows a large roundish neuroendocrine tumor (*nT*) of the pancreatic body with smooth borders and homogeneous echotexture. **c** EUS shows a small roundish and echopoor insulinoma (*I*) of pancreatic body with smooth borders and homogeneous echotexture (*sa*, splenic artery; *sv*, splenic vein). **d** EUS shows a small neuroendocrine tumor (*nT*) of the pancreatic body with irregular borders. **e,f** CE-EUS of the same case, the lesion in B mode (*arrow*) and in contrast harmonic analysis (*thick arrow*); baseline (**e**) and arterial phase (**f**): the lesion shows rapid and homogeneous enhancement in the arterial phase

precise localization of endocrine tumors because their size can be smaller than 10 mm and differential diagnosis with peripancreatic lymph nodes is mandatory. Typical EUS features of these rare pancreatic tumors are roundish, well-demarcated hypoechoic masses with homogeneous echopatterns (Fig. 3.4). Rarely, they appear as isoechoic or as hyperechoic, inhomogeneous lesions with irregular margins. A cystic pattern is the least common and may be unilocular, septated, microcystic, or mixed solid-cystic.

An intense vascularity can be displayed on EUS color Doppler, and a strong enhancement can be observed after administration of a contrast agent. Moreover CE-EUS can display a heterogeneous echopattern with filling defects, which has been significantly associated with malignant endocrine tumors [45].

On EUS elastography, neuroendocrine tumors show an intense blue coloration suggestive of hard tissue and a malignant pattern [24].

In a retrospective series of 41 patients with pancreatic endocrine tumors, EUS showed high sensitivity (95.1%) compared with multidetector CT (80.6%) and transabdominal US (45.2%) [45].

3.5.5 Pancreatic Metastasis

The pancreas is seldom a target for metastasis. On EUS, metastases appear as hypoechoic, roundish lesions with smooth margins, and a hyperechoic pattern can also be observed (Fig. 3.5). They are usually distinguished from primary pancreatic lesions based on EUS-FNA and the clinical history. In doubtful cases, CEUS shows a hyperenhancement pattern, reflecting hypervascular-

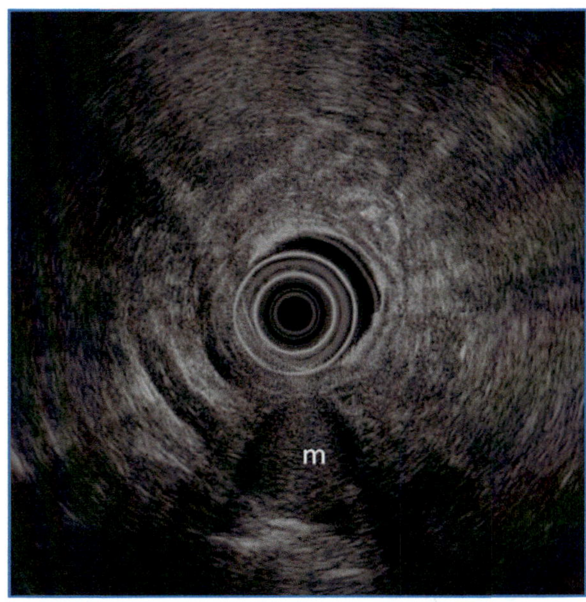

Fig. 3.5 Pancreatic metastasis: EUS shows a roundish echopoor metastasis (*m*) from renal carcinoma to pancreatic body

ity. A hypoenhanced pattern has been reported for colonic metastases. EUS elastography displays metastasis as hard blue lesions with a pattern that is similar to that of pancreatic adenocarcinoma [24].

3.5.6 Acute Pancreatitis

Due to its high diagnostic accuracy EUS can play a crucial role in the diagnosis of a suspected acute biliary pancreatitis (ABP) or an otherwise unexplained acute pancreatitis (Fig. 3.6). EUS has evolved in recent years

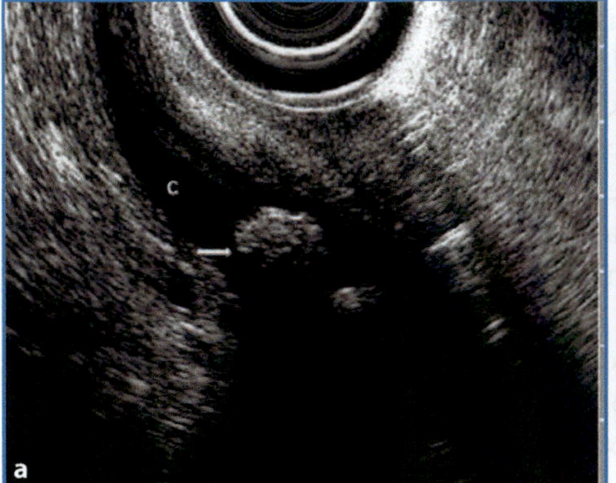

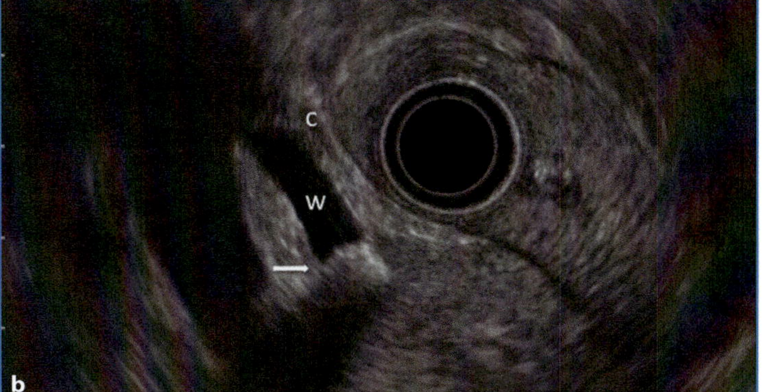

Fig. 3.6 a,b Acute pancreatitis. **a** EUS is able to detect the presence of a choledochal (*c*) stone (*arrow*) in a suspected acute biliary pancreatitis. **b** In this patient with recurrent acute pancreatitis EUS reveals the presence of a stone (*arrow*) in the Wirsung (*c*, common bile duct)

into an important diagnostic tool in biliary obstruction, as accurate as ERCP in detecting choledocholithiasis. The high resolution of EUS (0.1 mm) accounts for its particular sensitivity in detecting small stones (5 mm or less), regardless of bile duct diameter. Moreover, skilled endosonographers can easily detect stones and ERCP can be performed in the same endoscopic session with no added risk of sedation.

Cost-benefit analyses weighing costs and outcomes of EUS to ERCP revealed EUS screening for choledocholithiasis the more advantageous strategy in severe ABP with both lower costs, fewer ERCP and procedure related complications [46].

Although ERCP is an established procedure for early treatment of ABP and it has been used as the criterion standard in all studies, it is not a perfect criterion standard, as it presented a higher number of false positive readings and a higher rate of failure than EUS. Moreover, the higher positive predictive value of EUS than ERCP in detecting biliary stones should assign ERCP to selected patients with ABP and the negative predictive value similar for both procedures should suggest an alternative strategy based on EUS-first without the risks that ERCP carries [47].

Lastly, it should be recalled that pancreatic adenocarcinoma, or metastases or lymphoma or intraductal papillary mucinous tumor or, though more rarely, neuroendocrine tumors can cause acute pancreatitis as first symptom; due to the high diagnostic accuracy of EUS for the detection of a pancreatic lesion, an acute pancreatitis should not be defined as idiopathic unless EUS has been performed.

3.5.7   Chronic Pancreatitis

The EUS features for diagnosing chronic pancreatitis have evolved over the years. The earlier classification grouped parenchymal and ductal changes in the score, without weighing the importance of some criteria. The most recent scoring system is the Rosemont classification, which includes three major and six minor criteria [48]. Although a multicenter study comparing interobserver agreement between the standard and Rosemont classifications failed to find a significant increase in interobserver agreement with these new criteria, they do appear more suited to recognizing early pancreatitis [49].

According to the Rosemont classification, the following EUS findings are suggestive of chronic pancreatitis [48]:

- Parenchymal hyperechoic foci ≥2 mm in length and width with shadowing (major criterion) or without shadowing (minor criterion);
- Hyperechoic stranding ≥3 mm in length in at least two different directions (minor criterion);
- Presence of cysts (minor criterion);
- Parenchymal lobularity with honeycombing (major criterion) or without honeycombing (minor criterion). Lobules are well-circumscribed, ≥5-mm structures with an enhanced rim and a relatively hypoechoic center, and honeycombing indicates the presence of ≥3 contiguous lobules;
- Main pancreatic duct dilatation (minor criterion) with irregular contour (minor criterion) and hyperechoic margin (minor criterion);
- Main pancreatic duct calculi (major criterion);
- Dilated side branches (minor criterion): ≥3 tubular anechoic structures each measuring ≥1 mm in width, budding from the main pancreatic duct.

The findings of chronic pancreatitis can evolve with the progression of the disease (Fig. 3.7). The gland can appear normal in size, enlarged or atrophic. Focal chronic pancreatitis appears on EUS as a focal hypoechoic lesion with irregular margins, resembling pancreatic cancer. Many studies have attempted to identify EUS criteria to distinguish benign lesions from malignant lesions, but a correct diagnosis is not possible with EUS alone. The presence of EUS features of chronic pancreatitis in the surrounding parenchyma could indicate a benign lesion, but pancreatic cancer can develop from chronic pancreatitis. Histology is considered to be the criterion standard, and as mentioned above, EUS-FNA performance is inferior in this setting.

CE-EUS could be an additional tool for differentiating malignant lesions from focal chronic pancreatitis when EUS-FNA is negative. Pseudotumoral nodules in chronic pancreatitis can show a hyperenhanced or isoenhanced pattern after SonoVue injection [22].

In a recent prospective series of 54 patients with chronic pancreatitis and pancreatic cancer, the accuracy of the combined use of contrast-enhanced power Doppler and EUS sonoelastography to differentiate pancreatic focal lesions was evaluated. After SonoVue injection, focal lesions in chronic pancreatitis appear hypervascular with a mixed pattern (blue-green) on EUS-elastography in 95% of the cases, whereas only 24% of pancreatic cancer cases show these features [22].

Autoimmune pancreatitis is a particular type of chronic pancreatitis which is a relatively rare disease

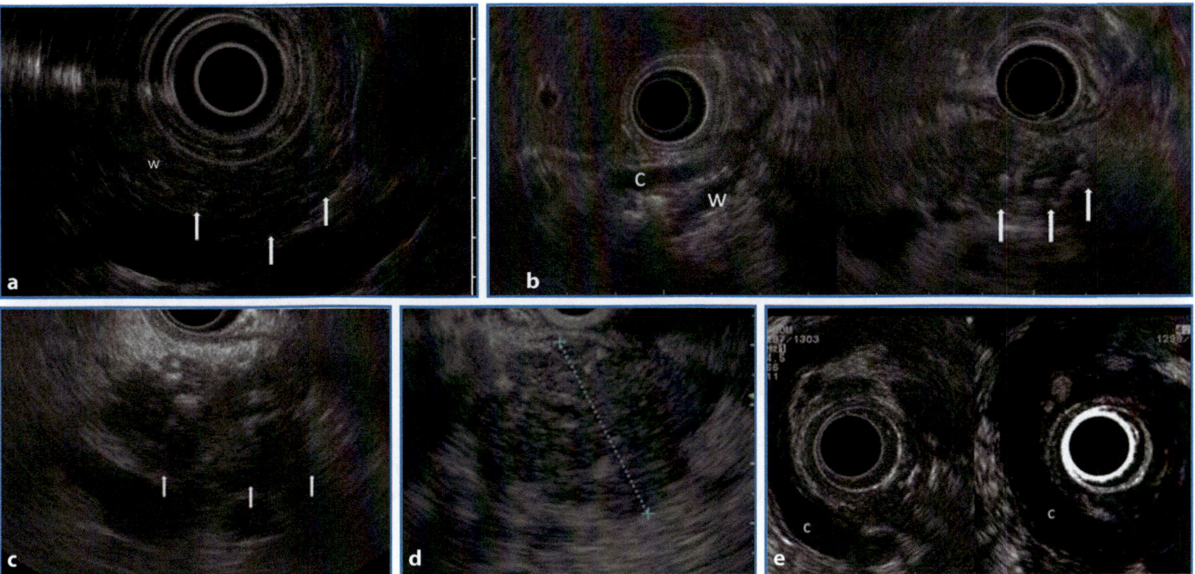

Fig. 3.7 a-e Chronic pancreatitis. **a** Early EUS signs of chronic pancreatitis are represented by the increased echogenicity of the interlobular septa (*arrows*) (*w*, Wirsung). **b** In chronic pancreatitis EUS shows the thickened wall of the duct of Wirsung (*w*), and multiple calcifications (*arrows*) of the pancreatic body (*c*, common bile duct). **c** EUS shows a markedly inhomogeneous pancreatic body, with irregular borders and gross calcifications (*arrows*) **d** Autoimmune pancreatitis: EUS shows a substantially enlarged pancreatic gland (*between calipers*), with preserved echotexture. **e** Autoimmune pancreatitis with biliary involvement: EUS shows the diffuse thickening of the bile duct (*c*) wall, which shows rapid and persistent contrast enhancement

that can affect the pancreas focally or diffusely. The predominant EUS feature of the diffuse form of autoimmune pancreatitis is a diffuse pancreatic enlargement with a hypoechoic pattern [50]. In the early stage of the disease, parenchymal lobularity and a hyperechoic pancreatic duct margin are recognized as typical EUS findings; reduced echogenicity, hyperechoic foci and hyperechoic strands have been found in early and advanced stages of autoimmune pancreatitis [51]. The focal form of autoimmune pancreatitis is characterized by a solitary, irregular, hypoechoic lesion, which is generally located in the head of the pancreas. The main pancreatic duct can be compressed by the enlarged parenchyma, normal-sized or dilated in the case of focal autoimmune pancreatitis. The common bile duct can show a thickened wall and dilatation. The involvement of the peripancreatic vessels and the presence of enlarged lymph nodes are additional possible EUS findings of this disease [50]. Even in this setting, a reliable diagnosis is achieved with a combination of imaging and histologic features; further aid can be provided using EUS-elastography [52, 53], which shows a homogeneous stiffness pattern of the focal lesions and of the remaining parenchyma in patients with autoimmune pancreatitis.

3.6 Therapeutic Interventional EUS

In recent years, a prototype forward-viewing linear echoendoscope has been developed to overcome the standard linear scope limitations, which are due to the acute angle between the needle and the gut wall, and to facilitate complex interventions, such as drainage of pseudocysts and neurolysis of the celiac plexus. A multicenter clinical trial compared EUS-guided drainage procedures in 58 patients who were randomized to the conventional, oblique-viewing scope or to the forward-viewing echoendoscope. This study failed to show differences in ease, safety and efficacy between the two echoendoscopes [54].

Drainage of pseudocysts is one of the established interventional EUS-guided procedures (Fig. 3.8), and it is actually considered the standard of care in tertiary centers. As described above, pseudocysts can complicate both acute and chronic pancreatitis. Indications for drainage included symptomatic pseudocysts and the presence of infection.

In the first phase of the examination, EUS evaluates the distance of the pseudocysts from the gastric or duo-

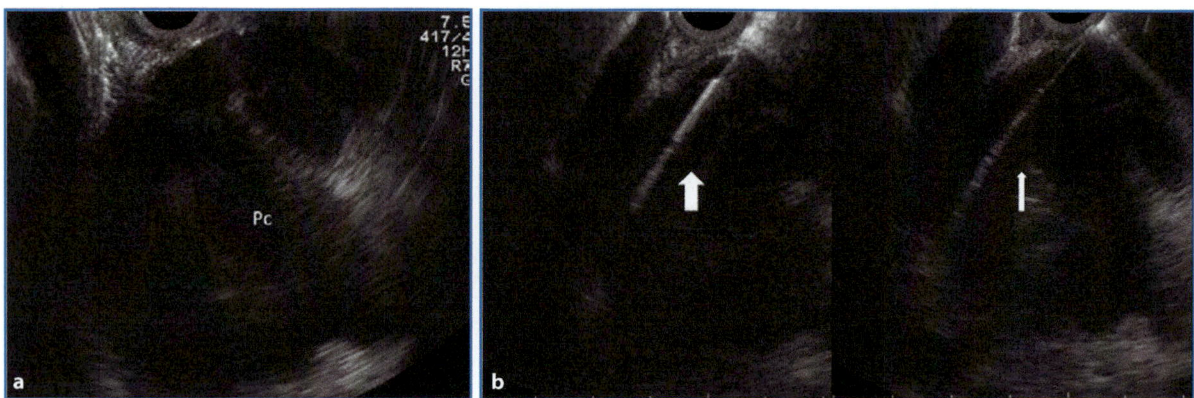

Fig. 3.8 a,b EUS-guided drainage of pseudocyst. **a** EUS shows the best site to puncture this large pseudocyst (*Pc*) where the distance from the stomach wall is minimal and there are no vessels interposed. **b** Under EUS guidance a 19-G needle (*thick arrow*) is inserted, and through this the guide wire (*arrow*) is left in the pseudocyst to pass thereafter the drainage catheter

denal wall, and with visualization of the interposed vessels using EUS color Doppler, a stent is placed in the pseudocysts without the use of duodenoscope.

The first randomized controlled trial comparing EUS-guided and open-surgical drainage in 36 patients with single pseudocysts >6 cm without signs of infection or necrosis was recently published as an abstract. There was no difference in recurrence at 18 months between the surgical and the endoscopic groups, and all procedures were performed without complications. Pain relief at 1 week was higher in the EUS group, and the EUS-guided procedure resulted in a significantly shorter hospital stay and lower costs [55].

EUS-guided celiac neurolysis is a safe and effective procedure for pain relief in chronic pancreatitis and pancreatic adenocarcinoma. It has replaced previous percutaneous techniques that were performed under CT or fluoroscopic guidance. Celiac ganglia are located anterior and lateral to the aorta at the level of the celiac artery. The right celiac ganglion is most commonly located 6 mm inferior to the celiac artery origin, whereas the left celiac ganglion is most commonly located 9 mm inferior to the celiac artery origin. EUS allows for real-time evaluation of the ganglia, which appear as hypoechoic, elongated structures.

In the case of pancreatic cancer, usually a long-acting anesthetic is injected first to reduce the pain due to the alcohol injection. In the case of chronic pancreatitis, a celiac block is obtained by injecting long-acting anesthetic and corticosteroids. A 19- or 22-gauge needle can usually be used, even if a dedicated 20-gauge needle with multiple side-holes is available. The entire solution can be injected into the area of the celiac artery, or half of the solution can be injected on one side of the celiac artery origin and half can be injected on the other side. During the injection, a hyperechoic blush can usually be observed. The most common side effects are transient diarrhea and hypotension, which are signs of the sympathetic block.

Potential candidates for celiac plexus neurolysis are patients with inoperable pancreatic cancer and pain requiring opioids. A higher rate of response is achieved when the procedure is performed early after pain onset, probably because at this stage, the origin of pain is essentially from the celiac plexus.

Data from patients undergoing celiac neurolysis [56, 57] after injections of solutions directly into their ganglia have shown pain relief in 94% of patients with pancreatic cancer and in 50% of patients with chronic pancreatitis, with better results after alcohol injection than after celiac plexus block [54]. An initial successful experience of celiac plexus neurolysis with a forward-viewing echoendoscope was recently reported by Eloubeidi in five patients [57].

In recent years interventional EUS has been used to treat pancreatic tumors. EUS-guided therapy of pancreatic carcinoma was attempted by injecting cytoimplant, an allogenic mixed-lymphocyte culture, into eight patients with unresectable cancer. Partial response was observed in two patients, with a median survival of 13.2 months [58]. In 2003, Hecht et al. reported the results of EUS-guided ONYX-015 injection in 21 patients with pancreatic cancer. ONYX-015 is an E1B-55-kDa gene–deleted adenovirus, which preferentially replicates in malignant cells. Side effects, such as sepsis and duodenal perforation, occurred without tumor regression in no patients at day 35. After combination with gemcitabine therapy, two patients showed partial response and two showed minor response. Six patients showed stable disease, whereas the disease progressed in eleven [59].

TNFerade is a replication-deficient adenovector containing the human tumor necrosis factor (TNF)-α gene, which is regulated by a radiation-inducible promoter. In 2006, a phase I trial using EUS-guided intratumoral injections of TNFerade combined with 5-FU and radiation showed mild toxicities, locoregional control of treated tumors and improved median survival; unfortunately, the phase III randomized controlled trial has not yet been published [60].

The last frontiers of EUS-guided treatment of tumors are brachytherapy with direct injection of radioactive seeds into the tumor [61] and the placement of gold fiducials for image-guided radiation therapy. In a recent study of 57 consecutive patients, the latter procedure was safe and effective in 50 cases without resorting to fluoroscopy [62].

Ethanol ablation of cystic tumors is safe and feasible, with resolution rates of 33% to 79% [63, 64]. During a long-term follow-up (median 26 months) in the study of Dewitt et al. [64], no recurrence was radiologically detected. Preliminary results with paclitaxel injection after ethanol lavage in 52 patients with pancreatic mucinous cysts showed complete resolution in 62% of the patients. Small cyst volume was a predictive factor for successful treatment [65].

References

1. Canto MI, Schulick RD, Kamel IR et al (2010) Screening for familial pancreatic neoplasia: a prospective, multicenter blinded study of EUS, CT, and secretin-MRCP (The NCI-Spore Lustgarten Foundation Cancer of the Pancreas CAPS 3 Study). Gastrointest Endosc 71:AB119
2. Siddiqui UD, Rossi F, Rosenthal LS et al (2009) EUS-guided FNA of solid pancreatic masses: a prospective, randomized trial comparing 22-gauge and 25-gauge needles. Gastrointest Endosc 70:1093-1097
3. Eloubeidi MA, Tamhane A, Lopes TL et al (2009) Cervical esophageal perforations at the time of endoscopic ultrasound: a prospective evaluation of frequency, outcomes, and patient management. Am J Gastroenterol 104:53-56
4. Wilson JA, Hoffman B, Hawes RH, Romagnuolo J (2010) EUS in patients with surgically altered upper GI anatomy. Gastrointest Endosc 72:947-953
5. ASGE Standards of Practice Committee, Anderson MA, Ben-Menachem T et al (2009) Management of antithrombotic agents for endoscopic procedures Gastrointest Endosc 70:1060-1070
6. Choi CW, Kim GH, Kang DH et al (2010) Associated factors for a hyperechogenic pancreas on endoscopic ultrasound. World J Gastroenterol 14:4329-4334
7. Lee SH, Ozden N, Pawa R et al (2010) Periductal hypoechoic sign: an endosonographic finding associated with pancreatic malignancy. Gastrointest Endosc 71:249-255
8. Puli SR, Singh S, Hagedorn CH et al (2007) Diagnostic accuracy of EUS for vascular invasion in pancreatic and periampullary cancers: a meta-analysis and systematic review. Gastrointest Endosc 65:788-797
9. Snady H, Bruckner H, Siegel J et al (1994) Endoscopic ultrasonographic criteria of vascular invasion by potentially resectable pancreatic tumors. Gastrointest Endosc 40:326–333
10. Rosch T, Dittler H-J, Strobel K et al (2000) Endoscopic ultrasound criteria for vascular invasion in the staging of cancer of the head of the pancreas: a blind reevaluation of videotapes. Gastrointest Endosc 52:469-477
11. Bach CM (2003) Melanoma of the skin. In: Greene FL, Page DL, Fleming ID et al. (eds) AJCC Cancer Staging Manual, Sixth Edition. New York, Springer-Verlag, pp 209-220
12. Tseng JF, Raut CP, Lee JE et al (2004) Pancreaticoduodenectomy with vascular resection: margin status and survival duration. J Gastrointest Surg 8:935-950
13. Nakao A, Takeda S, Sakai M et al (2004) Extended radical resection versus standard resection for pancreatic cancer: the rationale for extended radical resection. Pancreas 28:289-292
14. Catalano MF, Sivak MV, Rice T et al (1994) Endosonographic features predictive of lymph node metastasis. Gastrointest Endosc 40:442-446
15. Bhutani MS, Hawes RH, Hoffman BJ (1997) A comparison of echo features during endoscopic ultrasound (EUS) and EUS-guided fine-needle aspiration for diagnosis of malignant lymph node invasion. Gastrointest Endosc 45:474-479
16. Bhutani MS, Hawes RH, Baron PL et al (1997) Endoscopic ultrasound guided fine needle aspiration of malignant pancreatic lesions. Endoscopy 29:854-858
17. Agarwal B, Abu-Hamda E, Molke KL et al (2004) Endoscopic ultrasound-guided fine needle aspiration and multidetector spiral CT in the diagnosis of pancreatic cancer. Am J Gastroenterol 99:844–850
18. Buscarini E, De Angelis C, Arcidiacono PG et al (2006) Multicentre retrospective study on endoscopic ultrasound complications. Dig Liver Dis 38:762-767
19. Dietrich CF, Ignee A, Braden B et al (2008) Improved differentiation of pancreatic tumors using contrast enhanced endoscopic ultrasound. Clin Gastroenterol Hepatol 6:590-597
20. Hocke M, Schulze E, Gottschalk P (2006) Contrast-enhanced endoscopic ultrasound in discrimination between focal pancreatitis and pancreatic cancer. World J Gastroenterol 12:246-250
21. Napoleon B, Alvarez-Sanchez MV, Gincoul R et al (2010) Contrast-enhanced harmonic endoscopic ultrasound in solid lesions of the pancreas: results of a pilot study. Endoscopy 42:564-570
22. Saftoiu A, Iordache S, Gheonea DI et al (2010) Combined contrast-enhanced power Doppler and real-time sonoelas-

tography performed during EUS, used in the differential diagnosis of focal pancreatic masses Gastrointest Endosc 72:739-747

23. Giovannini M, Hookey LC, Bories E et al (2006) Endoscopic ultrasound elastography: the first step towards virtual biopsy? Preliminary results in 49 patients. Endoscopy 38:344–348
24. Giovannini M, Botelberge T, Bories E et al (2009) Endoscopic ultrasound elastography for evaluation of lymph nodes and pancreatic masses: a prospective multicentre study. World J Gastroenterol 15:1587-1593
25. Iglesias-Garcia J, Larino-Noia J, Abdulkader I et al (2010) Quantitative endoscopic ultrasound elastography: an accurate method for the differentiation of solid pancreatic masses. Gastroenterology 139:1172-1180
26. Rosch T, Braig C, Gain T et al (1992) Staging of pancreatic and ampullary carcinoma by endoscopic ultrasonography: comparison with conventional sonography, computed tomography, and angiography. Gastroenterology 102:188-199
27. Palazzo L, Roseau G, Gayet B et al (1993) Endoscopic ultrasonography in the diagnosis and staging of pancreatic adenocarcinoma: results of a prospective study with comparison to ultrasonography and CT scan. Endoscopy 25: 143-150
28. Müller MF, Meyenberger C, Bertschinger P et al (1994) Pancreatic tumors: evaluation with endoscopic US, CT, and MR imaging. Radiology 190:745-751
29. Marty O, Aubertin JM, Bouillot JL et al (1995) Prospective comparison of ultrasound endoscopy and computed tomography in the assessment of locoregional invasiveness of malignant ampullary and pancreatic tumors verified surgically. Gastroenterol Clin Biol 19:197-203
30. Mertz HR, Sechopoulos P, Delbeke D, Leach SD (2000) EUS, PET, and CT scanning for evaluation of pancreatic adenocarcinoma. Gastrointest Endosc 52:367-371
31. Rivadeneira DE, Pochapin M, Grobmyer SR et al (2003) Comparison of linear array endoscopic ultrasound and helical computed tomography for the staging of periampullary malignancies. Ann Surg Oncol 10:890-897
32. DeWitt J, Devereaux B, Chriswell M et al (2004) Comparison of endoscopic ultrasonography and multidetector computed tomography for detecting and staging pancreatic cancer. Ann Intern Med 141:753–763
33. Mansfield SD, Scott J, Oppong K et al (2008) Comparison of multislice computed tomography and endoscopic ultrasonography with operative and histological findings in suspected pancreatic and periampullary malignancy. Br J Surg 95:1512–1520
34. DeWitt J, Deveraux BM, Lehman GA et al (2006) Comparison of endoscopic ultrasound and computed tomography for the preoperative evaluation of pancretic cancer: a systematic review. Clin Gastroenterol Hepatol 4:717-725
35. Klapman JB, Chang KJ, Lee JG et al (2005) Negative predictive value of endoscopic ultrasound in a large series of patients with a clinical suspicion of pancreatic cancer. Am J Gastroenterol 100:2658–2661
36. Ramsay D, Marshall M, Song S et al (2004) Identification and staging of pancreatic tumours using computed tomography, endoscopic ultrasound and mangafodipir trisodium-enhanced magnetic resonance imaging. Australas Radiol 48:154–161
37. Soriano A, Castells A, Ayuso C et al (2004) Preoperative staging and tumor resectability assessment of pancreatic cancer: prospective study comparing endoscopic ultrasonography, helical computed tomography, magnetic resonance imaging, and angiography. Am J Gastroenterol 99:492–501
38. Kobayashi G, Fujita N, Noda Y et al (2011) Lateral spread along the main pancreatic duct in branch-duct intraductal papillary-mucinous neoplasms of the pancreas: usefulness of intraductal ultrasonography for its evaluation. Dig Endosc 23:62-68
39. Kubo H, Chijiiwa Y, Akahoshi K et al (2000) Intraductal papillary-mucinous tumours of the pancreas: differential diagnosis between benign and malignant tumours by endoscopic ultrasonography. Am J Gastroenterol 96:1429–1434
40. Sawai Y, Yamao K, Bhatia V et al (2010) Development of pancreatic cancers during long-term follow-up of side-branch intraductal papillary mucinous neoplasms. Endoscopy 42:1077-1784
41. Brugge WR, Lewandrowski K, Lee-Lewandrowski E et al (2004) Diagnosis of pancreatic cystic neoplasms: a report of the cooperative pancreatic cyst study. Gastroenterology 126:1330–1336
42. Thosani N, Thosani S, Qiao W et al (2010) Role of EUS-FNA-based cytology in the diagnosis of mucinous pancreatic cystic lesions: a systematic review and meta-analysis. Dig Dis Sci 55:2756-2766
43. Al-Haddad M, Gill KR, Raimondo M et al (2010) Safety and efficacy of cytology brushings versus standard fine-needle aspiration in evaluating cystic pancreatic lesions: a controlled study. Endoscopy 42:127-132
44. Chen CH, Yang CC, Yeh YH et al (2009) Reappraisal of endosonography of ampullary tumors: correlation with transabdominal sonography, CT, and MRI. J Clin Ultrasound 37:18-25
45. Ishikawa T, Itoh A, Kawashima H et al (2010) Usefulness of EUS combined with contrast-enhancement in the differential diagnosis of malignant versus benign and preoperative localization of pancreatic endocrine tumors. Gastrointest Endosc 71:951-959
46. Buscarini E, Tansini P, Vallisa D et al (2003) EUS for suspected choledocholithiasis: do benefits outweigh costs? A prospective, controlled study. Gastrointest Endosc 57:510-518
47. De Lisi S, Leandro G, Buscarini E (2011) Endoscopic ultrasonography versus endoscopic retrograde cholangiopancreatography in acute biliary pancreatitis: a systematic review. Eur J Gastroenterol Hepatol 23:367-374
48. Catalano MF, Sahai A, Levy M et al (2009) EUS-based criteria for the diagnosis of chronic pancreatitis: the Rosemont classification. Gastrointest Endosc 69:1251–1261
49. Stevens T, Lopez R, Adler DG et al (2010) Multicenter comparison of the interobserver agreement of standard EUS scoring and Rosemont classification scoring for diagnosis of chronic pancreatitis. Gastrointest Endosc 71:519-526
50. Buscarini E, De Lisi S, Arcidiacono PG et al (2011) Endoscopic ultrasonography findings in autoimmune pancreatitis. World J Gastroenterol 28:2080-2085
51. Kubota K, Kato S, Akiyama T et al (2009) A proposal for differentiation between early- and advanced-stage autoimmune pancreatitis by endoscopic ultrasonography. Digestive Endoscopy 21:162–169
52. Dietrich CF, Hirche TO, Ott M, Ignee A (2009) Real time

tissue elastography in the diagnosis of autoimmune pancreatitis. Endoscopy 41:718-720
53. Giovannini M (2007) Endosonography: new developments in 2006. Scientific World Journal 2:341-363
54. Voermans RP, Ponchon T, Larghi A et al (2010) Randomized controlled comparison of forward-viewing versus oblique-viewing EUS-scopes in drainage of pancreatic fluid collections. Gastrointest Endosc 71: AB135
55. Varadarajulu S, Trevino J, Wilcox CM et al (2010) Randomized trial comparing EUS and surgery for pancreatic pseudocyst drainage. Gastrointest Endosc 71:AB116
56. Levy MJ, Topazian MD, Wiersema MJ et al (2008) Initial evaluation of the efficacy and safety of endoscopic ultrasound-guided direct ganglia neurolysis and block. Am J Gastroenterol 103:98-103
57. Eloubeidi MA (2011) Initial evaluation of the forward-viewing echoendoscope prototype for performing fine-needle aspiration, Tru-cut biopsy, and celiac plexus neurolysis. J Gastroenterol Hepatol 26:63-67
58. Chang KJ, Nguyen PT, Thompson JA et al (2000) Phase I clinical trial of allogeneic mixed lymphocyte culture (cytoimplant) delivered by endoscopic ultrasound-guided fine-needle injection in patients with advanced pancreatic carcinoma. Cancer 88:1325-1335
59. Hecht JR, Bedford R, Abbruzzese JL et al (2003) A phase I/II trial of intratumoral endoscopic ultrasound injection of ONYX-015 with intravenous gemcitabine in unresectable pancreatic carcinoma. Clin Cancer Res 9:555-561
60. Farrell JJ, Senzer N, Hecht JR et al (2006) Long-term data for endoscopic ultrasound (EUS) and percutaneous (PTA) guided intratumoral TNFerade gene delivery combined with chemoradiation in the treatment of locally advanced pancreatic cancer (LAPC). Gastrointest Endosc 63:AB93
61. Jin Z, Du Y, Li Z et al (2008) Endoscopic ultrasonography-guided interstitial implantation of iodine 125-seeds combined with chemotherapy in the treatment of unresectable pancreatic carcinoma: a prospective pilot study. Endoscopy 40:314–320
62. Park WG, Yan BM, Schellenberg D et al (2010) EUS-guided gold fiducial insertion for image-guided radiation therapy of pancreatic cancer: 50 successful cases without fluoroscopy. Gastrointest Endosc 71:513-518
63. Gan SI, Thompson CC, Lauwers GY et al (2005) Ethanol lavage of pancreatic cystic lesions: initial pilot study. Gastrointest Endosc 61:746–752
64. DeWitt J, DiMaio CJ, Brugge WR (2010) Long-term follow-up of pancreatic cysts that resolve radiologically after EUS-guided ethanol ablation. Gastrointest Endosc 72:862-826
65. Oh HC, Seo DW, Song TJ et al (2011) Endoscopic ultrasonography-guided ethanol lavage with paclitaxel injection treats patients with pancreatic cysts. Gastroenterology 140:172-179

Percutaneous Ultrasound Guided Interventional Procedures in Pancreatic Diseases

4

Elisabetta Buscarini and Guido Manfredi

4.1　Introduction

Percutaneous interventional diagnostic and therapeutic procedures under ultrasound guidance are largely employed in pancreatic diseases. Diagnostic procedures include cytologic and/or histologic sampling with fine needles (diameter <1 mm) or coarse needles to sample pathologic tissue or fluids/collections for biochemical, cytologic and microbiologic examinations. Therapeutic procedures include the drainage of fluid collections by needle or catheter.

4.2　Examination Technique

4.2.1　Equipment

Two types of probes are typically used for interventional procedures: those with lateral devices and those with central support. Probes with lateral devices (Fig. 4.1) are the most commonly used and are characterized by a needle that is always visualized in oblique tracks so that the target is met in the safest possible way. Probes with central support have a noncontinuous transducer crystal and central support with a centrally mounted guide kit. With these probes, both vertical and oblique tracks can be used with a variable angle of incidence, depending on the available options. The guide kits are different in the caliber of needles (usually ranging from 22 to 14 gauge (G)) and have a modifiable angle based on the target organ.

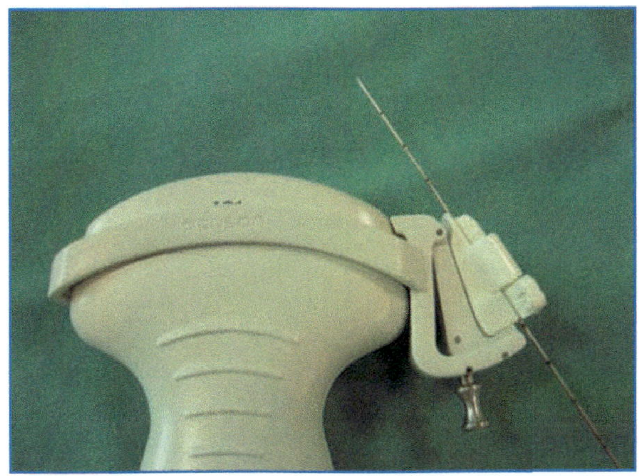

Fig. 4.1 Probe with lateral device for ultrasound guided percutaneous fine needle aspiration (FNA)

The needles used in diagnostic interventional procedures are different for cytologic versus tissue sampling. Needles for cytology aspiration (fine needle aspiration – FNA) generally have a caliber less than 1 mm with a removable inner stylet. For histologic sampling there are two types of needles with different mechanisms: the Menghini-type needle or end-cutting needle (Fig. 4.2) and the Tru-cut-type needle or side-cutting needle (Fig. 4.3). The Menghini-type needle takes a small portion of the pancreatic lesion via a suction mechanism, whereas the Tru-cut-type needle uses a guillotine mechanism.

4.2.2　Procedure

When performing biopsy with a cytology needle, the skin of the patient must be accurately disinfected with iodine. A fine cytology needle can be inserted directly into the skin and subcutaneous tissue (usually without

E. Buscarini (✉)
Department of Gastroenterology
Maggiore Hospital, Crema, Italy
e-mail: ebuscarini@rim.it

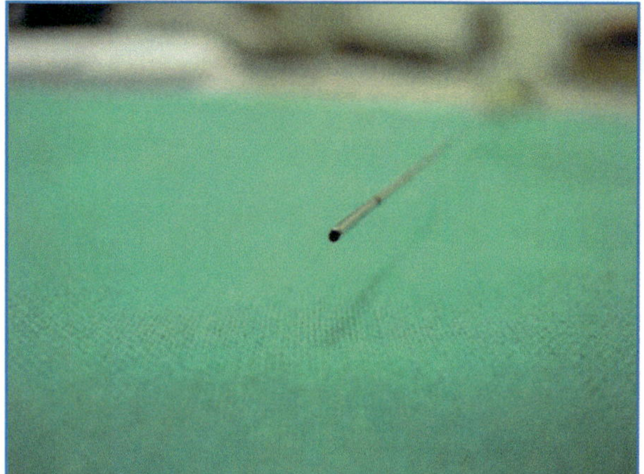

Fig. 4.2 Menghini-type needle or end-cutting needle

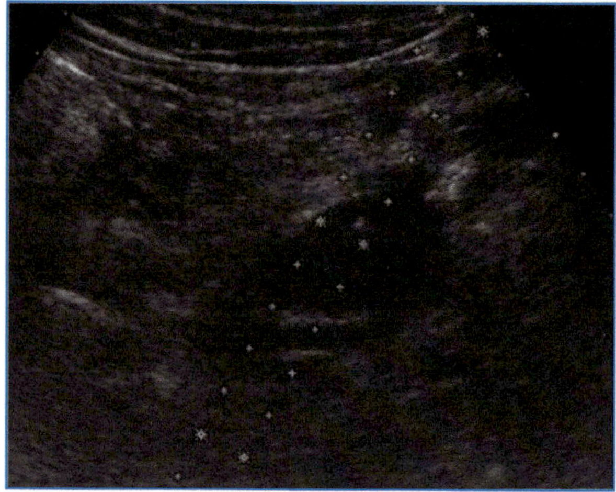

Fig. 4.4 Percutaneous ultrasound guided percutaneous FNA of a pancreatic head mass with the tip of the needle well visible along the track as a hyperechoic dot within the lesion

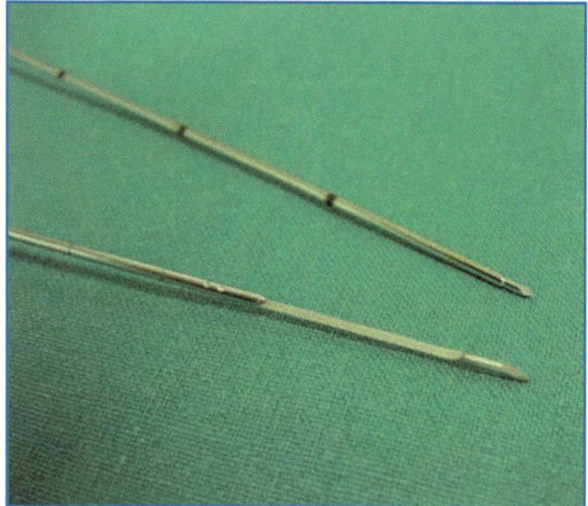

Fig. 4.3 Tru-cut-type needle or side-cutting needle

local anesthesia) and then directed to the target. It is very important that the tip of the needle be seen at US during the biopsy (Fig. 4.4). Color-Doppler preoperative evaluation is mandatory to identify major peripancreatic vessels confirming the safety of the track (Fig. 4.5). When the needle tip is in the correct position, the inner stylet is removed. The needle is connected to a 10-mL syringe that is attached to a special aspiration handle; suction is applied, and the needle is moved up and down three to four times. Before the needle is withdrawn, the syringe piston needs to be released to avoid contamination of the sample with cells from other organs/tissues. The collected material is placed onto slides. The cytologist onsite immediately checks the adequacy of the obtained sample, to avoid additional

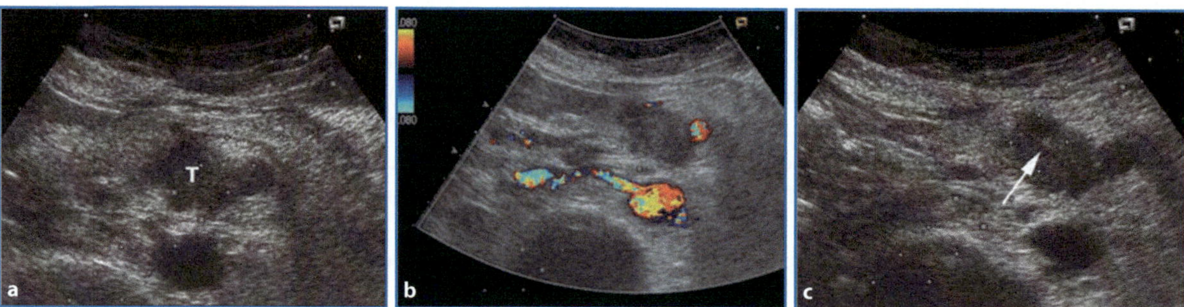

Fig. 4.5 a-c Percutaneous ultrasound guided percutaneous FNA of a pancreatic head mass (*T* in **a**). **b** Color-Doppler evaluation of the track with better identification of superior mesenteric artery and gastroduodenal artery involved by the tumor. **c** Along the track between the two arteries percutaneous ultrasound guided FNA of the pancreatic head mass is performed with the tip of the needle well visible (*arrow*) within the lesion

biopsy passes and repeat procedures for the patients.

When performing biopsy with a cutting needle, 2–3 mL of 1% lidocaine is injected into the skin and into the muscle layer along the prefixed puncture line. The Menghini needle is introduced up to the superior border of the lesion, and then suction is applied to the syringe and the needle is advanced rapidly for 2–3 cm and then retracted. The Tru-cut needle is also positioned at the proximal border of the target; the internal cannula is advanced, the tissue is trapped in the notch and is then cut by the advanced outer sheath.

Post-biopsy control involves observing the patient's vital parameters for at least 4 hours after the procedure, especially in cases in which a large needle is used. After this period of rest, in the absence of any problems, the patient can be discharged.

4.3 Patient Preparation

The patients must comply with the following blood-clotting criteria:
- Prothrombin activity ≥50%
- International normalized ratio (INR) <1.5
- Platelet count ≥50,000/mm^3

A proper discontinuation of aspirin and anticoagulants, possibly with appropriate replacement with low-molecular weight heparins according to the patient thromboembolic risk is mandatory before a biopsy. Written informed consent must be obtained from the patient.

4.4 Diagnostic Procedures

Diagnostic invasive procedures should be performed only if the diagnosis is of some benefit to the patient and cannot be achieved with noninvasive or less invasive methods.

4.4.1 Indications

Accepted indications of pancreatic US-guided biopsy are currently limited to the following:

- pancreatic cancer deemed non-resectable on the basis of imaging and eligibility for chemotherapy or radiotherapy; a pathologic diagnosis is a mandatory prerequisite;
- suspicion of a rare malignant disease (lymphoma; metastasis), which could not be characterized using endoscopic ultrasonography (EUS) (and other imaging techniques), and EUS-guided biopsy;
- difficult/impossible characterization of a focal pancreatitis [1, 2].

4.4.2 Results

Based on one preliminary study, US-guided fine-needle biopsy (FNB) of the pancreas was considered to be highly accurate [3], but 10 years later in a larger series, the same authors showed that the technique was effective in the identification of cancer (PPV = 98%) but was less satisfactory for the exclusion of malignancy (NPV = 69%) [4].

In 1998, a large series of US-guided FNBs of the pancreas was published, showing the effectiveness and safety of the procedure. The study demonstrated no significant difference in the values of diagnostic accuracy among three biopsy modalities: cytology, histology and cytology plus histology (Table 4.1) [5]. These results were consistent with those of previous papers (which included a total of 300 patients) on the same issue, as reviewed by the same authors. Moreover, Di Stasi et al. [5] observed that the effectiveness of US-guided FNB in diagnosing different pancreatic diseases was similar to that found in other studies of focal liver lesions [6]. Interestingly, a recent paper confirmed that the sensitivity, specificity and accuracy of US-guided cytologic or histologic FNB in patients with pancreatic cancer were similar and compared favorably to biopsies in patients with liver metastases [7].

Recently, the results obtained from a large single-center study (545 consecutive patients) [2] showed that US-guided FNB is safe and accurate for the diagnosis of focal pancreatic lesions (Table 4.2), even in cases of neuroendocrine tumor, where diagnostic accuracy was previously considered low [5].

Table 4.1 Series of 510 patients with pancreatic masses, either benign or malignant: cytologic and histologic examinations [5]

	Cytology (287 pts)	Histology (95 pts)	Cytology + histology (128 pts)
Sensitivity	87%	94%	94%
Specificity	100%	100%	100%
Diagnostic accuracy	91%	90%	95%

Table 4.2 Results of fine needle aspiration of 545 pancreatic lesions [2]

Nondiagnostic procedures	6.6%
Sensitivity	99.4%
Specificity	100.0%
Uneventful procedures	98.5%
Minor complications	1.5%

Although fine-needle aspiration results may lack sensitivity, this technique is also recommended for the diagnosis of cystic lesions and provides additional information to imaging results [8]. In this sense, there is general agreement that negative results of a pancreatic biopsy (cytologic or histologic examination) should be carefully evaluated [2, 5]. In any case, the analysis of cystic fluid (obtained under US or EUS guidance) markedly improves the overall diagnostic capability [9-12]; levels of CEA, CA19-9 and pancreatic enzymes are necessary to distinguish between benign lesions, pseudocysts and malignant tumors.

Pancreatic sampling can be performed with EUS guidance. This method has shown higher accuracy than US or computed tomography (CT) for pancreatic lesions <3 cm [13]. A randomized trial, however, found that EUS-guided FN cytology sampling was numerically (but not statistically) superior to CT/US-guided biopsy [14]. According to other studies [15], the diagnostic accuracy and safety of US-guided fine-needle aspiration favors its use over EUS-FNA for unresectable pancreatic tumors.

4.5 Therapeutic Procedures

Therapeutic invasive procedures should ensure the best possible result or a result equal to the one envisaged by a more invasive procedure.

4.5.1 Indications

The main indications for percutaneous treatment are symptomatic and/or infected pancreatic fluid collections; however, to date, no prospective controlled studies have compared the various therapeutic approaches (percutaneous, endoscopic and surgical) [16]. For pancreatic infections with symptomatic fluid collections or abscesses, drainage is the first line of treatment (Fig. 4.6). Catheters of various calibers can be used (generally from 8 to 14 French, i.e. from 2.7 to 4.7 mm).

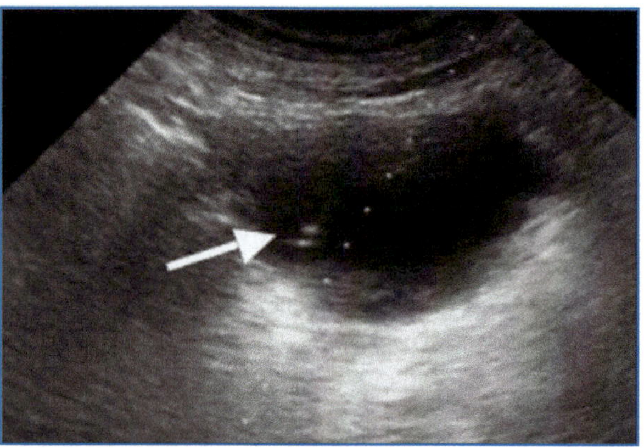

Fig. 4.6 Percutaneous catheter drainage of a large pancreatic collection. The catheter is visible within the collection (*arrow*)

4.5.2 Catheter Insertion Techniques

Methods for inserting catheters into a fluid collection are divided into the trocar technique and the Seldinger technique.

4.5.2.1 Trocar Technique
A catheter mounted on a trocar is directly positioned in the lesion (Fig. 4.7). After 1% lidocaine injection into the abdominal wall at the prefixed entry point, a small skin incision is performed to insert the trocar under US guidance. When the catheter is in the correct position, the inner stylet of the trocar is retracted, the flow of the fluid is controlled and then the trocar can be removed.

4.5.2.2 Seldinger Technique
After local anesthesia and skin incision, an 18–20-gauge needle is inserted into the fluid collection under US guidance, and a guidewire, which can be subsequently withdrawn, can easily pass through the needle. The catheter (with preliminary use of dilators of increasing caliber when required) is advanced over the guide wire up to the collection cavity and fluid is drained. The Seldinger technique is preferred when larger catheters are employed. Inadvertent catheter withdrawal is prevented by using a pigtail-shaped catheter or J-shaped tip; the catheter, however, must be externally fixed by suturing it to the patient's skin. When drainage output becomes minimal and the cavity remains clearly reduced or collapsed (as confirmed with US control), the catheter is removed.

Table 4.3 Numbers and percentages of complications reported in 33 series of patients (in total 2533 patients) who underwent pancreatic biopsy [30]

	Mortality	Minor complications	Major complications
Number	1	22	12
%	0.039	0.86	0.47

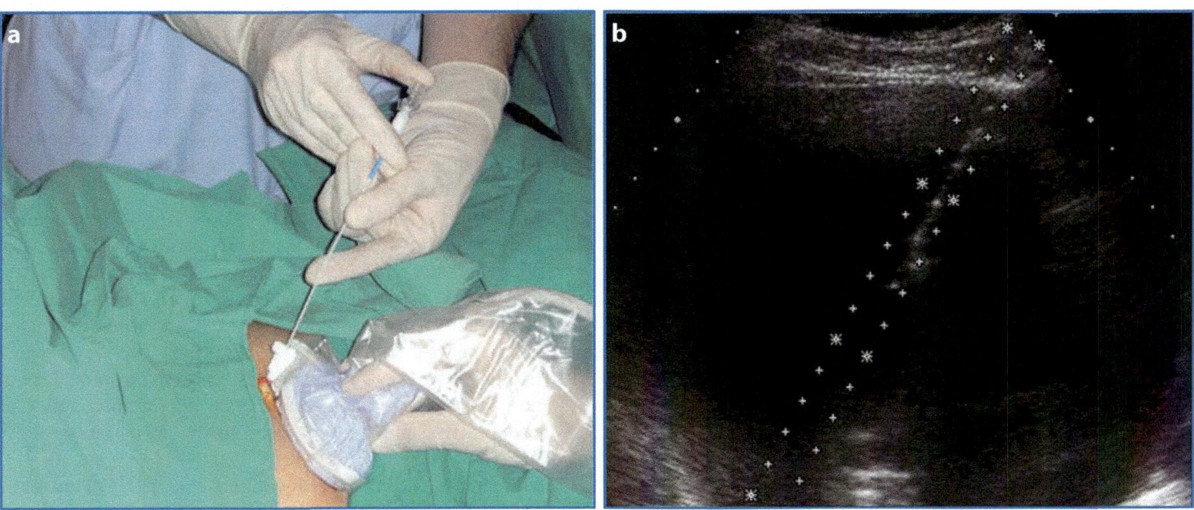

Fig. 4.7 a,b Trocar technique (**a**) for percutaneous ultrasound-guided catheter insertion in a large pancreatic collection (**b**)

4.5.3 Results

To drain pseudocysts, large-bore catheters should be used because of the presence of fibrin plugs and necrotic debris. Long periods of time, which may be months in some cases, are generally required to cure pseudocysts with percutaneous drainage. In 13 series [17-29], a total of 308 patients underwent US-guided percutaneous drainage of pancreatic fluid collections, with success rates of 32 to 94%.

4.6 Complications

Complications can be defined as unfavorable and unexpected events that occur because of an invasive procedure, in spite of the technical accuracy of the procedure. They can occur both in diagnostic and therapeutic procedures. The prevalence of the complications associated with pancreatic biopsy has been evaluated in an analysis of 33 series reported in the literature [30], as summarized in Table 4.3.

To correctly target the problem of death after pancreatic biopsy, it is necessary to recall four sporadic cases (case reports) [31-34] and two cases that were described in two abdominal FNB complication surveys [35, 36]. It is important to stress that fatal complications are mainly due to severe pancreatitis, after the puncture of a normal pancreas because of the wrong presumed diagnosis of a tumor.

A feared complication is so-called *tumor seeding*, which describes the dragging of a critical number of tumor cells along the needle track, their deposition in tissue or organs and subsequent tumor growth. This process can occur over a few months or may require two years or more. The incidence of needle tract seeding in abdominal percutaneous diagnostic procedures seems to be very low (between 0.003 and 0.009%), but the exact percentage is not easily determined because follow-up is often inadequate [37]. However, a high incidence of tumor seeding after pancreas tumor biopsy is possible based on nine case reports of seeding after pancreatic cancer biopsies [37]. However, in two large case series of pancreas biopsies, no cases of tumor seeding occurred [2, 5].

Complications of pancreatic fluid collection using percutaneous drainage may occur, and because some of these procedures are performed on severely ill patients, it is not easy to distinguish between procedure-related complications and natural disease courses. Nevertheless, major complications were found in 23% of 378 patients (literature review), with no mortality [30]. However, one case that resulted in death has been reported after fine-needle aspiration of a pseudocyst, due to septic shock [38].

4.7 Tips, Recommendations and Comments

Experimental studies on biopsy needles show no influence of needle caliber on the induction of bleeding [30], whereas a higher risk of bleeding with cutting needles compared to aspiration needles was suggested. However, based on large surveys on procedure complications, no conclusive data have emerged with regard to bleeding [35-44].

The number of complications can depend on the number of performed passes [36, 37]. With cytologic sampling, we recommend immediate verification of specimen adequacy with onsite cytology [2]; if immediate assessment is not possible, we recommend the performance of a maximum of two passes for each lesion, as the diagnostic yield does not improve with more passes [45, 46]. To avoid the risk of injury to a vascular structure, a color-Doppler US (Fig. 4.5) must be performed before the biopsy. Severe pancreatitis may occur after the biopsy of a normal pancreas, and puncture of a fluid collection presents a possible risk of sepsis.

References

1. Hartwig W, Schneider L, Diener MK et al (2009) Preoperative tissue diagnosis for tumors of the pancreas. Br J Surg 96:5-20
2. Zamboni GA, D'Onofrio M, Idili A et al (2009) Ultrasound guided percutaneous fine-needle aspiration of 594 focal pancreatic lesions. Am J Roentgenol 193:1691-1695
3. Hancke S, Holm HH, Koch F (1975) Ultrasonically guided percutaneous fine needle biopsy of the pancreas. Surg Gynecol Obstet 140:361-364
4. Hancke S, Holm HH, Koch F (1984) Ultrasonically guided puncture of solid pancreatic mass lesions. Ultrasound Med Biol 10:613-615
5. Di Stasi M, Lencioni R, Solmi L et al (1998) Ultrasound-guided fine needle biopsy of pancreatic masses: results of a multicenter study. Am J Gastroenterol 93:1329-1333
6. Buscarini L, Fornari F, Bolondi L et al (1990) Ultrasound guided fine-needle biopsy of focal liver lesions. Technique, diagnostic accuracy and complications. J Hepatol 11:344-348
7. Matsubara J, Okusaka T, Morizane C et al (2008) Ultrasound guided percutaneous pancreatic tumor biopsy in pancreatic cancer: a comparison with metastatic liver tumor biopsy, including sensitivity, specificity and complications. J Gastroenterol 43:225-232
8. Garcea G, Ong SL, Rajesh A et al (2008) Cystic lesion of the pancreas. A diagnostic and management dilemma. Pancreatology 8:326-351
9. Lewandrowski KB, Southern JF, Pins MR et al (1993) Cyst analysis in differential diagnosis of pancreatic cysts. A comparison of pseudocysts, serous cystoadenomas, mucinous cystic neoplasms and mucinous cystic adenocarcinomas. Ann Surgery 217:41-47
10. Sperti C, Pasquali C, Guolo P et al (1996) Serum tumor markers and cyst fluid analysis are useful for diagnosis of the pancreatic cystic tumors. Cancer 78:237-243
11. Carlson SK, Johnson CD, Brandt KR et al (1998) Pancreatic cystic neoplasms: the role and sensitivity of needle aspiration and biopsy. Abdom Imaging 23:387-393
12. Brugge WR, Lewandrowski K, Lee-Lewandrowski E et al (2004) Diagnosis of pancreatic cystic neoplasms: a report of cooperative pancreatic cyst study. Gastroenterology 126:1330-1336
13. Volmar KE, Vollmer RT, Jowell PS et al (2005) Pancreatic FNA in 1000 cases: a comparison of imaging modalities. Gastrointest Endosc 61:854-861
14. Horwhat JD, Paulson EK, McGrath K et al (2006) A randomized comparison of EUS-guided FNA versus CT or US-guided FNA for the evaluation of pancreatic mass lesions. Gastrointest Endoscop 63:966-975
15. Levy MJ (2006) Know when to biopsy 'em, know when to walk away. Gastrointest Endosc 63:630-634
16. Habashi S, Draganov PV (2009) Pancreatic pseudocyst. World J Gastroenterol 15:38-47
17. Gerzof SG, Robbins AH, Birkett DH (1979) Percutaneous catheter drainage of abdominal abscesses guided by ultrasound and computed tomography. Am J Roentgenol 133:1-8
18. Karlson KB, Martin EC, Fankuchen EI (1982) Percutaneous drainage of pancreatic pseudocysts and abscesses. Radiology 142:619-624
19. vanSonnenberg E, Wittich GR, Casola G et al (1985) Complicated pancreatic inflammatory disease: diagnostic and therapeutic role of interventional radiology. Radiology 155:335-340
20. Steiner E, Mueller PR, Hahn PF et al (1988) Complicated pancreatic abscesses: problems in interventional management. Radiology 167:443-446
21. Freeny PC, Lewis GP, Traverso LW, Ryan JA (1988) Infected pancreatic fluid collections: percutaneous catheter drainage. Radiology 167:435-441
22. Stanley JH, Gobien RP, Schabel SI et al (1988) Percutaneous drainage of pancreatic and peripancreatic fluid collections. Cardiovasc Inter Rad 1:21-25
23. vanSonnenberg E, Wittich GR, Casola G et al (1989) Percutaneous drainage of infected and non-infected pancreatic pseudocysts: experience in 101 cases. Radiology 170:757-761
24. Adams DB, Harvey TS, Anderson MC (1990) Percutaneous catheter drainage of infected pancreatic and peripancreatic fluid collections. Arch Surg 125: 1554-1557

25. Lee MJ, Rattner DW, Legemate DA et al (1992) Acute complicated pancreatitis: redefining the role of interventional radiology. Radiology 183:171-174
26. Migaleddu W, Strusi G, Fais G, Canalis GC (1995) Percutaneous drainage with vacuum aspiration of pancreatic pseudocysts. Eur Radiol 5:501-503
27. Davies RP, Cox MR, Wilson TG et al (1996) Percutaneous cystogastrostomy with a new catheter for drainage of pancreatic pseudocysts and fluid collections. Cardiovasc Inter Rad 19:128-131
28. vanSonnenberg E, Wittich GR, Chon KS et al (1997) Percutaneous radiologic drainage of pancreatic abscesses. Am J Roentgenol 168:979-984
29. Freeny PC, Hauptmann E, Althaus SJ et al (1998) Percutaneous CT-guided catheter drainage of infected acute necrotizing pancreatitis: techniques and results. Am J Roentgenol 170:969-975
30. Buscarini E, Di Stasi M (1996) Complications of abdominal interventional ultrasound. Poletto Ed., Milan, pp. 24, 77
31. Evans WK, Ho CS, McLoughlin MJ, Tao LC (1981) Fatal necrotizing pancreatitis following fine-needle aspiration biopsy of the pancreas. Radiology 141:61-62
32. Mueller PR, Miketic LM, Simeone JF et al (1988) Severe acute pancreatitis after percutaneous biopsy of the pancreas. Am J Roentgenol 151:493-494
33. Levin DP, Bret PM (1991) Percutaneous fine needle aspiration biopsy of the pancreas resulting in death. Gastrointest Radiol 16:67-69
34. Moulton JS, Moore PT (1993) Coaxial percutaneous biopsy technique with automated biopsy devices: value in improving accuracy and negative predictive value. Radiology 186:515-522
35. Smith EH (1984) The hazards of fine needle aspiration biopsy. Ultrasound Med Biol 10:629-634
36. Smith EH (1991) Complications of percutaneous abdominal fine needle biopsy. Radiology 178:253-258
37. Buscarini L (1998) Complications of abdominal interventional ultrasound: the dissemination risk. JEMU 19:149-152
38. Ulich TR, Layfield LJ (1985) Fatal septic shock after fine needle aspiration of a pancreatic pseudocyst. Acta Cytol 29:879-881
39. Scott Gazelle G, Haaga JR, Rowland DY (1992) Effect of needle gauge, level of anticoagulation, and target organ on bleeding associated with aspiration biopsy. Radiology 183:509-513
40. Livraghi T, Damascelli B, Lombardi G, Spagnoli I (1983) Risk in fine needle abdominal biopsy. J Clin Ultrasound 11:77-81
41. Weiss H, Duntsch U, Weiss A (1998) Risiken der Feinnadelpunktion. Ergebnisse einer Umfrage in der BRD (DEGUM-Umfrage). Ultraschall Med 9:121-127
42. Fornari G, Civardi G, Cavanna L et al (1989) Complications of ultrasonically guided fine-needle abdominal biopsy. Results of a multicenter Italian study and review of the literature. The Cooperative Italian Study Group. Scand J Gastroenterol 24:949-955
43. Weiss H (1994) Komplikationen der Feinnadel Punktion. DEGUM Umfrage 2. Bildgebung Imaging 61[suppl 2]:25-28
44. Nolsoe C, Nielsen L, Torp-Pedersen S, Holm HH (1990) Major complications and deaths due to interventional ultrasonography: a review of 8,000 cases. JCU 18:179-184
45. Livraghi T, Lazzaroni S, Civelli L et al (1997) Risk conditions and mortality rate of abdominal fine needle biopsy. J Intervent Radiol 10:57-64
46. Civardi G, Fornari F, Cavanna L et al (1988) Value of rapid staining and assessment of ultrasound-guided fine needle aspiration biopsies. Acta Cytol 32:552-554

Intraoperative Ultrasonography of the Pancreas

5

Mirko D'Onofrio, Emilio Barbi, Riccardo De Robertis, Francesco Principe, Anna Gallotti and Enrico Martone

5.1 Introduction

Intraoperative ultrasonography (IOUS) still remains a useful and occasionally a problem-solving technique in pancreatic diseases, even though its role has recently been downsized owing to preoperative imaging advances [1]. Since its introduction in the 1980s, progressive technical developments have led to an increase in the diagnostic accuracy of IOUS. The availability of scanners that provide the depiction of fine anatomic details and the detection of small lesions in real-time with excellent spatial and contrast resolution allow the widespread application of this imaging method [1, 2]. Moreover, IOUS is able to clearly show lesions not detectable with other preoperative imaging modalities, and to accurately define the extension of the tumor and its relationship with vessels, sometimes determining significant changes in the therapeutic management of patients [3-5]. In addition, its ability in guiding interventional procedures (i.e. biopsy, duct cannulation and drainage of abscesses or cysts) has been widely reported [2, 6]. Lastly, its impact has significantly increased since both the development of mini-invasive laparoscopic approaches, due to the impossibility for the surgeon to visually and manually inspect the affected organ and the retroperitoneum, and the recent introduction of alternative palliative treatments under IOUS-guidance [7, 8].

5.2 Technical Background

The pancreatic IOUS examination requires the use of sterilized high multifrequency dedicated transducers (usually from 3-5 to 8-10 MHz) that allow the selection of the best frequency for each organ and disease. To enable an approach as easy and as accurate as possible, probes with particular shapes have to be used, especially to evaluate the deepest regions, such as the pancreatic tail and the posterior aspect of the right liver lobe. I-shaped or flat-T probes and cylindrical or sector probes are generally utilized. The former are usually preferred for scanning large flat organ surfaces (i.e. the liver and the pancreas), whereas the latter are used to scan smaller structures (i.e. blood vessels and bile ducts) because of their front-viewing. The I-shaped transducers (Fig. 5.1) allow easier exploration of the whole pancreatic gland, especially of the tail, being easier to move and providing

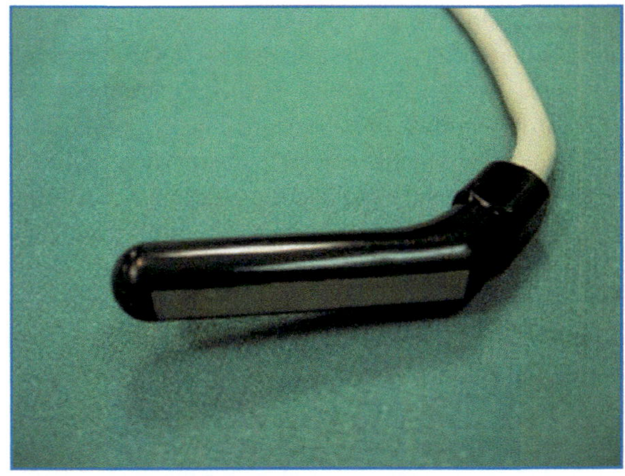

Fig. 5.1 I-shaped IOUS probe

M. D'Onofrio (✉)
Department of Radiology
G.B. Rossi University Hospital, Verona, Italy
e-mail: mirko.donofrio@univr.it

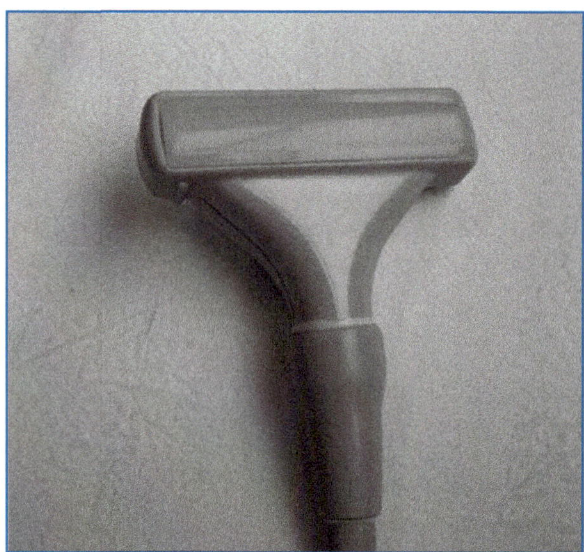

Fig. 5.2 T-shaped IOUS probe

immediate transition from transversal to longitudinal scans, compared to flat-T probes (Fig. 5.2). Furthermore, other more dedicated transducers have been developed. For example, Kaneko et al. reported the application of a 7.5 MHz annular array probe able to generate good quality longitudinal images useful in the determination of the extent of intraductal papillary mucinous neoplasms (IPMN) [9]. All modern systems provide the application of harmonic and Doppler evaluation and dedicated software for a contrast-enhanced study (CEUS) after microbubbles injection [1, 2].

As previously mentioned, recent technologic advances and technical developments have extended the role of minimally invasive surgery and treatment options. The laparoscopic approach for several pancreatic diseases has been receiving increasing interest in recent years [7, 10, 11]. Dedicated sterilized instruments are obviously required. For an accurate description of this relatively new surgical approach the revision of the literature is recommended. On the other hand, radiofrequency ablation (RFA) of pancreatic tumors is nowadays an IOUS-guided procedure performed during laparotomy in open surgery. IOUS covers the mandatory role of staging, evaluation of feasibility, guidance and monitoring of the RFA procedure [8, 12, 13]. A detailed description of the technique, its indications, feasibility and complications are not among the aims of this chapter and for an accurate comprehension the reader should refer to the literature.

5.3 Protocols

After Kocher's maneuver which consists of the transection of the gastrocolic ligament and mobilization of the duodenum and the pancreas, IOUS can be performed by moving the probe in both transverse and longitudinal planes carefully exploring the entire parenchyma. The first approach consists of a transverse scan of the body-tail of the gland; then the head and the body should be serially studied also in the longitudinal plane [1, 2]. Placing the probe either directly on the surface of the organ or with a minimal fluid interface can avoid interference by the abdominal wall or the gas-filled bowel and significantly improve image quality [2, 14]. Each examination has to follow four fundamental steps: (1) detection of the lesion; (2) evaluation of its relationship with the main pancreatic duct; (3) assessment of its potential resectability, mainly focusing on the relationship with the main peri-pancreatic vascular structures; and (4) liver staging [1-3]. In patients with a resectable pancreatic tumor, liver lesions which are questionable or not identified at preoperative imaging studies should undergo fine-needle aspiration (FNA) under IOUS-guidance to achieve a final diagnosis. IOUS has been reported to add 10 to 15 minutes to operating time [6].

5.4 Clinical Applications

The clinical role of pancreatic IOUS can be divided into three applications: lesion detection, lesion staging and lesion treatment.

5.4.1 Lesion Detection

IOUS is primarily utilized for lesion detection (Fig. 5.3) in hyper-functioning (syndromic) endocrine tumors, often multifocal as for the insulinoma, to exclude the co-existence of synchronous lesions hidden at preoperative imaging [1]. As the technique is able to describe fine details, several studies reported its capability in detecting small tumors ranging from 86-95% to 100%, higher than that described for US, computed tomography (CT) and magnetic resonance imaging (MRI), which fail to reveal the majority of insulinomas [15-18]. Therefore, IOUS and regional localization are recommended for insulinoma if preoperative imaging is equivocal [18].

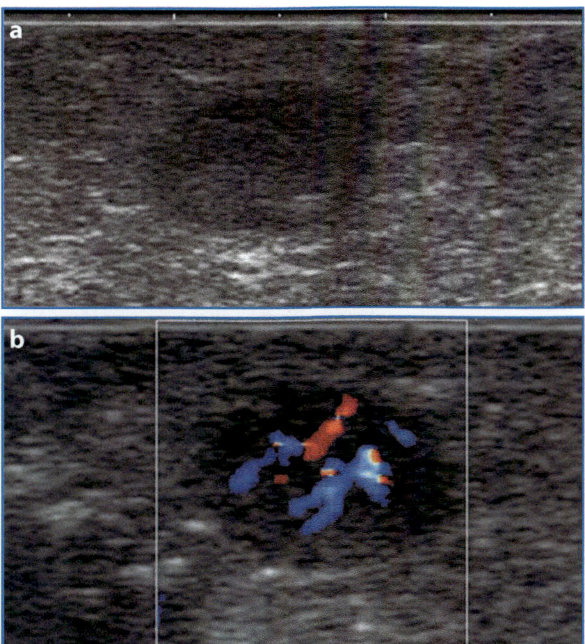

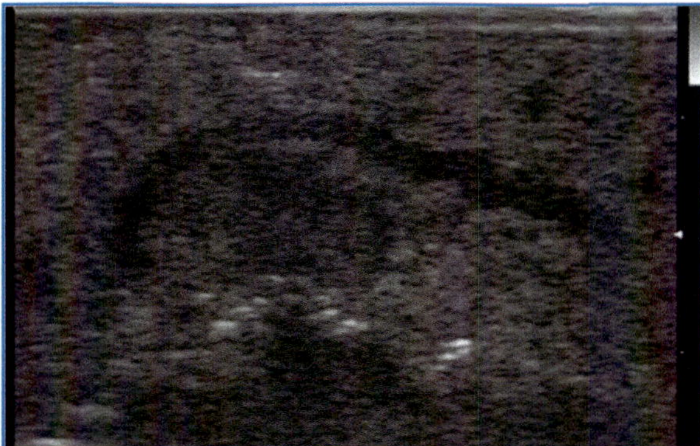

Fig. 5.4 Pancreatic insulinoma. Small hypoechoic nodule detected at the pancreatic body located dorsally to the main pancreatic duct that results minimally involved and upstream slightly dilated

Fig. 5.3 a,b Pancreatic insulinoma. Hypoechoic nodule smaller than 1 cm with well-defined margins detected intraoperatively in the pancreatic head (**a**). Intralesional vessels are visible at color-Doppler imaging (**b**)

5.4.2 Lesion Staging

IOUS plays an important role in accurately performing the staging of a pancreatic tumor. Lesion staging is based on the evaluation of its borders to correctly define their relations with the main pancreatic duct and the main peripancreatic vascular structures, as well as on the whole liver study excluding distant spread. Both local and distant staging influence the therapeutic strategy. First, small lesions far from the main pancreatic duct should be enucleated as these have a low risk of fistulization. Enucleation decreases the operative time and may be performed with less tissue trauma and greater sparing of pancreatic parenchyma [19-22]. Clearly, this aspect is crucial dealing with small endocrine tumors. After detection of small pancreatic nodule IOUS has the role of judging the relations between the lesion and the pancreatic duct (Fig. 5.4). Second, the resectability of a pancreatic mass depends on the relations between the lesion and the adjacent vascular structures and is based on the absence of distant metastases. The involvement of arterial vessels (all but the gastroduodenal and splenic arteries) is an absolute

contraindication for surgery, while venous involvement is a relative one [23]. Preoperative imaging modalities mostly allow accurate local staging, however sometimes an obvious cleavage between the tumor and vessel walls is not clearly depicted. IOUS is recommended in all these cases [24]. Three possible scenarios can be observed: (1) a clear distance between tumor and vessel walls (Fig. 5.5a) owing to the presence of normal parenchyma or preserved perivisceral perivascular fat; (2) a tumor strictly tangent to the vessel wall (Fig. 5.5b) without any echogenic interface between them; (3) a lesion evidently abutting the vessel lumen (Fig. 5.5c), with clear vascular invasion (Fig. 5.5d). Liver staging is often adequately obtained by CEUS, CT and MRI. In some instances however, IOUS is able to show very small focal liver lesions (Fig. 5.6), most often located marginally, hidden at preoperative imaging modalities [1, 25]. In an evaluation of liver lesions with IOUS, CT and MRI, Zacherl et al. [26] confirmed that IOUS is crucial in tumor staging, providing new information on location, number and topographic features of the liver metastases in about 30% of cases, with a significant influence on surgical treatment. However, in a comparison between IOUS and MRI with hepatospecific contrast agent for the detection of liver lesions, Sahani et al. [27] hypothesized that the advantage of IOUS was due to the minor technologic developments of the techniques required to perform the examination.

5.4.3 Lesion Treatment

Therapeutic procedures under IOUS-guidance are the last, but not the least clinical application of intraopera-

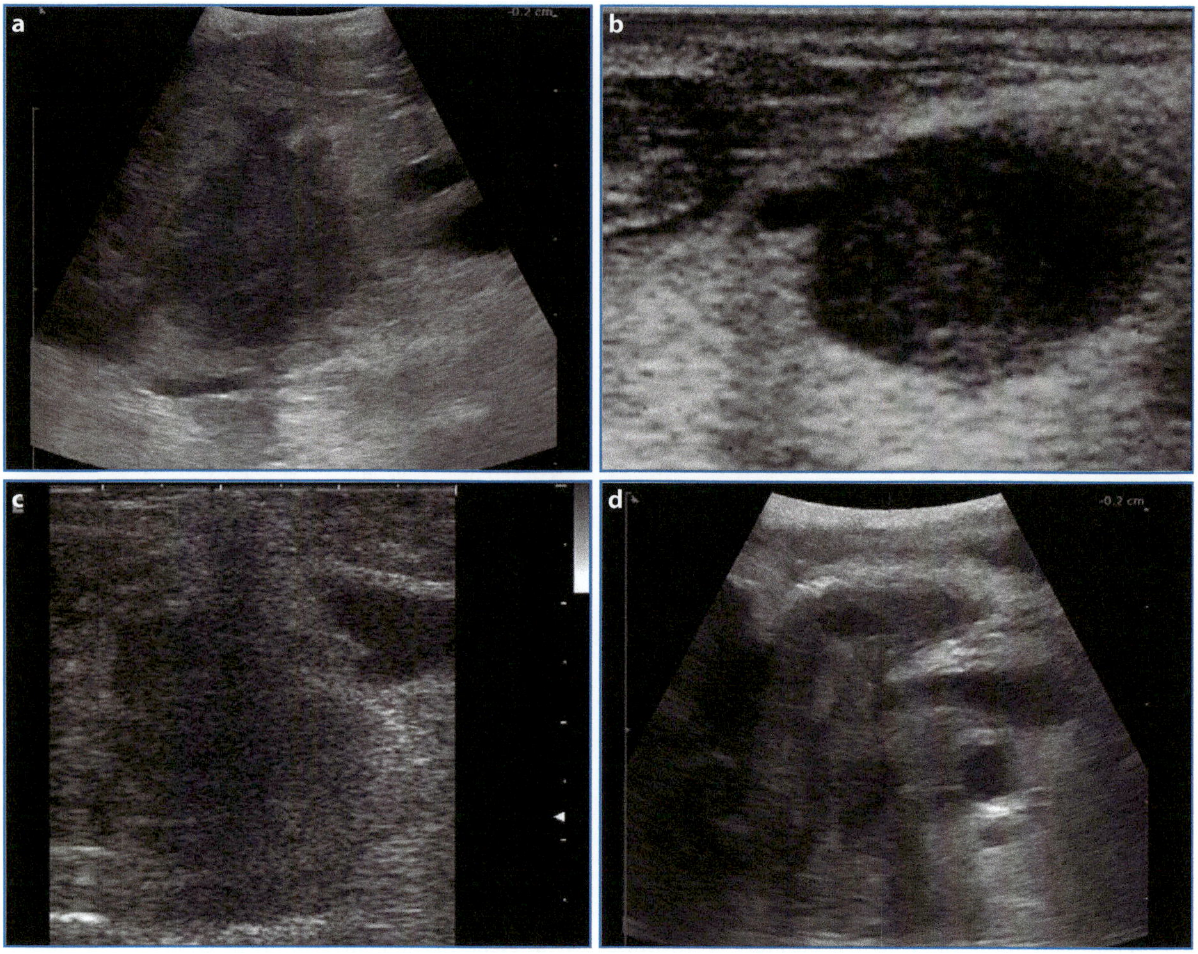

Fig. 5.5 a-d Pancreatic masses: IOUS local staging. **a** Pancreatic head mass not involving the main vessels. **b** Small hypoechoic mass not separated from the gastroduodenal artery resulting for a very small tract in direct contact with the lumen of the artery. **c** Pancreatic head hypoechoic mass not separated from the superior mesenteric vein with a small neoplastic portion within the lumen of the vein. The wall of the vein appears irregular with deformation of the vessel. **d** Pancreatic head mass involving the main vessels

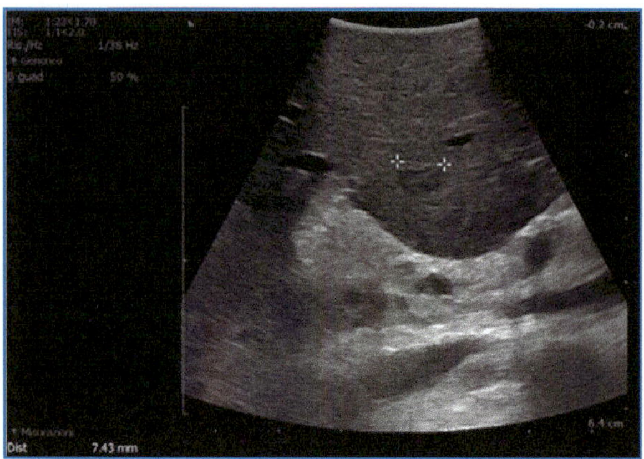

Fig. 5.6 Liver metastasis. Very small (<1 cm) liver metastatic lesion detected at IOUS appearing as a hypoechoic nodule (*caliper*)

tive ultrasound. Since its introduction, IOUS has been used to guide biopsies, fine-needle aspirations and interventional procedures (i.e. duct cannulation and drainage of abscesses or cysts) [2, 6]. In more recent years, the introduction of innovative therapeutic techniques based on IOUS-guidance gave it a new function. First, recent advances in operative techniques and instrumentation have empowered surgeons to virtually perform all procedures in the pancreas, under minimally invasive approaches [7]. Indications for laparoscopic pancreatic surgery include distal pancreatectomy, with or without preserving the spleen, Whipple procedure and the treatment of complications of acute and chronic pancreatitis [28, 29]. In experienced hands, a minimally invasive approach reduces the postoperative hospital

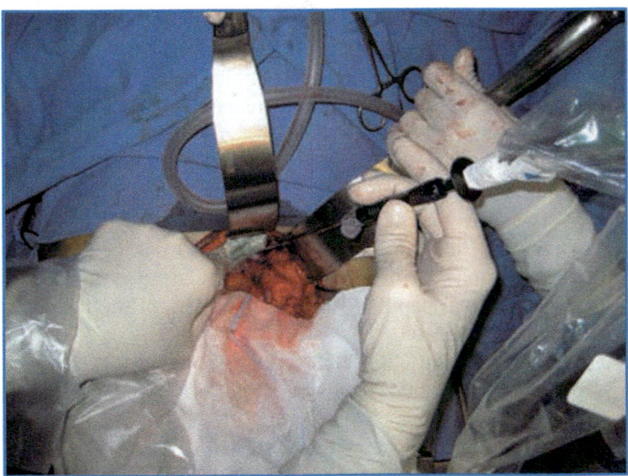

Fig. 5.7 Radiofrequency ablation of unresectable non-metastatic pancreatic adenocarcinoma. Pre-procedure IOUS evaluation and needle insertion under IOUS guidance

procedure without any risk of damage to the contiguous vascular and digestive structures, especially the duodenum. Tumor shape and diameters technically influence the procedure (approach, choice of needle and opening of the electrodes). Moreover, real-time IOUS is used to guide and monitor the treatment (Fig. 5.8). Some studies have focused on the feasibility and complications of RFA, and none of these reported major intraoperative complications [30-34]. Therefore, RFA seems to be a well-tolerated, feasible, potentially safe and promising option in patients with locally advanced non-resectable and non-metastatic pancreatic cancer, with immediate postoperative pain relief. Mini-invasive laparoscopic or percutaneous approaches, as happen in other districts, are expected.

5.5   Laparoscopic Ultrasound

stay and expedites recovery. Moreover, it has been reported in the literature that staging laparoscopy and laparoscopic US avoids unnecessary laparotomy in approximately one-fifth of patients with pancreatic cancer [29]. Second, as mentioned above, a new palliative treatment option for advanced pancreatic cancers consists of RFA. This is restricted to locally advanced, non-resectable but non-metastatic lesions and leads to tumor reduction, improving the quality of life of patients [8]. Nowadays RFA is an IOUS-guided procedure performed during laparotomy in open surgery (Fig. 5.7). IOUS should confirm the safety and feasibility of the

Laparoscopic US probes are specific (Fig. 5.9) for the use through the laparoscopic access ports. The frequencies of the transducer probe range from 5 to 10 MHz with the possibility of color and power Doppler imaging. Standardization of the screening technique is necessary to achieve good reproducible results [35]. Evaluation of the target area must be complete, and the organ should be studied by multiplanar scans. The use of color Doppler can greatly enhance the examination [36]. Regarding clinical results, in the experience of Doucas et al. [37] laparoscopic US altered the management of the patient thought to have a resectable pancreatic tumor in

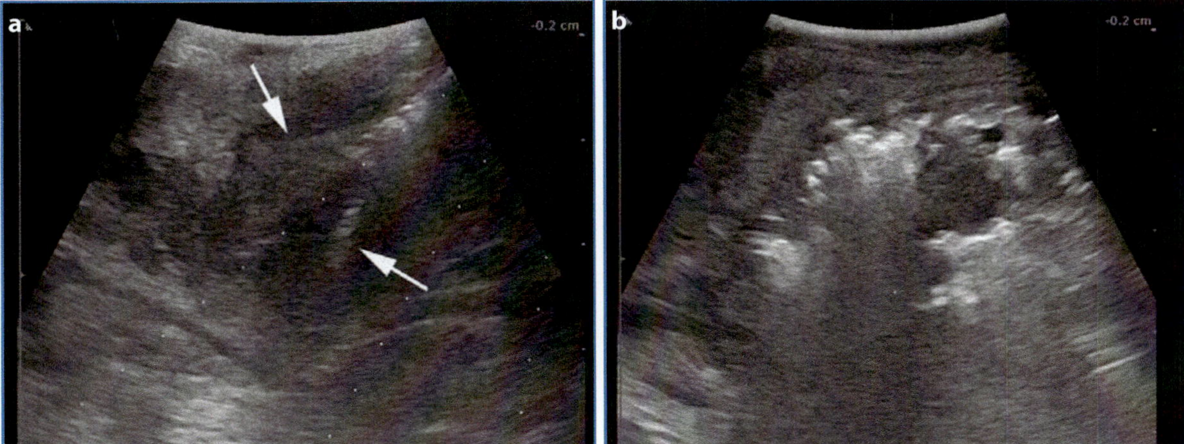

Fig. 5.8 a,b Radiofrequency ablation of unresectable non-metastatic pancreatic adenocarcinoma. **a** IOUS guidance and control of needle placement after electrodes (*arrows*) opening. **b** Post-procedure IOUS control with hyperechoic (*gas*) aspect of the ablated area

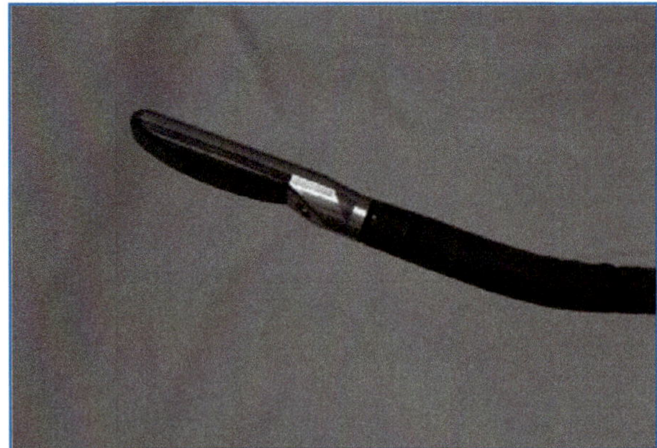

Fig. 5.9 Laparoscopic US probe

44% of cases. This result was then confirmed in the meta-analysis performed by Hariharan et al. [38] demonstrating the utility of the laparoscopic approach in potentially resectable cancers of pancreaticobiliary origin. The conclusion of this meta-analysis was: the continuous evolution of imaging modalities will hopefully be able to identify the unresectable disease (particularly liver and peritoneal metastasis) and render staging laparoscopy, an invasive investigation, obsolete in the near future. In current clinical practice, staging laparoscopy appears beneficial for patients with pancreatic and biliary cancers for detection of peritoneal disease and small, surface liver metastasis, which are currently below the threshold of imaging modalities. Staging laparoscopy should be adopted in routine clinical practice and algorithms designed for its judicious use [38].

References

1. D'Onofrio M, Vecchiato F, Faccioli N et al (2007) Ultrasonography of the pancreas. 7. Intraoperative imaging. Abdom Imaging 32:200-206
2. Sun MR, Brennan DD, Kruskal JB et al (2010) Intraoperative ultrasonography of the pancreas. Radiographics 30:1935-1953
3. Long EE, Van Dan J, Weistein S et al (2005) Computed tomography, endoscopic, laparoscopic, and intra-operative sonography for assessing respectability of pancreatic cancer. Surg Oncol 14:105-113
4. Benson MD, Gandhi MR (2000) Ultrasound of the hepatobiliary-pancreatic system. World J Surg 24:166-170
5. Guimaraes CM, Monteiro Correira M, Baldesserotto M et al (2004) Intraoperative ultrasonography of the liver in patients with abdominal tumors: a new approach. J Ultrasound Med 23:1549-1555
6. Machi J, Oishi AJ, Furumoto NJ et al (2004) Intraoperative ultrasound. Surg Clin North Am 84:1085-1111
7. Butturini G, Crippa S, Bassi C et al (2007) The role of laparoscopy in advanced pancreatic cancer diagnosis. Dig Surg 24:33-37
8. D'Onofrio M, Barbi E, Girelli R et al (2010) Radiofrequency ablation of locally advanced pancreatic adenocarcinoma: an overview. World J Gastroenterol 16:3478-3483
9. Kaneto T, Nakao A, Inoue S et al (2001) Intraoperative ultrasonography by high-resolution annular array transducer for intraductal papillary mucinous tumors of the pancreas. Surgery 129:55-65
10. Kooby DA, Chu CK (2010) Laparoscopic management of pancreatic malignancies. Surg Clin North Am 90:427-446. Review
11. Ammori BJ (2003) Pancreatic surgery in the laparoscopic era. JOP 4:187-192
12. Hadjicostas P, Malakounides N, Varianos C et al (2006) Radiofrequency ablation in pancreatic cancer. HPB (Oxford) 8:61-64
13. Tang Z, Wu YL, Fang HQ et al (2008) Treatment of unresectable pancreatic carcinoma by radiofrequency ablation with 'cool-tip needle': report of 18 cases. Zhonghua Yi Xue Za Zhi 88:391-394. Chinese
14. Luck AJ, Maddern GJ (1999) Intraoperative abdominal ultrasonography. Br J Surg 86:5-16
15. Prokesch RW, Chow LC, Beaulieu CF et al (2002) Local staging of pancreatic carcinoma with multi-detector row CT: use of curved planar reformations initial experience. Radiology 225:759-765
16. D'Onofrio M, Mansueto G, Falconi M et al (2004) Neuroendocrine pancreatic tumor: value of contrast-enhanced ultrasonography. Abdom Imaging 29:246-258
17. D'Onofrio M, Mansueto G, Vasori S et al (2003) Contrast-enhanced ultrasonographic detection of small pancreatic insulinoma. J Ultrasound Med 22:413-417
18. Hiramoto JS, Feldstein VA, LaBerge JM et al (2001) Intraoperative ultrasound and preoperative localization detects all occult Insulinomas. Arch Surg 136:1020-1025; discussion 1025-1026
19. Falconi M, Zerbi A, Crippa S et al (2010) Parenchyma-preserving resections for small nonfunctioning pancreatic endocrine tumors. Ann Surg Oncol 17:1621-1627
20. Zhao YP, Zhan HX, Zhang TP et al (2011) Surgical management of patients with insulinomas: Result of 292 cases in a single institution. J Surg Oncol 103:169-174
21. Dedieu A, Rault A, Collet D et al (2011) Laparoscopic enucleation of pancreatic neoplasm. Surg Endosc 25:572-576
22. Casadei R, Ricci C, Rega D et al (2010) Pancreatic endocrine tumors less than 4 cm in diameter: resect or enucleate? a single-center experience. Pancreas 39:825-828
23. Minniti S, Bruno C, Biasiutti C et al (2003) Sonography versus helical CT in identification and staging of pancreatic ductal adenocarcinoma. J Clin Ultrasound 31:175-182
24. D'Onofrio M, Gallotti A, Pozzi Mucelli R (2010) Imaging techniques in pancreatic tumors. Expert Rev Med Devices 7:257-273
25. Kane RA (2004) Intraoperative ultrasonography: history, current state of the art, and future directions. J Ultrasound Med 23:1407-1420
26. Zacherl J, Scheuba C, Imhof M et al (2002) Current value of

intraoperative sonography during surgery for hepatic neoplasms. World J Surg 26:550-554

27. Sahani DV, Kalva SP, Tanabe KK et al (2004) Intraoperative US in patients undergoing surgery for liver neoplasms: comparison with MR imaging. Radiology 232:810-814

28. Mori T, Abe N, Sugiyama M et al (2005) Laparoscopic pancreatic surgery. J Hepatobiliary Pancreat Surg 12:451-455

29. Ammori BJ (2003) Pancreatic surgery in the laparoscopic era. JOP 4:187-192

30. Girelli R, Frigerio I, Salvia R et al (2010) Feasibility and safety of radiofrequency ablation for locally advanced pancreatic cancer. Br J Surg 97:220-225

31. Wu Y, Tang Z, Fang H et al (2006) High operative risk of cool-tip radiofrequency ablation for unresectable pancreatic head cancer. J Surg Oncol 94:392-395

32. Limmer S, Huppert PE, Juette V et al (2009) Radiofrequency ablation of solitary pancreatic insulinoma in a patient with episodes of severe hypoglycemia. Eur J Gastroenterol Hepatol 21:1097-1101

33. Carrafiello G, Laganà D, Recaldini C et al (2008) Radiofrequency ablation of a pancreatic metastasis from renal cell carcinoma: case report. Surg Laparosc Endosc Percutan Tech 18:64-66

34. Siriwardena AK (2006) Radiofrequency ablation for locally advanced cancer of the pancreas. JOP 7:1-4

35. Jakimowicz JJ (2006) Intraoperative ultrasonography in open and laparoscopic abdominal surgery: an overview. Surg Endosc 20[Suppl 2]:S425-S435. Review

36. Smulders JF, Jakimowicz JJ (1995) Color Doppler application in laparoscopic intraoperative ultrasonography. Surg Techn Intern 4:184-187

37. Doucas H, Sutton CD, Zimmerman A et al (2007) Assessment of pancreatic malignancy with laparoscopy and intraoperative ultrasound. Surg Endosc 21:1147-1152

38. Hariharan D, Constantinides VA, Froeling FE et al (2010) The role of laparoscopy and laparoscopic ultrasound in the preoperative staging of pancreatico-biliary cancers—A meta-analysis. Eur J Surg Oncol 36:941-948. Review

Pancreatic Anatomy, Variants and Pseudolesions of the Pancreas

6

Emilio Barbi, Salvatore Sgroi, Paolo Tinazzi, Stefano Canestrini, Anna Gallotti and Mirko D'Onofrio

6.1 Introduction

For many years the pancreas was left unexplored by radiologic research except indirectly and for more important diseases, such as calcifications in chronic pancreatitis on plain film radiography, gastric and duodenal imprint of largest masses on the barium meal study or the neoplastic involvement of peri-pancreatic vessels on the angiographic study.

Since the early 1980s the diffusion of ultrasound (US), computed tomography (CT) and magnetic resonance imaging (MRI) has allowed direct visualization of the gland, even in normal conditions, with gradual improvement of anatomic details which have currently reached high levels of precision.

6.2 Pancreatic Anatomy

The pancreas is a compound gland (both exocrine and endocrine) connected to the digestive system which empties its secretions into the lumen of the duodenum.

6.2.1 Site

The pancreas is located in the upper part of the abdomen, where it lies within the anterior pararenal compartment of the retroperitoneum (Figs. 6.1-6.3) [1-3]. Centrally it lies on the front side of the first two lumbar vertebrae and may also lie on the last dorsal vertebra, with the interposition of the abdominal aorta on the left and the inferior vena cava on the right. Laterally it is located on the lower boundary of the diaphragmatic crura, where these insert in the spinal column, with the interposition of peritoneal fat. On the right it is surrounded by the duodenal C-loop, on the left it reaches the splenic hilum, while in front it is covered by the stomach.

6.2.2 Shape, Volume and Consistency

The pancreas has a stretched shape, with a transversal location and slightly flattened anteroposteriorly. Its shape is not symmetrical because its right part is voluminous but short, passing over the midline just for a few centimeters, while the left part is thin, long (1:2) and extends further laterally. On the whole the head accounts for 60–70% of the gland.

The pancreas consists of small lobules, each drained by small pancreatic ducts which increase in diameter to eventually merge into two main pancreatic ducts.

The pancreas is prone to remarkable volume changes, depending on age, sex and kind of constitution (Fig. 6.4). Its mean length is 16-20 cm, mean height 4-5 cm and thickness 2-3 cm. It grows quickly during the childhood and adolescence, reaching its maximum size around 40 years of age; after 50 years of age it begins a gradual process of senile regression. Generally the pancreas is larger in men than in women, more voluminous than average in the obese and the endomorph, and the opposite in the ectomorph. Its weight varies between 30 and 100-150g depending on the volume.

Its color is white-grey, but it becomes flush during digestion, because of increased blood flow. In normal conditions the pancreas is friable, such that sutures barely hold unless attached to the connective tissues.

E. Barbi (✉)
Department of Radiology
Hospital "Casa di Cura Pederzoli",
Peschiera del Garda (VR), Italy
e-mail: emilioba@infinito.it

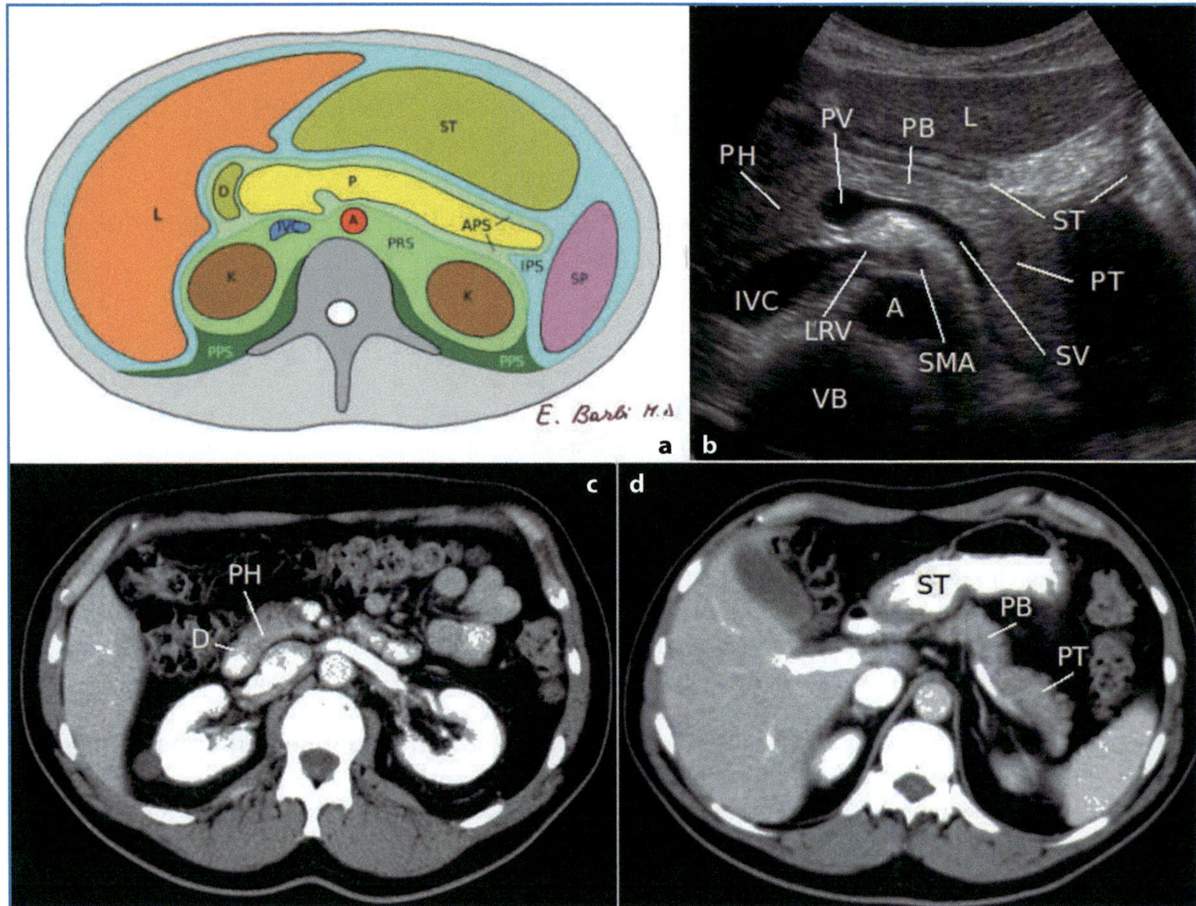

Fig. 6.1 a-d Axial anatomy of the pancreas (*P*). **a** Anatomic features of the pancreas and its relations with the surrounding organs. The anterior pararenal space (*APS*, light green) in front; the perirenal space (*PRS*, medium green) and the posterior pararenal space (*PPS*, dark green) behind; the intraperitoneal space (*IPS*, sky blue) anterior and lateral. **b** US of the pancreas: head (*PH*), body (*PB*) and tail (*PT*). **c,d** CT of the pancreas passing through the head (*PH*), without visualization of the body-tail (**c**), or passing through the body-tail, without visualization of the head (**d**). (*A*, aorta; *D*, duodenum; *IVC*, inferior vena cava; *K*, kidney; *L*, liver; *LRV*, left renal vein; *PV*, portal vein; *SMA*, superior mesenteric artery; *SP*, spleen; *ST*, stomach; *SV*, splenic vein; *VB*, vertebral body

On the other hand it becomes very hard in chronic pancreatitis, in tumors and after radiotherapy, all these conditions characterized by a marked increase in the fibrous component.

6.2.3 Subdivision

The pancreas is classically divided into four (or five) main portions with no clear distinction between them. The head (Figs. 6.5, 6.6) is located on the right side, is short, squat but voluminous and well developed in the three axes compared to the other portions. It is the most caudal part of the pancreas, completely surrounded by the duodenal C-loop on its lateral side.

The uncinate process is a small appendix placed inferiorly and medially compared to the head, to which it belongs. It develops differently in different subjects. It is the most caudal and deep part of the pancreas, lying between the mesenteric vessels anteriorly and the inferior vena cava posteriorly.

The isthmus (Fig. 6.7) is the connection between head and body and is marginally thinner than its contiguous parts. Its backside is marked by the portal vein and the mesenteric-portal confluence.

The body (Figs. 6.8-6.10) is centrally placed, slightly flattened anteroposteriorly and more developed craniocaudally. It is the most superficial part of the pancreas, because it is pushed forward by the vertebral column.

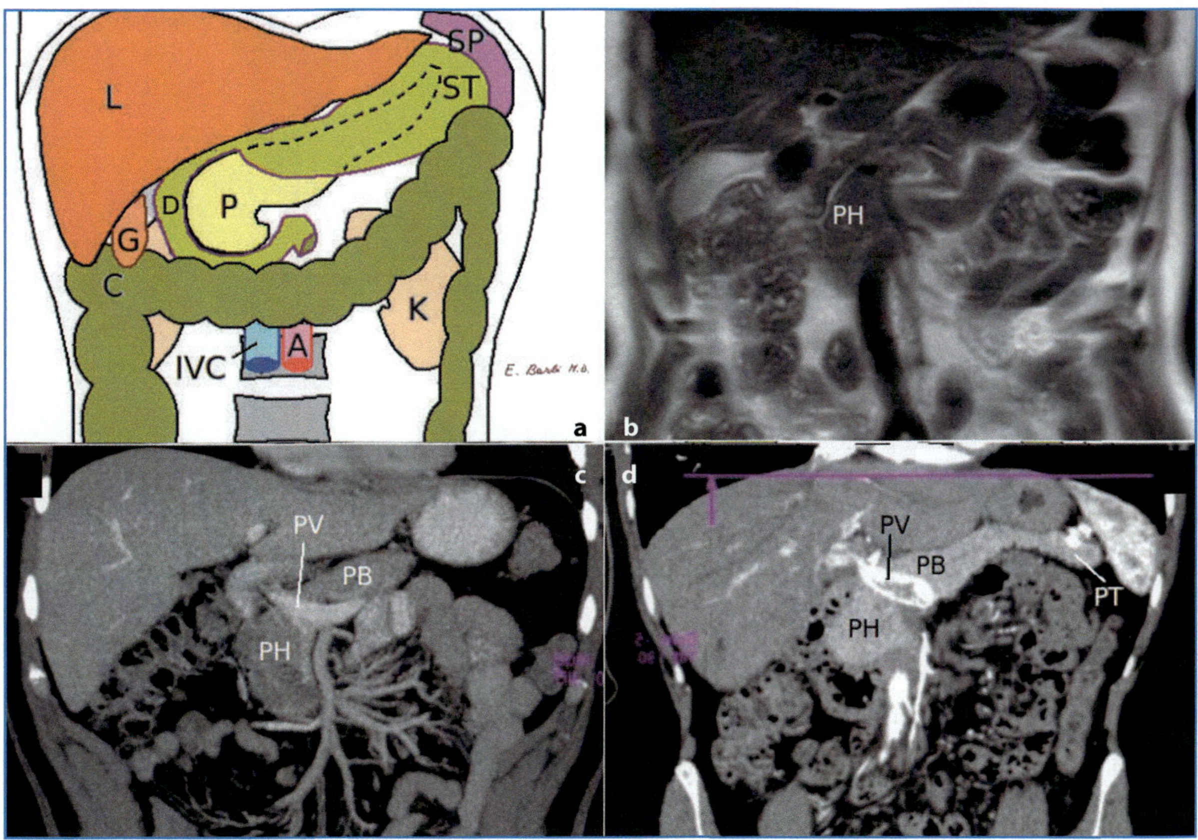

Fig. 6.2 a-d Coronal anatomy of the pancreas (*P*). **a** Anatomic features of the pancreas and its relations with the surrounding organs. The pancreatic gland is located below the liver (*L*), partially covered by the stomach (*ST*) and the transverse colon (*C*) in front. The head is surrounded on three sides by the duodenal C-loop (*D*); the aorta (*A*) and the inferior vena cava (*IVC*) lie behind. The tail reaches the hilum of the spleen (*SP*). **b** MRI of the pancreas, passing through the head (*PH*), without visualization of the body-tail. **c** CT of the pancreas, passing through the head-body (*PH*, *PB*), without visualization of the tail. **d** CT curved reconstruction along the major axis of the gland, allowing the visualization of the entire gland, from the head (*PH*) to the tail (*PT*). (*G*, gallbladder; *K*, kidney; *PV*, portal vein)

The tail (Figs. 6.11, 6.12) constitutes the left side of the gland and tapers toward its distal extreme. It is the only part of the gland partially surrounded by peritoneum in its distal tract toward the splenic hilum (Fig. 6.1a), therefore it may be partially moved by variations in posture.

6.2.4 Microscopy

Unlike the kidneys or the liver, the pancreas is lacking a real capsule and this fact probably justifies the early spread of neoplastic and inflammatory processes to the surrounding structures. It is moreover bound by soft connective tissue which branches in intraglandular ramifications.

Functionally the pancreas is a compound gland with a major exocrine part and a minor endocrine one [4]. The exocrine component of the gland is quantitatively predominant (98-99%) and constituted by two different cell populations. The acinar (serous) cells produce enzymes for the digestion of proteins (trypsin and chymotrypsin are the two most important), fats (lipase) and carbohydrates (amylase, also produced by the parotid gland). These enzymes are produced as inactive precursors and are activated in the intestinal lumen. The potential dysfunctional intraglandular activation can cause autodigestion processes of large portions of the pancreas, as occurs in severe acute pancreatitis. The inactive enzymes are carried from the gland acini to the duodenum by a complex ductal system, consti-

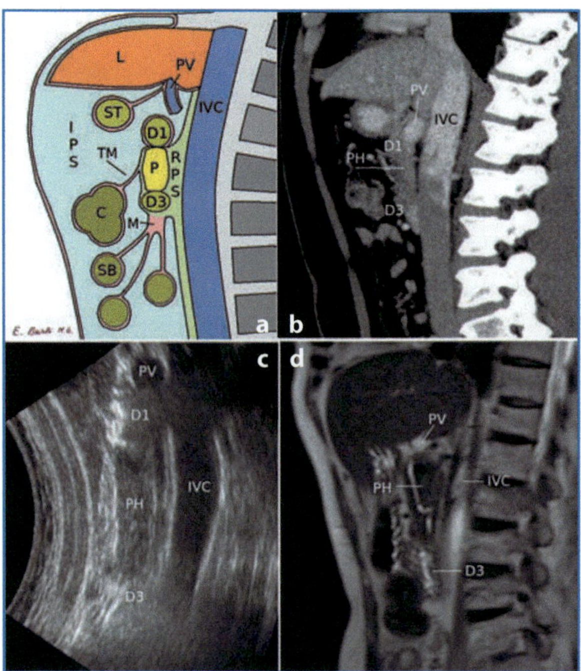

Fig. 6.3 a-d Sagittal anatomy of the pancreas (*P*). **a** Anatomic features of the pancreatic head and its relations with the surrounding organs. The head of the pancreas takes up the most anterior part of the retroperitoneal space (*RPS*), in front of the inferior vena cava (*IVC*), above and below the first and the third duodenal portion (*D1* and *D3*). It fits the colon (*C*) through the transverse mesocolon (*TM*) ventrally and the small bowel (*SB*) through the mesentery (*M*) below; anteriorly the intraperitoneal space (*IPS*, in sky blue). **b** CT of the pancreatic head (*PH*). **c** US of the pancreatic head (*PH*). **d** MRI of the pancreatic head (*PH*). (*L*, liver; *PV*, portal vein)

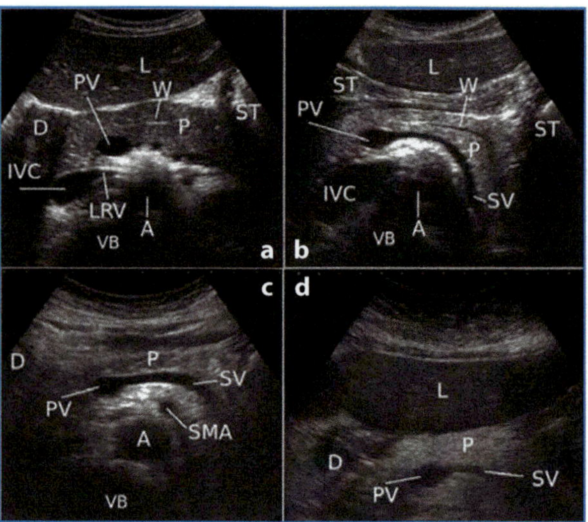

Fig. 6.4 a-d Anatomic variants of the pancreas (*P*). **a** A globular normotrophic gland in a 10 year-old child. **b** A well-represented gland isoechoic to the liver (*L*) in a normotype young adult. **c** A hypotrophic gland in an elderly subject. **d** A hyperechoic globular gland in an obese young adult. (*A*, aorta; *D*, duodenum; *IVC*, inferior vena cava; *LRV*, left renal vein; *PV*, portal vein; *SMA*, superior mesenteric artery; *ST*, stomach; *SV*, splenic vein; *VB*, vertebral body; *W*, duct of Wirsung)

tuted by ducts of increasing caliber (second order ducts), which in the end flow into two main ducts, the duct of Wirsung and the duct of Santorini (Fig. 6.13).

The ductal (mucinous) cells of the pancreas not only constitute the epithelial covering of the excretory ducts but also serve an important secretory function, producing a large quantity of water and bicarbonates (1-2 L/day) in order to neutralize the acidity of the gastric juice in the duodenum. Despite accounting for only 10% of the exocrine glandular component of the pancreas, the neoplastic degeneration of this kind of cell is responsible for almost 90% of all malignant exocrine pancreatic tumors.

The endocrine component of the gland (1-2%) consists of cellular collections termed islets of Langerhans, which are mostly found in the tail and the periductal region. It produces an overall number of at least twenty hormones, most of which are issued directly into the bloodstream, reaching the liver through the portal vein, where they perform their function, whereas a smaller part is directly emptied into the pancreatic ducts. The endocrine gland component consists of four cell populations:

- Alpha cells (20%) are responsible for synthesizing and secreting glucagon peptide hormone, which elevates the glucose level in the blood by moving glycogen from the liver, balancing in this way the insulin effect. It also affects fat and pancreatic metabolism;
- Beta cells (70%) produce insulin, a well-known hormone that increases glucose consumption by the muscles, the fat tissue and the liver. It also acts on lipid metabolism by increasing fat storage in the tissues and on protein metabolism by performing an anabolic action. As is well known, sudden onset of idiopathic diabetes in adults with no family history can be sustained by a pancreatic tumor with consequent upstream obstructive atrophy and digestive disorders because of inadequate exocrine production;
- Delta cells (5%) are responsible for producing somatostatin, a hormone that influences sphincter of Oddi tone, inhibiting the production of insulin and

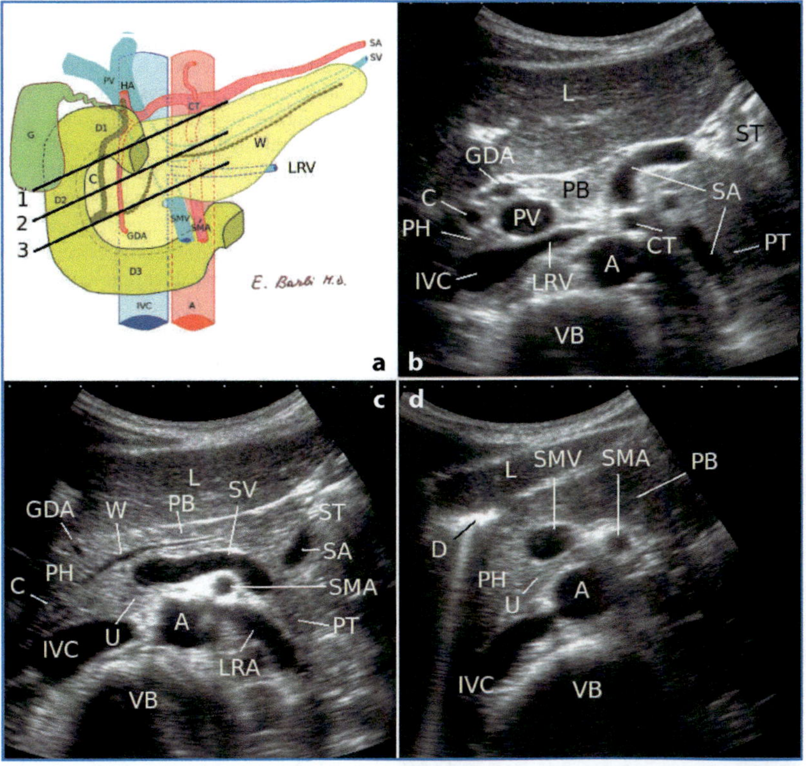

Fig. 6.5 a-d Pancreatic head (*PH*): axial planes. **a** Anatomic features and its relations with the surrounding structures. **b-d** US craniocaudal scans along planes 1, 2 and 3 reported in **a**, respectively. (*A*, aorta; *C*, main bile duct (choledochus); *CT*, celiac trunk; *D*, duodenum (first, second and third portion respectively *D1*, *D2* and *D3*); *G*, gallbladder; *GDA*, gastroduodenal artery; *HA*, hepatic artery; *IVC*, inferior vena cava; *L*, liver; *LRA*, left renal artery; *LRV*, left renal vein; *PB*, pancreatic body; *PT*, pancreatic tail; *PV*, portal vein; *SMA*, superior mesenteric artery; *SMV*, superior mesenteric vein; *ST*, stomach; *SA*, splenic artery; *SV*, splenic vein; *U*, uncinate process; *VB*, vertebral body; *W*, duct of Wirsung)

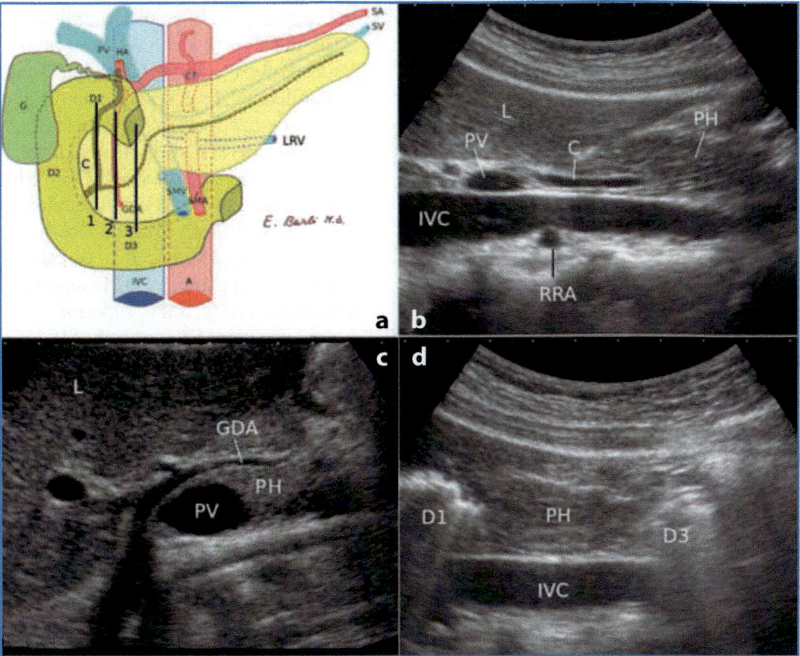

Fig. 6.6 a-d Pancreatic head (*PH*): sagittal planes. **a** Anatomic features and its relations with the surrounding structures. **b-d** US lateromedial scans along planes 1, 2 and 3 reported in **a**, respectively. (*A*, aorta; *C*, main bile duct (choledochus); *CT*, celiac trunk; *D*, duodenum (first, second and third portion respectively *D1*, *D2* and *D3*); *G*, gallbladder; *GDA*, gastroduodenal artery; *HA*, hepatic artery; *IVC*, inferior vena cava; *L*, liver; *LRV*, left renal vein; *PV*, portal vein; *RRA*, right renal artery; *SMA*, superior mesenteric artery; *SMV*, superior mesenteric vein; *SA*, splenic artery; *SV*, splenic vein)

glucagon as well as pancreatic exocrine secretion in general. A synthetic analogue of somatostatin, octeotride, characterized by a greater half-time than somatostatin, is used in neuroendocrine tumors of the pancreas for its antisecretory effects;

• PP cells (5%) produce the pancreatic polypeptide

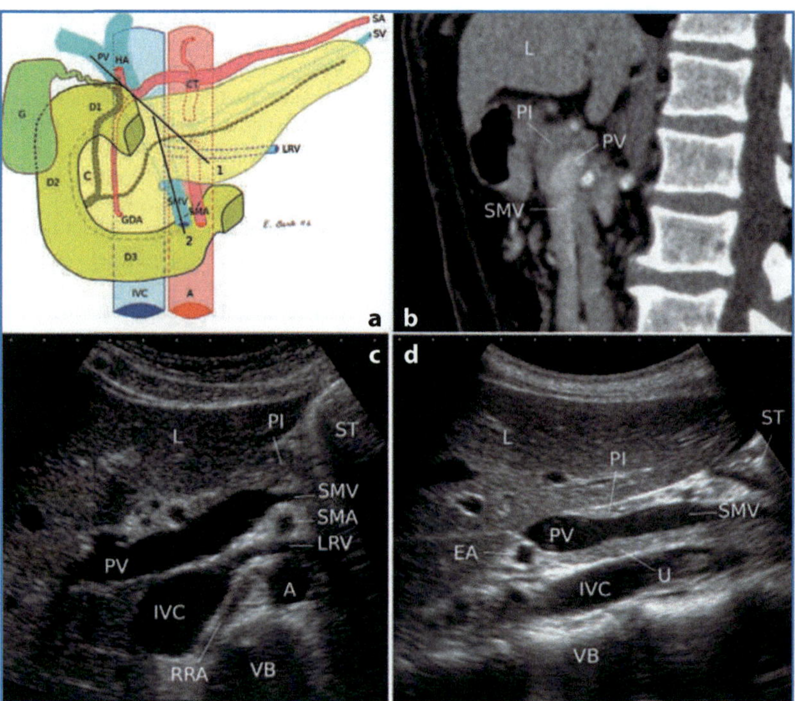

Fig. 6.7 a-d Pancreatic isthmus (*PI*): sagittal planes along the vascular portal-mesenteric axis. **a** Anatomic features and its relations with the surrounding structures. **b** CT scan passing through the portal-mesenteric confluence. **c,d** US scans along the portal vein (*PV*) and the superior mesenteric vein (*SMV*), corresponding to planes 1 and 2 in **a**, respectively. (*A*, aorta; *C*, main bile duct (choledochus); *CT*, celiac trunk; *D*, duodenum (first, second and third portion respectively *D1*, *D2* and *D3*); *G*, gallbladder; *GDA*, gastroduodenal artery; *HA*, hepatic artery; *IVC*, inferior vena cava; *L*, liver; *LRV*, left renal vein; *RRA*, right renal artery; *SMA*, superior mesenteric artery; *ST*, stomach; *SA*, splenic artery; *SV*, splenic vein; *U*, uncinate process; *VB*, vertebral body)

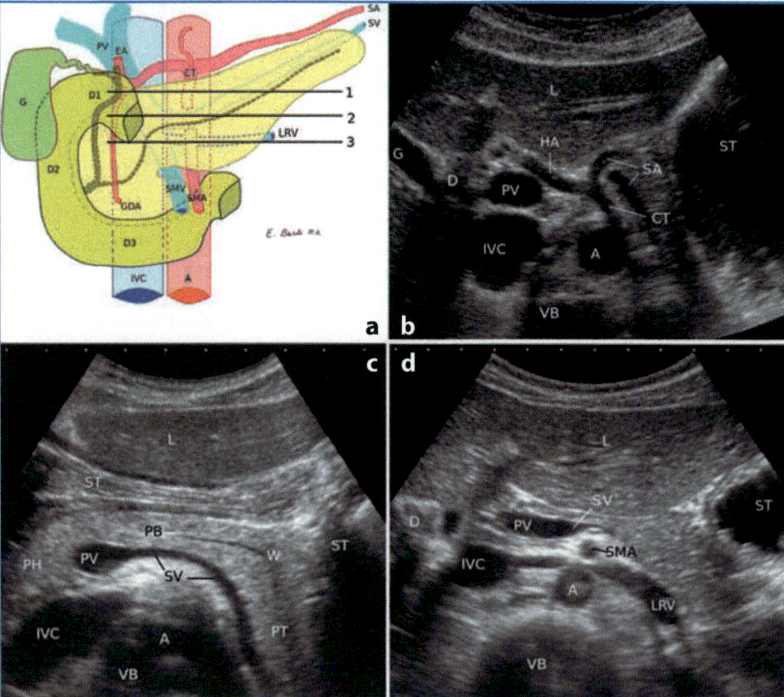

Fig. 6.8 a-d Pancreatic body (*PB*): axial planes. **a** Anatomic features and its relations with the surrounding structures. **b-d** US craniocaudal scans along planes 1, 2 and 3 reported in **a**, respectively. (*A*, aorta; *CT*, celiac trunk; *D*, duodenum (first, second and third portion respectively *D1*, *D2* and *D3*); *G*, gallbladder; *GDA*, gastroduodenal artery; *HA*, hepatic artery; *IVC*, inferior vena cava; *L*, liver; *LRV*, left renal vein; *PB*, pancreatic body; *PH*, pancreatic head; *PV*, portal vein; *PT*, pancreatic tail; *SA*, splenic artery; *SMA*, superior mesenteric artery; *SMV*, superior mesenteric vein; *ST*, stomach; *SV*, splenic vein; *VB*, vertebral body; *W*, duct of Wirsung)

and also perform an inhibitory action on exocrine pancreatic secretion.

Contrary to what was thought in the past, the coexistence of the two glandular components is not a chance occurrence. A strict control on the exocrine component by the endocrine one has in fact been demonstrated through the direct release of the above mentioned hormones both in the ductal system and in the local micro-

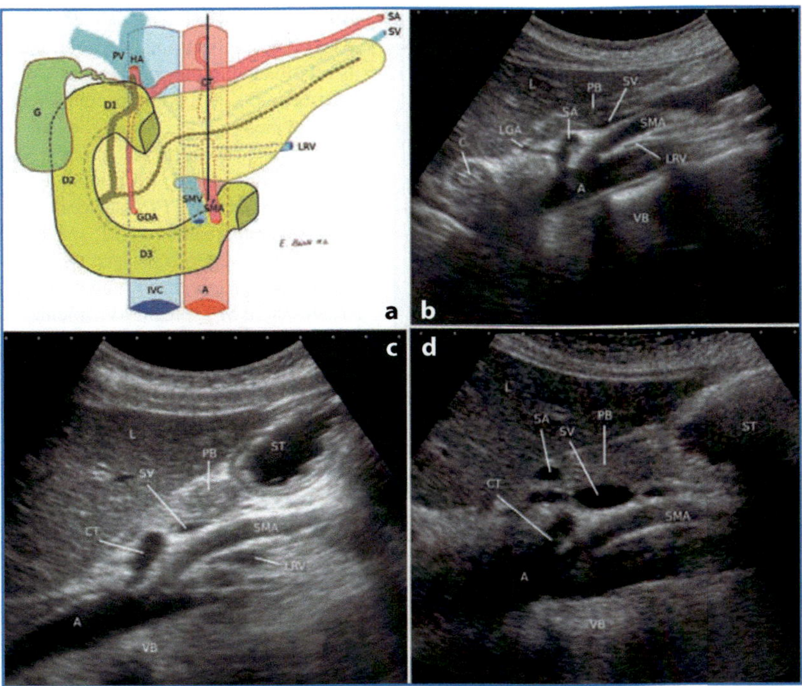

Fig. 6.9 a-d Pancreatic body (*PB*): sagittal planes. **a** Anatomic features and its relations with the surrounding structures. **b-d** US scans along the aortic (*A*) axis. (*C*, cardias; *CT*, celiac trunk; *D*, duodenum (first, second and third portion respectively *D1*, *D2* and *D3*); *G*, gallbladder; *GDA*, gastroduodenal artery; *HA*, hepatic artery; *IVC*, inferior vena cava; *L*, liver; *LGA*, left gastric artery; *LRV*, left renal vein; *PV*, portal vein; *SA*, splenic artery; *SMA*, superior mesenteric artery; *SMV*, superior mesenteric vein; *ST*, stomach; *SV*, splenic vein; *VB*, vertebral body)

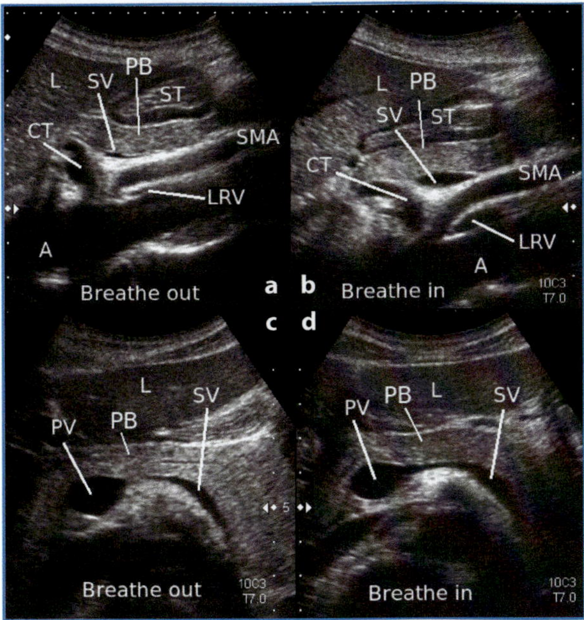

Fig. 6.10 a-d Pancreatic body (*PB*): variations of the retropancreatic vascular axes with breathing, on the sagittal (**a,b**) and axial (**c,d**) planes. During forced expiration (**a,c**) the venous return to the right atrium is improved providing a consequent emptying of both the splenic vein (*SV*) and the left renal vein (*LRV*). In contrast, during deep inspiration, the venous return to the heart is hampered leading to a consequent hyperdistension of both the splenic and the left renal veins, and a lowering of the diaphragm and the liver. Moreover, a concomitant slight lowering of the pancreas can improve the visualization of the gland by using the hepatic acoustic window, especially in the presence of abundant tympanites. (*A*, aorta; *CT*, celiac trunk; *L*, liver; *LRV*, left renal vein; *PB*, pancreatic body; *PV*, portal vein; *SMA*, superior mesenteric artery; *ST*, stomach; *SV*, splenic vein)

circulation (paracrine action) [4]. The functional interaction of the two systems explains how the inadequate production of insulin in a patient with type 1 diabetes is often associated with digestive disorders secondary to deficient exocrine production of bicarbonate and amylase, even under secretin stimulation and despite the absolute integrity of the exocrine glandular component.

6.3   Imaging: US, CT and MRI

Each of the three main modalities – US, CT and MRI – has inherent strengths and weaknesses, so that none of them alone can be preliminarily regarded as conclusive in all circumstances. On the contrary, very often,

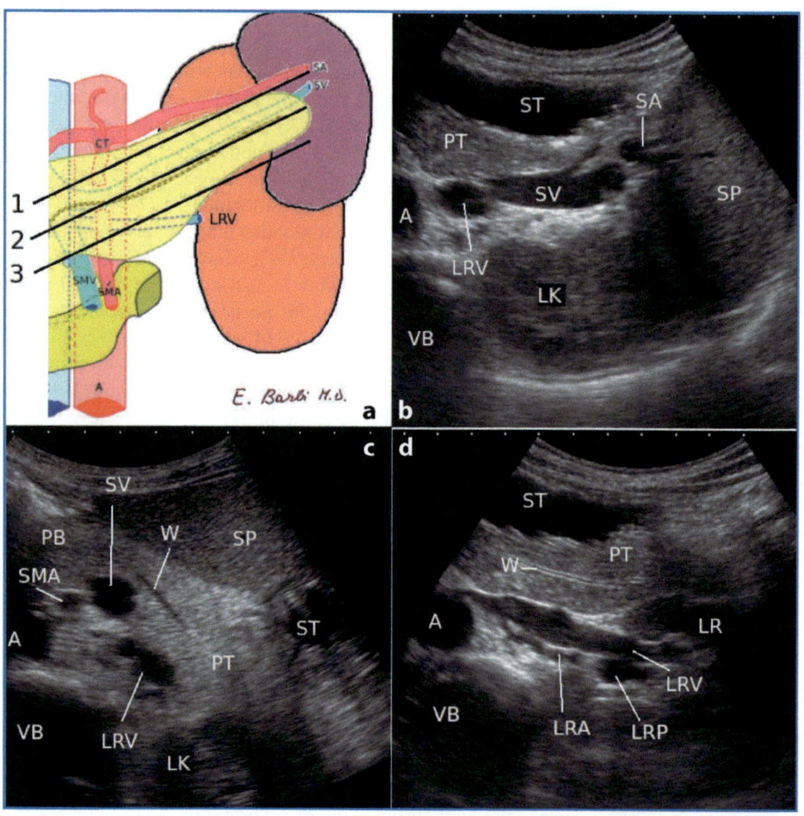

Fig. 6.11 a-d Pancreatic tail (*PT*): axial planes. **a** Anatomic features and its relations with the surrounding structures. **b-d** US craniocaudal scans along planes 1, 2 and 3 reported in **a** respectively. (*A*, aorta; *CT*, celiac trunk; *LK*, left kidney; *LRP*, left renal pelvis; *LRV*, left renal vein; *PB*, pancreatic body; *PT*, pancreatic tail; *SA*, splenic artery; *SMA*, superior mesenteric artery; *SMV*, superior mesenteric vein; *ST*, stomach; *SP*, spleen; *SV*, splenic vein; *VB*, vertebral body; *W*, duct of Wirsung)

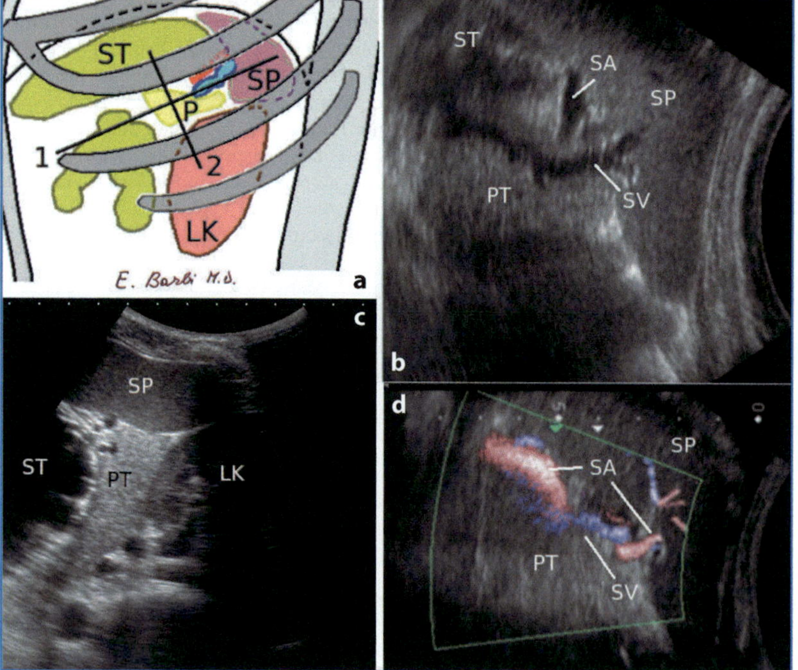

Fig. 6.12 a-d Pancreatic tail (*PT*): left intercostal approach. **a** Anatomic features and its relations with the surrounding structures. **b** US axial plane parallel to the ribs (plane 1 in **a**): the tail of the pancreas (*PT*) reaches the hilum of the spleen (*SP*) together with the splenic vessels. **c** US coronal plane perpendicular to the costal axes (plane 2 in **a**); the tail of the pancreas (*PT*) is circumscribed by the stomach (*ST*) above, the left kidney (*LK*) below and the spleen behind. **d** As shown in **b**, the splenic vessels are better evaluated on color-Doppler study. (*SA*, splenic artery; *SV*, splenic vein)

when studying the pancreas their combined use allows the best diagnostic result to be obtained.

US is well-known as an inexpensive, widely available, safe and dynamic (real time observation) imaging

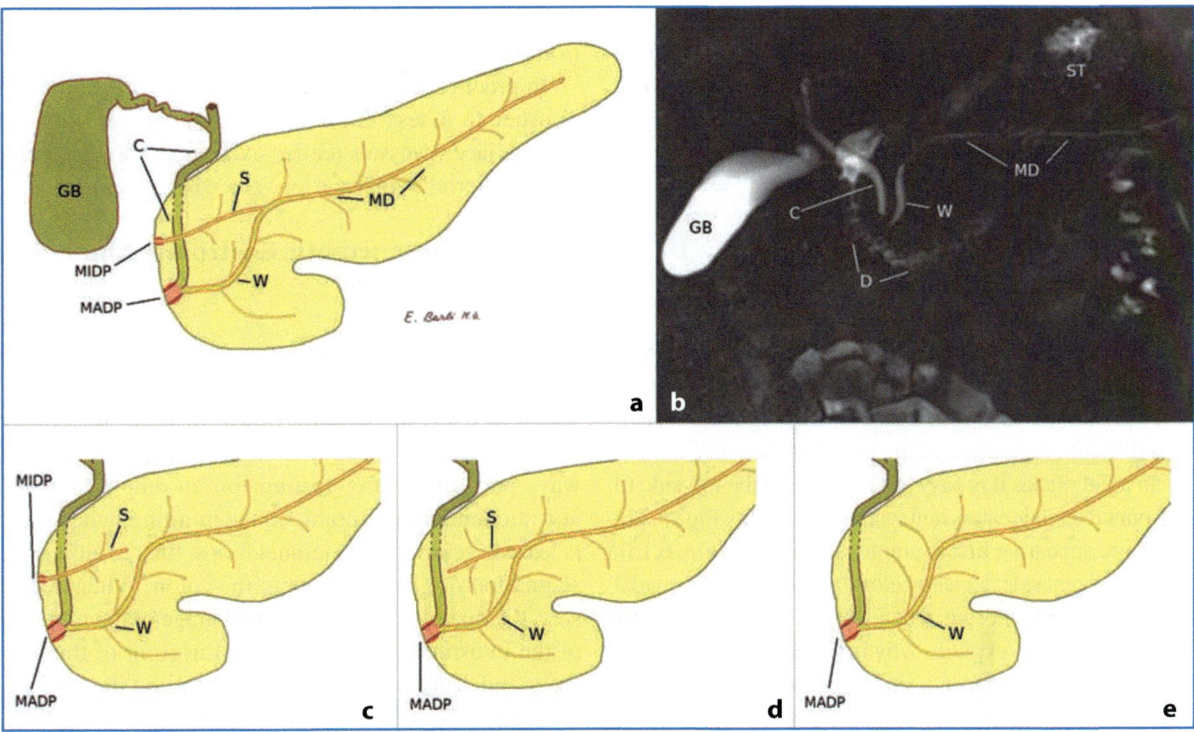

Fig. 6.13 a-e Ductal system of the pancreas. **a** Typical anatomic features of the ductal system: the main duct (*MD*) consists of the duct of Wirsung (*W*) which flows into the duodenum (*D*) through the major papilla (*MADP*) together with the main bile duct (*C*); duct of Santorini (*S*) remains as an accessory duct and flows into the duodenum through the minor papilla (*MIDP*). **b** MRCP: typical MR outline of the ductal system, corresponding to the scheme reported in **a**. **c** Anatomic variant consisting of an isolated duct of Santorini, without communication with the main duct, with independent outlet in the minor papilla. **d** Anatomic variant consisting of duct of Santorini as an accessory branch of the main duct. **e** Anatomic variant without duct of Santorini. (*D*, duodenum; *GB*, gallbladder; *ST*, stomach)

modality provided with high spatial and contrast resolution which are further increased by the use of second generation contrast media. If correctly performed it is the best imaging modality to carry out most of the interventional procedures and can be effectively used intraoperatively, both for diagnostic and for therapeutic procedures, such as the recent radiofrequency ablation (RFA) applications. Unfortunately it is sometimes compromised by an excessive tympanites, overly thick subcutaneous fat, or by the alteration of anatomic planes, as occurs after surgery, inflammation or radiotherapy.

Unlike US, CT provides the best results in obese subjects, with abundant fat surrounding the various organs. The current multidetector technology, as well as improving the power of spatial resolution and shortening examination time, enables acquisition of volumetric data and direct image reconstruction in any spatial plane, thus removing the previous limitation of single detector machines. The procedure also includes the

mandatory use of ionizing radiation, of iodinated contrast media and it can be affected by poor contrast resolution making a reliable solid/liquid typing of small lesions difficult.

MRI offers good spatial and contrast resolution, the latter further increased by paramagnetic contrast media and can be used for biochemical evaluation (diffusion weighted sequences).

Particularly useful is magnetic resonance cholangiopancreatography (MRCP) which, thanks to specific sequences and special reconstruction algorithms, provides an excellent view of the pancreas ductal system and the adjacent biliary tree (Fig. 6.13b). This has significantly reduced the diagnostic use of endoscopic retrograde cholangiopancreatography (ERCP), avoiding the potential complications (acute pancreatitis). Unfortunately MRI is still strongly influenced by motion artifacts; moreover it cannot be performed in patients with pacemaker or suffering from claustrophobia (unless the examination is performed with the patient deeply sedated). Moreover, MRI does not allow the visualization of intraglandular and/or intraductal calcifications, which are instead clearly visible in both US and CT.

6.4 Pancreatic Imaging

The anatomic features of the pancreas set out above certainly represent a conditioning factor with regard to its imaging study, although in different ways among the various methods. The pancreas is tilted and curved in all the three planes of space which makes its overall representation difficult, regardless of the imaging modality used.

In axial planes it is easy to observe that the left side of the pancreas is located higher than the right (Fig. 6.2a), therefore appearing first in craniocaudal scans (Fig. 6.1d), while the right side, located below, appears at more caudal levels (Fig. 6.1c), often when the left side has already disappeared. This explains why in CT and MRI the entire gland does not appear in a single direct axial plane, so it may be necessary to resort to slightly oblique planes.

In coronal planes the central part of the pancreas is the most anterior, being pushed ventrally from the vertebral column and great vessels, abdominal aorta and inferior vena cava, while its two sides lie more posterior, especially the left side (Fig. 6.1a). Also in this case CT and MRI do not allow the gland to be displayed in its entirety in a single coronal plane (Fig. 6.2b,c). The best view of the gland – even partially– is achieved with oblique coronal planes (more back to the left), or better with curved coronal plane reconstructions anterior to the spine and the major abdominal vessels (Fig. 6.2d) [5, 6].

At US the coronal approach to the pancreas is affected by the considerable distance of the gland from the cutaneous plane; in fact the only part of the pancreas which is easily visible in the coronal plane is the tail, with coronal scans adjacent to the splenic hilum (Fig. 6.12a,c). In sagittal planes only a very small portion of the parenchyma is visualized, whereas the gland has a predominant cross development (Figs. 6.6, 6.7, 6.9).

At the level of the tail and the body the pancreas shows a very small sagittal section, with oval shape more extended in the craniocaudal and less represented in the anteroposterior direction.

At the level of the head the area displayed in the section is much greater and is bent backwards in its posterior and inferomedial part, where the uncinate process arises. This is a small offshoot, medially directed, between mesenteric vessels anteriorly and inferior vena cava posteriorly.

In practice these scanning planes are useful mainly in order to assess the relations of the gland with the large adjacent vessels (celiac axis, superior mesenteric vessels, portal vein, inferior vena cava and aorta).

6.4.1 Peripancreatic Gastrointestinal Structures

This certainly is the most unfavorable element for US imaging, because of the barrier effect caused by intestinal gas over the acoustic beam. In order to remedy this problem, the US examination of the pancreas is always performed after fasting (on an empty stomach and duodenum), preferably in the morning, when there is less stretching of the jejunal loops, thus avoiding the stagnation of gas and feces in the colon. When necessary, the operator should take advantage of the mobility of the intestinal structures located in front of the pancreas and seek to move them by changing the position and respiration of the patient. The left lobe of the liver, lowered in deep inspiration, can be used as an acoustic window, especially to study the body-tail region, in obese patients (Figs. 6.4d, 6.10).

In certain cases it is possible to use the stomach filled with water as an acoustic window, after an appropriate waiting period for degasing, particularly to study the body-tail region (Figs. 6.8b, 6.11b,d), combining this with standing or semi-erect position, although in practice this procedure is nowadays less applied, because of the poor and inconsistent results. In practice, if there are permanent technical limitations to the US investigation, it is better to use different imaging methods.

CT and MRI themselves are limited by the proximity of the duodenal C-loop and stomach, due to both density values being almost superimposable and the motion artifacts that these structures may cause. In practice these limitations can be overcome by relaxation of these intestinal structures, with water or better still with ionic or paramagnetic contrast agents, depending on the method.

6.4.2 Peripancreatic Vascular Structures

The vascular structures are extensively prepared to wrap the entire pancreatic gland, from which they can be distinguished through their enhancement, however obtained (with iodinated contrast medium in CT, with paramagnetic contrast medium in MRI). In this setting

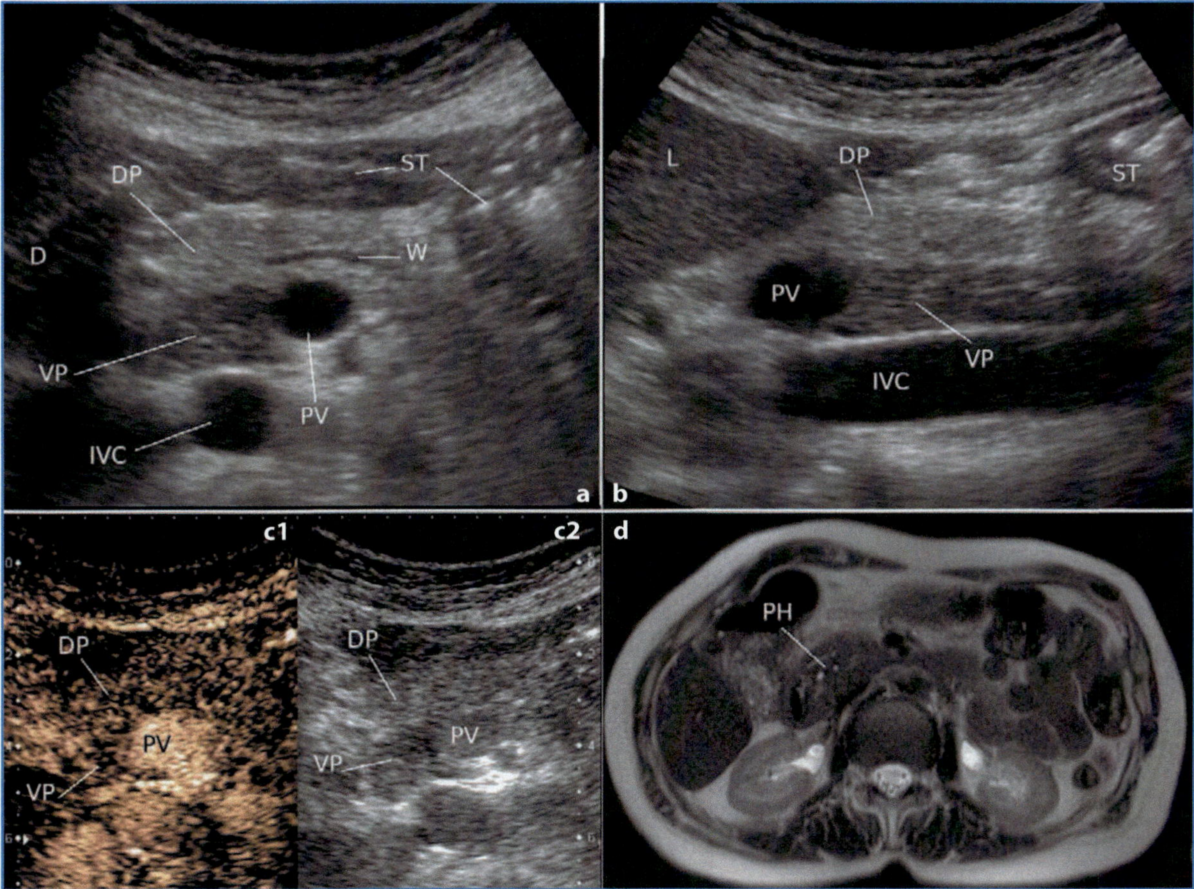

Fig. 6.14 a-d Artifact of the pancreatic head resembling a pseudolesion: different echogenicity of the ventral and dorsal pancreas. **a,b** US scans in the axial (**a**) and sagittal (**b**) planes passing through the pancreatic head. A hypoechoic area with sharp borders in the ventral pancreas (*VP*) compared to the dorsal pancreas (*DP*); a slight dilation of the duct of Wirsung (*W*) can also be seen. **c** Contrast enhanced US (CEUS) of the pancreatic head (**c1** venous contrast enhanced phase compared with **c2** matching image without contrast medium). The pseudolesion of the pancreatic head shows similar enhancement to the contiguous normal gland, thus excluding neoplastic origin. **d** MRI with contrast medium: axial scan. Normal pancreatic head (*PH*), without any focal mass. (*D*, duodenum; *IVC*, inferior vena cava; *L*, liver; *PV*, portal vein; *ST*, stomach)

US has the advantage of a possible immediate appeal to the broad Doppler applications (color Doppler, pulsed and power Doppler) (Fig. 6.12d), increasingly sophisticated and able to meet each specific need, or related to the recent use of US contrast agents, coupled with electronic subtraction algorithms, able to selectively enhance the circulation districts reached by the contrast agent (Fig. 6.14c).

6.4.3 Ductal System

Because of the small diameter of the ducts the pancreas ductal system cannot be visualized under normal conditions, especially at CT without contrast agent. In this sense US is less influenced, thanks to its high contrast resolution, which is easily able to differentiate solid/liquid between parenchyma and ductal content and to directly visualize the normal duct wall. US instead suffers from the angle of incidence of the US beam related to the ductal walls, whereas the perpendicular incidence allows the best visualization of the main pancreatic duct, as for the body, while a more oblique incidence determines a lower reflection of the US beam and a worse view of the ducts, as happens for the head and the tail (Figs. 6.4a,b, 6.5c, 6.8c, 6.10c, 6.11c,d, 6.16c,d). In order to improve the visualization of the ductal system other means are required.

The temporary pharmacologic dilatation of the ductal

system by the intravenous infusion of secretin, a hormone that increases glandular secretion and Oddi sphincter tone at the same time, causes its temporary overdistension and is a good way of obtaining an enhancement of the pancreatic excretory system for some time [5-7]. This technique, especially used in the past in US, CT and MRI, but almost abandoned partly due to the associated high costs, had the purpose of obtaining functional information about the secretory activity of the gland, since the appearance of a good glandular dilatation was a good sign of effective secretory response. In contrast, a lack of change compared to the measured caliber at rest was indicative of a reduced secretory response, generally indicative of the fibrous replacement of the glandular component, as occurs in chronic pancreatitis.

The artificial increase in contrast between gland and ducts is the second option pursued to improve the visualization of the ductal system. This technique is most useful in CT (more than any other technique characterized by low contrast resolution), whereby the intravenous infusion of iodinated contrast agent tends to increase the density values of glandular component (highly vascular), while leaving the low density values of the ducts filled with pancreatic juice unchanged. The US technique uses the same trick, not only to better highlight the ductal system, but also to emphasize intraglandular cysts, which being filled with fluid particles are difficult to assess. In addition it is more able to differentiate intraductal or intracystic vegetating lesions from simple debris, since the microcirculation of the former takes up the US contrast medium and thus enhances their echogenicity, while with debris and corpuscular content there is no contrast medium uptake, and they become anechoic with subtraction algorithms and remain so throughout the entire examination.

The use of specific cholangiographic sequences (CWMR) is able to highlight with very strong signal the structures containing non-moving liquid, present in a given volume, almost totally erasing the surrounding anatomic structures (Fig. 6.16b). These applications which as stated above have largely limited the diagnostic indications of the ERCP, both on the biliary and pancreatic side, have at the pancreatic level the advantage of matching the image of the duct, i.e. the *content*, with the *container*, that is the gland surrounding it, allowing the direct assessment of masses and their obstructive/infiltrative effect on the excretory system. It also should be noted that the CWMR has brought to the attention of pancreas experts a world previously almost unknown and the exclusive prerogative of the ERCP world, the world of intraductal tumors [8, 9].

6.5   Ultrasound Pancreatic Anatomy

The pancreas is generally well detected by US, despite the above mentioned constraints, related to both the gland position and patient constitution. Under normal conditions the pancreas shows regular and homogeneous echogenicity, usually equal to or slightly greater than in the liver (Fig. 6.4a-c). Changes in echogenicity, such as its increase in obese, diabetic and dyslipidemic patient are common, in analogy and combination with what happens in the liver (Fig. 6.4d).

Its volume is also subject to discrete changes related to both age and trophism, with a generally more bulky pancreas in the obese and endomorph patient compared to the ectomorph patient.

Each glandular area is usually studied with a specific US approach. The pancreatic head is bordered on three sides by the duodenal C-loop, name derived from the fact that the duodenum embraces the pancreatic head in the shape of the letter C (Fig. 6.2a). At US the duodenal C-loop may appear distended by gas or liquid or contracted, depending on its content. In the first case it gives the typical hyperechoic reverberation artifact (Figs. 6.5d, 6.6d), while in the latter it has an anechoic corpuscular component, constantly stirred by peristalsis (Fig. 6.14a). The normal appearance is usually given by the peristaltic alternation of the two phases, a finding which is even more definite when the stomach is filled with water.

The cranial surface of the head is bounded by the duodenal bulb, with close but not tight contact, considering that the duodenal bulb, unlike the pancreas, is almost completely enveloped by the peritoneum. The gastroduodenal artery, the first branch of the division of the common hepatic artery, runs in the space between the bulb and the pancreas, descending on the anterior side of the head (Fig. 6.5a-c, 6.6a,c); duodenum and pancreas adhere further the passage of this vessel.

The lateral surface of the head is closely related to the second duodenal part, into which both the two main pancreatic ducts (of Wirsung and Santorini, through the papilla major and minor respectively) and the bile duct flow, the latter usually with the duct of Wirsung (Fig. 6.13).

Due to the special anatomic and functional complexity this area has been given the name of pancreatic *groove*. It corresponds to the duodenal-pancreatic close board, from the knee above to the third duodenal portion, and also includes the common bile duct and the papilla. It is a common site for the spread of disease processes, starting from the duodenum-bile duct-papillar area to the pancreas (cystic duodenal dystrophy, common bile-duct tumors and inflammations, papillitis, etc.) and the other way round (groove pancreatitis, annular pancreas with duodenal stenosis, aberrant pancreas, etc.) [5, 10].

The lower side of the head is surrounded by the third part of the duodenum. In this area the pancreas, from the outside to the middle, gradually begins to lose the close contact with the duodenum.

The medial surface of the pancreatic head is related to the right edge of the superior mesenteric vein below and the border of the portal vein above, which runs in a retropancreatic course (Figs. 6.5, 6.7). This vascular limit is very well recognized on US, constituting one of the fundamental sonographic landmarks. On the posteromedial surface of the pancreatic head there is the uncinate process, a small glandular appendix that lies between the inferior vena cava and the superior mesenteric vein ending in contact with the superior mesenteric artery (Fig. 6.5c,d).

The back side is separated from the inferior vena cava only by two thin sheets adhering to each other (the fibrous lamina of Treitz), the embryonic remains of two peritoneal layers of the primitive mesogastrium (Fig. 6.6d). These two peritoneal layers, covered with connective tissue are easily separable and this feature is very successfully used in radical surgery to obtain the mobilization of the duodenal-pancreatic block and its forward tipping, known as the *Kocker maneuver*. The free portion of the bile duct runs on the posterior surface of the head, becoming then intrapancreatic, before piercing the second part of the duodenum (Fig. 6.6b).

The anterior surface of the pancreatic head is covered by the posterior parietal peritoneum (Fig 6.1a), whose double reflection forms the transversal mesocolon (Fig. 6.3a). It should be recalled that this structure can easily be a medium for the spread of inflammatory or neoplastic processes [11].

These bands generally are not visible on US because of little or no difference in echogenicity between them and the surrounding fat, although they are usually observable on CT and MRI [2].

The pancreatic isthmus is very short (1 cm) and corresponds to the width of the mesenteric-portal axis, which runs downwards and backwards with its conflu-

ence also including the splenic vein coming from the left (Fig. 6.7). Its limitations with the head and the body are fictitious.

The pancreatic body originates at the medial side of the splenoportal axis and it has not a clear limit with the tail (Figs. 6.8, 6.9).

The cranial surface is crossed at the middle third by the celiac axis, from which arises the splenic artery to the left, the common hepatic artery to the right and the left gastric artery above (Figs. 6.8a,b, 6.9).

The lower side is perpendicularly crossed at the middle by the superior mesenteric artery (Figs. 6.8a,d, 6.9). Longitudinally to the axis of the body also runs the left renal vein, which empties into the inferior vena cava after its course between the aorta posteriorly and the superior mesenteric artery anteriorly (aortomesenteric compass) (Figs. 6.8a,d, 6.9). It is in contact with the duodenojejunal angle of Treitz, constituting, with the superior mesenteric artery, the root of the mesentery, directed downward and to the left.

The posterior surface transversally crosses the aorta, from which it is separated by the lamina of Treitz. It is accompanied by the splenic vein, which runs longitudinally to its major axis, towards the mesenteric-portal confluence (Figs. 6.8, 6.9).

The front side is in contact with the rear wall of the stomach, by the interposition of the omental bursa (Figs. 6.1, 6.2, 6.8-6.10). Below the stomach lies the transverse colon, whose listing on the posterior abdominal wall is just above the angle of Treitz, at the anteroinferior margin of the pancreatic body [12].

The pancreatic tail extends laterally and cranially almost up to the splenic hilum, receiving a small part of the peritoneal lining. It lies behind the gastric fundus and splenic flexure of the colon which under normal conditions hinder the anterior US approach. It also lies very close to the adrenal gland and the upper pole of the left kidney (Figs. 6.1, 6.2, 6.11, 6.12).

The ductal system of the pancreas normally consists of the main duct of Wirsung, with a relatively large gauge (2–3mm) which increases towards the head and extends the entire length of the gland, and the accessory duct of Santorini, usually limited to the cephalic portion and more cranial than the Wirsung (Fig. 6.13).

The duct of Wirsung pierces the duodenum at the level of the papilla major, together with the common bile duct, gathering just before its end a small accessory branch from the uncinate process.

The duct of Santorini instead leads to the papilla

minor level, whose duodenal orifice is located approximately 2–3 cm above the previous one. The two ducts are generally in communication with each other, but the possible anatomic variations are numerous and frequent, such as lack of communication, agenesis and role reversal with the dominance of the Santorini (pancreas divisum) (Figs. 6.13c-e, 6.16) [13, 14].

A small interlobular ductal network (of second order) is a tributary of this ductal system. The Wirsung is generally viewable on US at the level of the head and body, both due to the larger caliber and the most favorable projective incidence, since its walls lie perpendicular to the US beam (Figs. 6.4b, 6.5c).

The Santorini is normally recognizable only in special conditions or when highly developed (Fig. 6.16). The other ducts, although not in ordinary conditions, may become visible when involved in intraductal cystic disease (IPMN).

6.6 Pancreatic Embryology and Anatomic Variants

A basic understanding of the embryologic development of the pancreas is essential for identifying the anatomic variants and developmental anomalies described below.

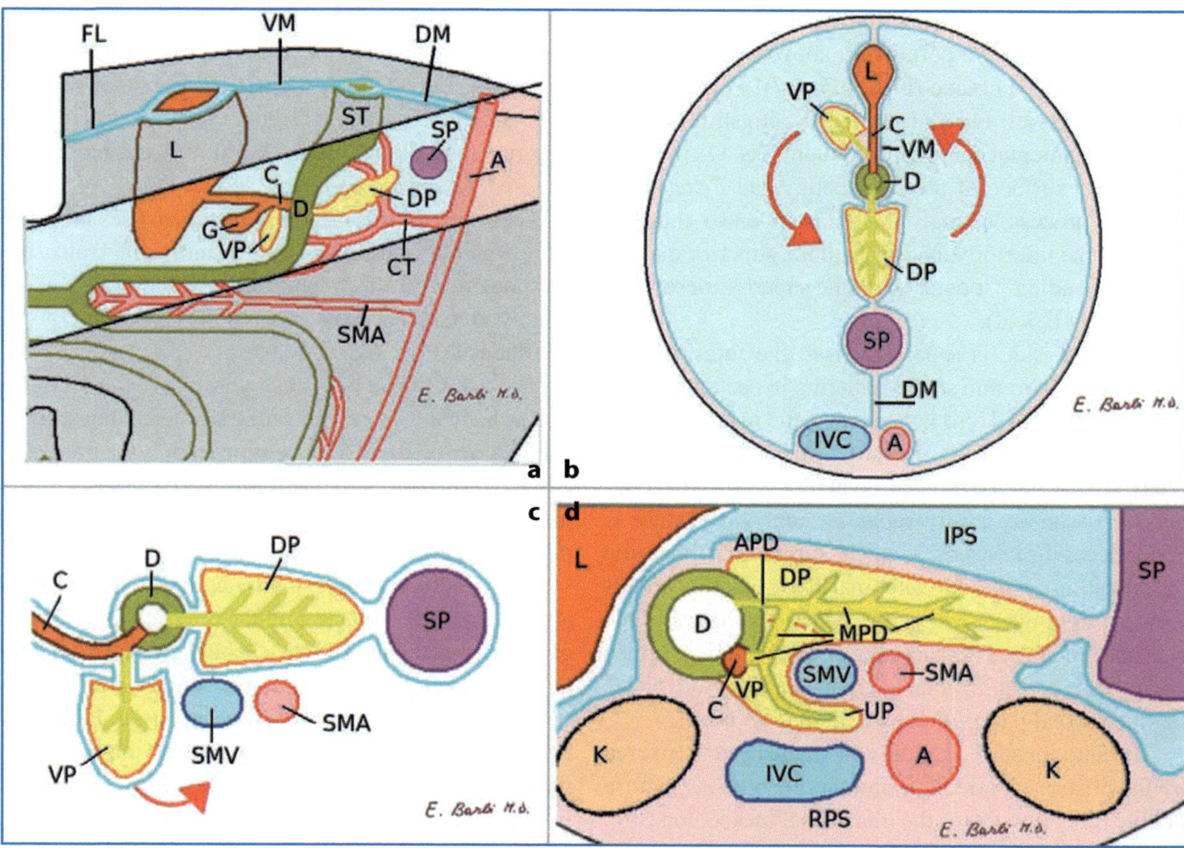

Fig. 6.15 a-d Embryologic development of the pancreas. **a,b** Anatomic pattern of the pancreatic-biliary-duodenal district in a five-week-old embryo: (**a**) sagittal plane; (**b**) axial plane, corresponding to the section shown in **a**. The dorsal pancreas (*DP*) is located on the midline, at the back of the duodenum (*D*), contained in the dorsal mesogastrium (*DM*) with the spleen (*SP*); the ventral pancreas (*VP*) is located on the midline, in front of the duodenum (*D*), contained in the ventral mesogastrium (*VM*) with the gallbladder (*G*) and the main bile duct. **c,d** In the following weeks the dorsal pancreas rotates 90° moving to the left with the spleen. At the same time the ventral pancreas rotates 270° around the duodenum first on the right, than backwards and finally leftwards, in the end being placed below and behind the dorsal bud and finally merging together. A part of the ventral bud forms the uncinate process (*UP*) which embraces the superior mesenteric vein (*SMV*) from behind. The ducts of the two pancreatic buds join together and that of the ventral pancreas (Wirsung) becomes dominant (*MPD*) in respect to the duct of Santorini (*APD*). The main bile duct (*C*) follows the ventral pancreas during its rotation around the duodenum. (*A*, aorta; *CT*, celiac trunk; *FL*, falciform ligament; *IPS*, intraperitoneal space; *IVC*, inferior vena cava; *K*, kidney; *L*, liver; *RPS*, retroperitoneal space; *SMA*, superior mesenteric artery; *ST*, stomach)

6.6.1   Embryologic Development

The pancreas originates from two distinct buds arising from the primitive intestine, called respectively ventral pancreas and dorsal pancreas, located on opposite sides of the duodenum (Fig. 6.15).

The dorsal pancreas develops earlier (4th week of embryonic life), is more cranially located and reaches a discrete size. It is initially located on the posterior side of the duodenum (hence its name). During development the rotation process of the digestive tract takes it side-ways and to the left, placing it behind the stomach [3, 15]. Its relations with the spleen are very close, since they develop in the same structure (dorsal mesogastrium) (Fig. 6.15). It has its own very long excretory duct, precursor of the Santorini duct, flowing into the duodenum, through what will then become the papilla minor.

The ventral pancreas starts to develop later. It is located further down and is smaller than the dorsal pancreas. Initially it is ventrally located compared to the duodenum, in a mirror position in respect to the dorsal pancreas. During its development the ventral pancreas

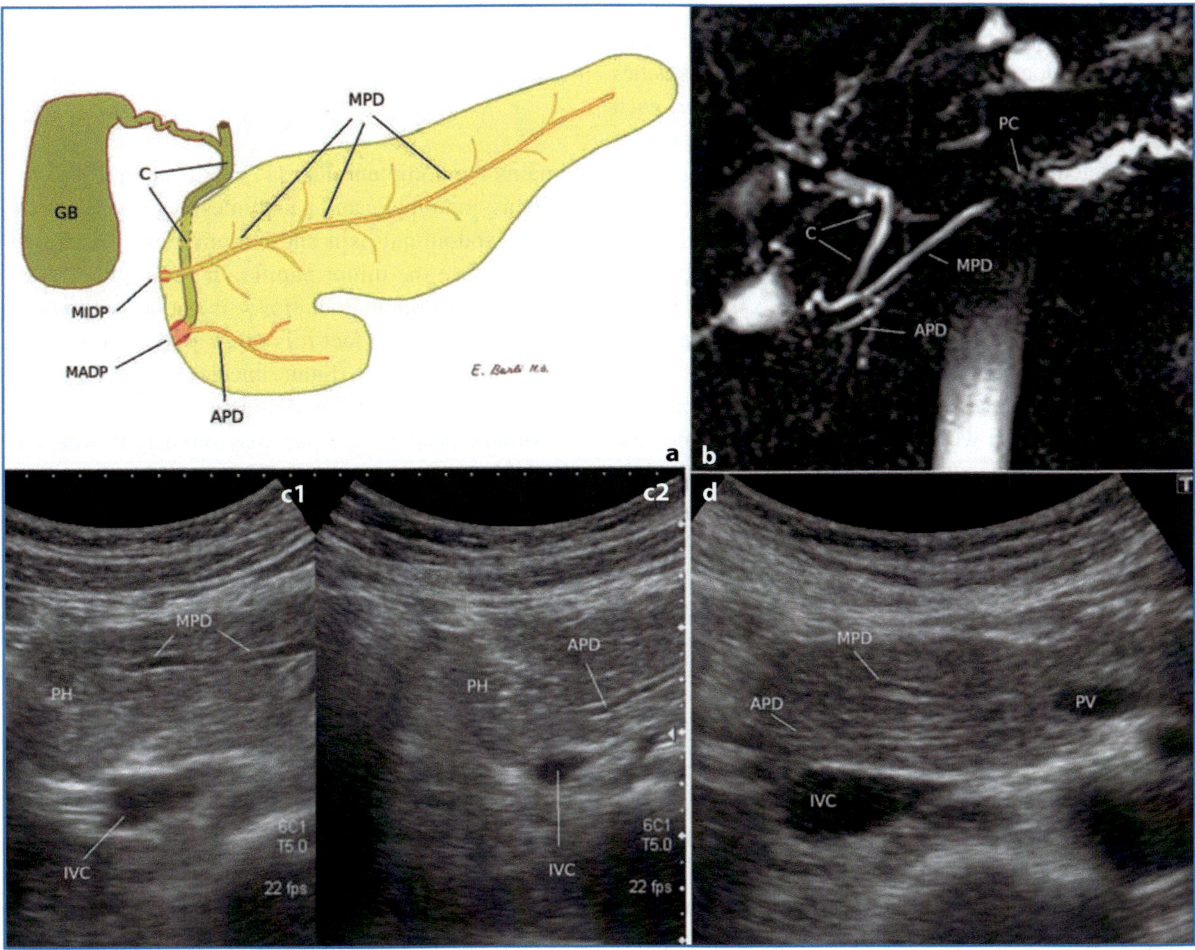

Fig. 6.16 a-d Pancreas divisum. **a** Anatomic features. The persistence of a main duct (*MPD*) in continuity with Santorini's duct which flows into the duodenum through the minor papilla (*MIDP*) is due to the lack of fusion between the two pancreatic ducts. The duct of Wirsung remains a short accessory duct (*APD*) which flows into the duodenum together with the main bile duct (*C*) through the major papilla (*MADP*). **b** MRCP of pancreas divisum. Both ducts are recognizable, the more caudal one appearing thin and short and the more cranial one longer and larger in diameter. A focal stricture at the body is documented with an upstream dilation of the main duct owing to a small pancreatic cancer (*PC*). **c** US in the axial plane at the level of the pancreatic head (*PH*). Both ducts are independently identifiable, with the duct of Santorini (*MPD*) more superficial (**c1**) and the duct of Wirsung (*APD*) deeper (**c2**). **d** US in the axial plane at the level of the pancreatic head. Both ducts are visualized in the same scan. (*GB*, gallbladder; *IVC*, inferior vena cava; *PV*, portal vein)

is subject to a rotation of 270° around the vertical axis of the digestive tract, which moves it first to the right, then posteriorly and finally to the left, to be finally placed immediately below the dorsal pancreas (Fig. 6.15) [3, 15]. It has a slightly squat shape, less stretched, with a short excretory duct, the future Wirsung duct, which flows into the duodenum through what will become the major papilla. Since it originates from the same cell group forming the main biliary tree (hepatopancreatic ring), the excretory duct of the ventral pancreas is closely linked to the common bile duct, sharing with it not only the common duodenal mouth in the papilla major but also the Oddi sphincter complex.

Regarding the fusion of the two pancreatic buds, once the rotation is completed, the two pancreas sketches are very close but still distinct from each other, each with its own excretory duct. The development process is completed with the merger of the two glandular buds into a single structure, in which the dorsal outline forms the top of the head, the isthmus, the body and the tail, while the bottom of the head and the uncinate process originate from the ventral outline (Fig. 6.15d) [3, 15]. Also the two excretory ducts join together, not far from their mouth into the duodenum, taking a horizontal "Y" aspect on the whole. The duct of the ventral portion, which was shorter, with its development becomes the dominant one, both in terms of length and caliber, while the distal portion of the dorsal excretory duct becomes progressively thinner, becoming the accessory duct, sometimes losing the connection with the main duct, other times losing the duodenal outlet in the papilla minor (Fig. 6.13) [16].

6.6.2 Anatomic Variants

Anomalies of the pancreas can be distinguished in anomalies of fusion (pancreas divisum, complete or incomplete), migration (annular pancreas and ectopic pancreas) and duplication (number and shape) [13].

Pancreas divisum is the most common anomaly of the pancreas, being reported in 4%-10% of the population (Fig. 6.16) [5-7, 13-16]. This anomaly consists of lack of fusion of the ventral and dorsal embryonic buds. In this way the duct of Wirsung results very thin and short, draining only the lower part of the pancreatic head. In contrast, the duct of Santorini remains long, dominant in size, with no communication with the Wirsung. In the incomplete forms a communication between the two ducts exists, although the Santorini

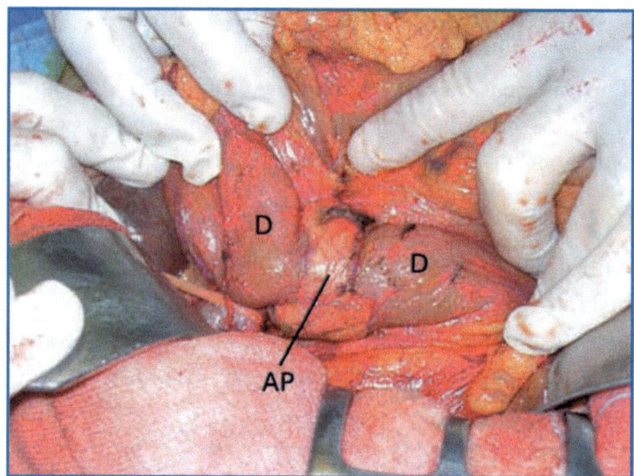

Fig. 6.17 Annular pancreas (*AP*) in adulthood. (*D*, duodenum)

remains the dominant duct [17]. This anomaly is generally asymptomatic and sometimes associated with recurrent abdominal pain and chronic pancreatitis, perhaps because the minor papilla, in which most of the produced pancreatic juice flows, is not large enough to support this role; in fact it is often associated with the onset of ductal ectasia (Santorinicele) [7, 16]. Diagnosis is based on ERCP or CWMR [18].

Annular pancreas is a pancreas anomaly in which the gland forms a stenotic ring surrounding the second part of the duodenum, resulting in its occlusion (Figs. 6.17, 6.18). In half of the cases it presents as a duodenal occlusion at birth, often associated with other intestinal malformations. In the other cases it may persist into adulthood, presenting with nonspecific digestive disorders, acute or chronic pancreatitis (15%-20%) (Figs. 6.17, 6.18). Also in this case the diagnosis is based on the appearance of the excretory ducts, displayed by ERCP or CWMR, which appear surrounding the duodenal lumen [13, 16, 17, 19].

Ectopic pancreas is relatively common (0.6%-14%), although often it is diagnosed not by imaging but suspected by endoscopy or in surgery and histologically confirmed (Fig. 6.19b). It consists of the presence of extrapancreatic glandular islets (0.5cm-2cm), which can be localized within the wall of the stomach (26%-38%), duodenum (28%-36%), jejunum (16%), ileum or Meckel diverticulum. More rarely it affects the colon, esophagus, gallbladder, biliary tract, liver, gut, mesentery, etc. It is usually small (0.5cm-2cm), localized in the submucosa, generally asymptomatic and when clinically evident this is because of its complications (stenosis, ulcers, bleeding, intussusception, etc.) [16, 20].

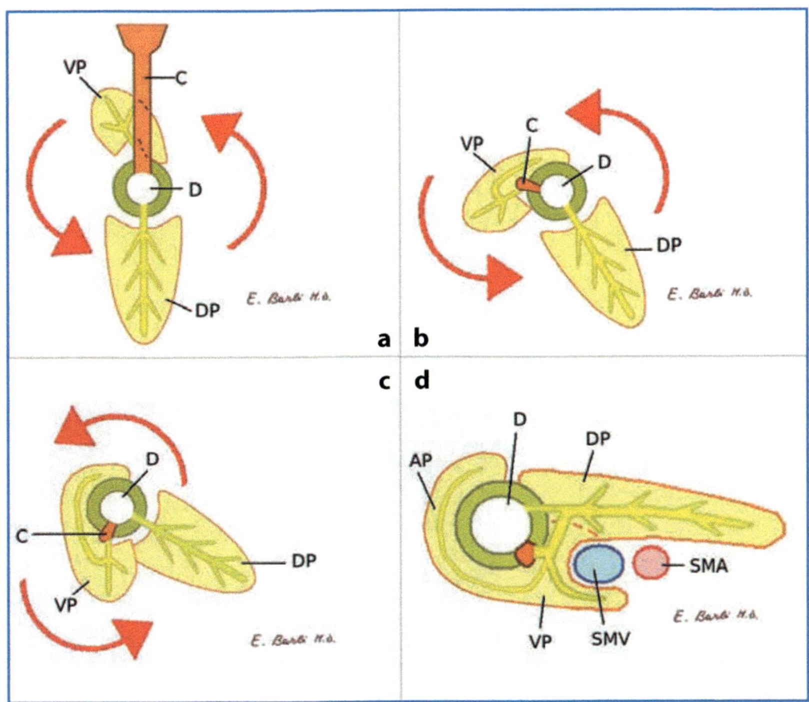

Fig. 6.18 a-d Embryologic hypothesis on the development of annular pancreas. A portion of the ventral pancreas (*VP*), instead of rotating 270° as described in Fig. 14a-d from its original anterior position (**a**) to the final one below and behind the dorsal bud (*DP*) (**d**), is thought to be anchored on the front side. This is thought to generate a pancreatic ring (*AP*) completely or incompletely surrounding the duodenal C-loop (*D*), sometimes causing a stenosis of the lumen as in early post-natal cases. **b,c** Intermediate stages of the rotation process of the ventral bud from the initial front position (**a**) to the left rear final site (**d**). (*C*, main bile duct (choledochus); *SMA*, superior mesenteric artery; *SMV*, superior mesenteric vein)

Agenesis of the dorsal pancreas is a rare malformation consisting of the absence of the glandular part derived from the dorsal bud, intended to form the most cranial part of the head and the body-tail. Therefore just a small gland forming the bottom of the head and the uncinate process is present (Fig. 6.19a) [15, 21]. It is usually associated with other malformations such as asplenia (spleen agenesis), polysplenia (many accessory spleens) and heterotaxy (situs ambiguus), i.e. the anomalous position of some organs. The associated cardiovascular anomalies are frequent [22, 23]. The suspicion of a pancreatic malformation, supposed on the basis of morphologic imaging techniques, should always be confirmed by ERCP or CWMR in order to directly visualize the excretory system anatomy and to exclude any sectorial atrophy, secondary to malignant obstructive disease [15, 21].

Truncated pancreas is similar to the previous malformation but with agenesis only of the body-tail (or just tail), and spleen [24, 25].

Reversed pancreas is present in the complete forms of situs viscerum inversus, in which all the abdominal organs are mirrored from their normal position: the pancreatic head located to the left (together with liver, biliary tree and duodenum), while the pancreatic tail to the right (together with the spleen) [25, 26].

Folded pancreas is another rare congenital anomaly,

described in association with heterotaxy. The entire pancreas is located to the left of the midline and bent onto itself at the level of the isthmus: it has been described in association with intestinal malrotation [25, 27].

The ductal system is often affected by minor anomalies, taking into account that the classic anatomic configuration, with bifid appearance of the Wirsung and the Santorini, is seen in 60% of cases [16]. In the other cases the duct of Santorini can be rudimentary or missing (25%-30%), dominant (1%) or *bend-shaped*, with a curving course embracing the duct of Wirsung [13]. More potential variants are the bifid duct, at the caudal level, or the leap of caliber at the junction of Wirsung with Santorini and uniform narrowing of the duct at the body-tail level. All these anomalies are well visualized with CWMR, as well as ERCP.

The biliary-pancreatic outlet is a frequent location of minor anatomic variants (1.5%-3%), the most important of which is the high merger of the common bile duct with the Wirsung, out of the duodenum, resulting in the formation of a common duct, even more than 1.5 cm long. In these cases idiopathic ectasia of the bile duct is common (33%-83%), possibly due to reflux disease and associated with increased incidence of biliary tumors. Once again these anomalies are well visualized by CWMR and ERCP [5, 16].

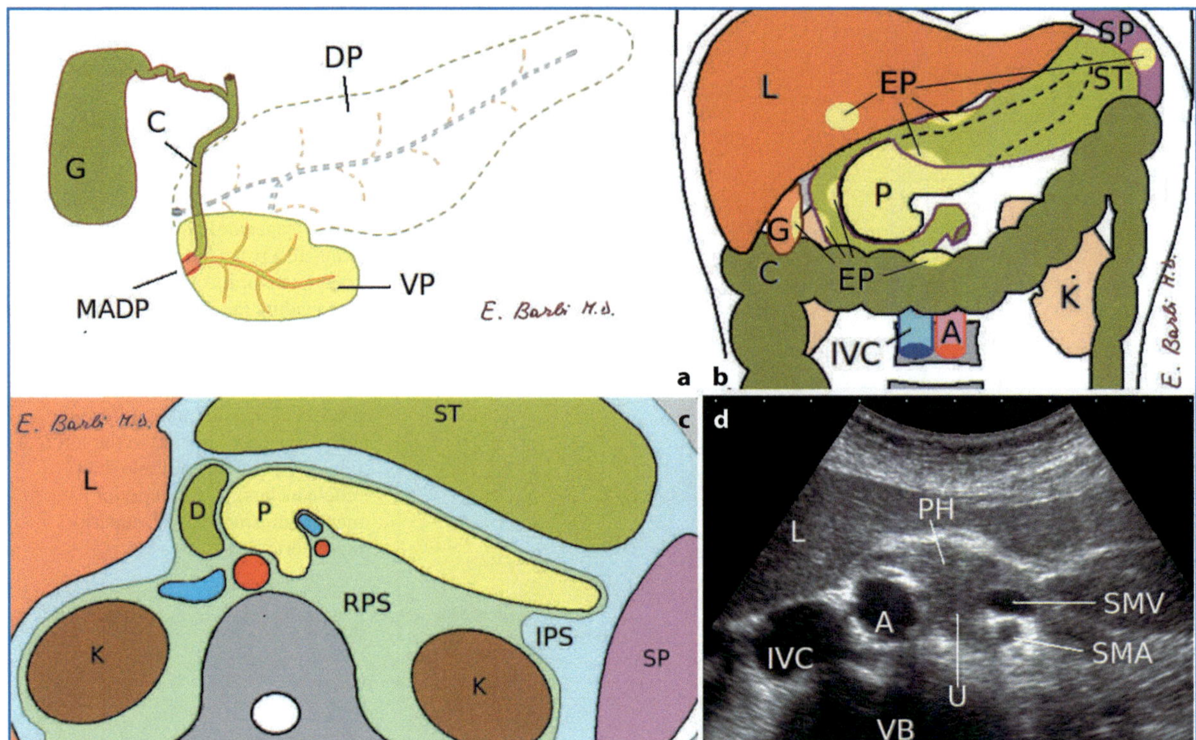

Fig. 6.19 a-d Malformations and anatomic variants of the pancreas. **a** Agenesis of the dorsal pancreas (*DP*), with development of the glandular component arising solely from the ventral bud (*VP*), consisting of the lower portion of the head and the uncinate process. **b** Ectopic pancreas: in addition to the normally located gland (*P*), one or more islets of pancreatic tissue (*EP, yellow*) can be present in ectopic location (stomach, duodenum, colon, gallbladder and bile ducts, liver, etc.). The islets of ectopic tissue are generally localized in the submucosa and show an excretory duct which empties the pancreatic juice into the intestinal lumen. **c,d** Left sided pancreas: anatomic features (**c**) and the US axial scan (**d**). The pancreas is supported by the aorta (*A*) shifted to the right with the inferior vena cava (*IVC*) so that the pancreatic head (*PH*) is moved in an anomalous position, to the left of the aorta rather than in front of the inferior vena cava. The uncinate process (*U*) is displaced between the aorta and the superior mesenteric vein (*SMV*) instead of between the inferior vena cava and the superior mesenteric vein. (*C*, main bile duct (choledochus); *D*, duodenum; *G*, gallbladder; *IPS*, intraperitoneal space; *K*, kidney; *L*, liver; *MADP*, main duodenal papilla; *RPS*, retroperitoneal space; *SMA*, superior mesenteric artery; *SP*, spleen; *ST*, stomach; *VB*, vertebral body)

6.7 Pancreatic Pseudolesions

Pseudolesions of the pancreas may result from changes in the volume and/or in the echogenicity of the gland. Reduction of the pancreatic volume is not necessarily a pathologic finding; in fact after forty years of age the gland starts a process of physiologic senile involution, with a progressive decrease in its thickness. Between fifty and sixty years of age the anteroposterior diameter of the head decreases from 3.5cm of the prosperous period of the young adult to 2.5cm; similarly the thickness of the body and the tail changes from about 2 cm to 1.5cm [16]. The widespread increase of pancreatic volume is not necessarily an expression of a disease, but it can often be observed in the overweight patient, in association with hepatosplenomegaly, as already mentioned (Fig. 6.4d).

Pancreatic echogenicity is considered normal if comparable or slightly higher than that of normal healthy liver. However this reference frequently fails because the liver could present increased echogenicity (steatosis), while the pancreas remains normal and thus less echogenic, or because the pancreas, together with the liver, increases its echogenicity because of fatty infiltration, as is often observed in the obese, in diabetics, in dysmetabolic patients, in cystic fibrosis, etc. (Fig. 6.4d).

Pancreatic pseudomasses may be frequently due to focal echogenicity alterations of the gland. Typical and quite common is the pseudomass of the head-uncinate process, actually supported by the lower echogenicity of the ventral pancreas compared to the dorsal pancreas, which is probably due to the different distribution of the local vasculature, similarly to what is frequently observed in typical areas of fatty liver, such as the peri-gallbladder and perihilar regions (Fig. 6.14) [5]. A further pitfall is the presence of pancreatic lobules with 1cm of diameter that can alter the profile of the gland simulating neoplastic nodules.

References

1. Gore RM, Balfe DM, Aizenstein RI, Silverman PM (2000) The great escape: interfascial decompression planes of the retroperitoneum. Am J Roentgenol 175:363-370
2. Korobkin M, Silverman PM, Quint LE, Francis IR (1992) CT of the extraperitoneal space: normal anatomy and fluid collections. Am J Roentgenol 159:933-941
3. Vikram R, Balachandran A, Bhosale PR et al (2009) Pancreas: peritoneal reflections, ligamentous connections, and pathways of disease spread. Radiographics 29:e34
4. Bertelli E, Bendayan M (2005) Association between endocrine pancreas and ductal system. More than an epiphenomenon of endocrine differentiation and development? J Histochem Cytochem 53:1071-1086
5. Hakimé A, Giraud M, Vullierme MP, Vilgrain V (2007) MR imaging of the pancreas. J Radiol 88:11-25
6. Kim HC, Yang DM, Jin W et al (2007) Multiplanar reformations and minimum intensity projections using multi-detector row CT for assessing anomalies and disorders of the pancreaticobiliary tree. World J Gastroenterol 13:4177-4184
7. Manfredi R, Costamagna G, Brizi MG et al (2000) Pancreas divisum and "santorinicele": diagnosis with dynamic MR cholangiopancreatography with secretin stimulation. Radiology 217:403-408
8. Peters HE, Vitellas KM (2001) Magnetic resonance cholangiopancreatography (MRCP) of intraductal papillary-mucinous neoplasm (IPMN) of the pancreas: case report. Magn Reson Imaging 19:1139-1143
9. Tollefson MK, Libsch KD, Sarr MG et al (2003) Intraductal papillary mucinous neoplasm: did it exist prior to 1980? Pancreas 26:e55-e58
10. Yu J, Fulcher AS, Turner MA, Halvorsen RA (2004) Normal anatomy and disease processes of the pancreatoduodenal groove: imaging features. Am J Roentgenol 183:839-846
11. Charnsangavej C, Dubrow RA, Varma DG (1993) CT of the mesocolon. Part 2. Pathologic considerations. Radiographics 13:1309-1322
12. Charnsangavej C, DuBrow RA, Varma DG et al (1993) CT of the mesocolon. Part 1. Anatomic considerations. Radiographics 13:1035-1045
13. Bang S, Suh JH, Park BK et al (2006) The relationship of anatomic variation of pancreatic ductal system and pancreaticobiliary diseases. Yonsei Med J 47:243-248
14. Yu J, Turner MA, Fulcher AS, Halvorsen RA (2006) Congenital anomalies and normal variants of the pancreaticobiliary tract and the pancreas in adults: part 2, Pancreatic duct and pancreas. Am J Roentgenol 187:1544-1553
15. Balakrishnan V, Narayanan VA, Siyad I et al (2006) Agenesis of the dorsal pancreas with chronic calcific pancreatitis. case report, review of the literature and genetic basis. JOP. J Pancreas (Online) 7:651-659
16. Mortelé KJ, Rocha TC, Streeter JL, Taylor AJ (2006) Multimodality imaging of pancreatic and biliary congenital anomalies. Radiographics 26:715-731
17. Rizzo RJ, Szucs RA, Turner MA (1995) Congenital abnormalities of the pancreas and biliary tree in adults. Radiographics 15:49-68; quiz 147-148
18. Shanbhogue AK, Fasih N, Surabhi VR et al (2009) A clinical and radiologic review of uncommon types and causes of pancreatitis. Radiographics 29:1003-1026
19. Fu PF, Yu JR, Liu XS et al (2005) Symptomatic adult annular pancreas: report of two cases and a review of the literature. Hepatobiliary Pancreat Dis Int 4:468-471
20. Jovanovic I, Knezevic S, Micev M, Krstic M (2004) EUS mini probes in diagnosis of cystic dystrophy of duodenal wall in heterotopic pancreas: a case report. World J Gastroenterol 10:2609-2612
21. Joo YE, Kang HC, Kim HS et al (2006) Agenesis of the dorsal pancreas: a case report and review of the literature. Korean J Intern Med 21:236-239
22. Kapa S, Gleeson FC, Vege SS (2007) Dorsal pancreas agenesis and polysplenia/heterotaxy syndrome: a novel association with aortic coarctation and a review of the literature. JOP 8:433-437
23. Varga I, Galfiova P, Adamkov M et al (2009) Congenital anomalies of the spleen from an embryological point of view. Med Sci Monit 15:RA269-RA276
24. Fulcher A, Tumer M (2002) Abdominal manifestations of situs anomalies in adults. Radiographics 22:1439-1456
25. Onder A, Okur N, Bülbülo□lu E, Yüzba□io□lu MF (2009) Cecal volvulus in situs inversus totalis accompanied with pancreatic malrotation. Diagn Interv Radiol 15:188-192
26. Sceusi EL, Wray CJ (2009) Pancreatic adenocarcinoma in a patient with situs inversus: a case report of this rare coincidence. World J Surg Oncol 7:98
27. Yu J, Turner MA, Fulcher AS, Halvorsen RA (2006) Congenital anomalies and normal variants of the pancreaticobiliary tract and the pancreas in adults: part 1, Biliary tract. Am J Roentgenol 187:1536-1543

Steffen Rickes and Holger Neye

7.1 Introduction

Ultrasonography (US) is a noninvasive imaging modality which is often the first imaging technique in the evaluation of patients with pancreatic diseases. It has undergone significant advances in recent years. In this chapter the value of US in the diagnosis of pancreatitis and pseudocysts will be described and discussed. The article is focused on B-mode US, Doppler sonography and contrast-enhanced ultrasound (CEUS).

7.2 Acute Pancreatitis

Acute pancreatitis is a common disease that affects about 300,000 patients per year in America with a mortality of about 7% [1]. The diagnosis is based on clinical and laboratory evaluation. The clinical course of acute pancreatitis varies from a mild transitory form to a severe necrotizing disease. Most episodes of acute pancreatitis are mild and self-limiting. Patients with mild pancreatitis respond well to medical treatment, requiring little more than intravenous fluid resuscitation and analgesia. In contrast, severe pancreatitis is defined as pancreatitis associated with organ failure and/or local complications such as necrosis, abscess formation, or pseudocysts. Severe pancreatitis can be observed in about 20% of all cases, and requires intensive care and sometimes surgical or radiologic intervention. Early

correct assessment of the etiology and the severity of acute pancreatitis allows distinct therapeutic algorithms and can result in better outcome [1]. Advances in imaging modalities have revolutionized the management of patients with acute pancreatitis over the past decade.

Contrast enhanced computed tomography (CT) is the criterion standard for diagnosing pancreatic necrosis and peripancreatic collections, as well as for grading acute pancreatitis by the Balthazar system [2]. In recent years the Balthazar grading system has been further developed into the so-called CT severity index (Table 7.1). This index is an attempt to improve the early prognostic value of CT by the intravenous administration of contrast medium. In this way also parenchymal necrosis of the pancreas can be diagnosed [3, 4]. The CT severity index can also be used for other imaging procedures.

Table 7.1 Computed tomography grading of severity of acute pancreatitis [2-4]. This system can also be used for other imaging modalities

Computed tomography grade		
(A) Normal pancreas		0
(B) Edematous pancreatitis		1
(C) B plus mild extrapancreatic changes		2
(D) Severe extrapancreatic changes including one fluid collection		3
(E) Multiple or extensive extrapancreatic changes		4
Necrosis		
None		0
<One third		2
>One third, <one half		4
>Half		6
CT severity index = CT grade+necrosis score		
	Complications	Deaths
0-3	8%	3%
4-6	35%	6%
7-10	92%	17%

S. Rickes (✉)
Department of Internal Medicine
AMEOS Hospital St. Salvator, Halberstadt, Germany
e-mail: rickes@medkl.salvator-kh.de

M. D'Onofrio (ed.), *Ultrasonography of the Pancreas*, © Springer-Verlag Italia 2012

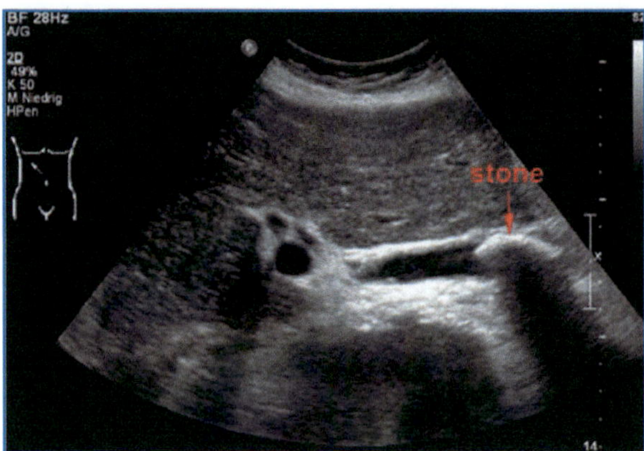

Fig. 7.1 Gallstone at the main bile duct at transabdominal US

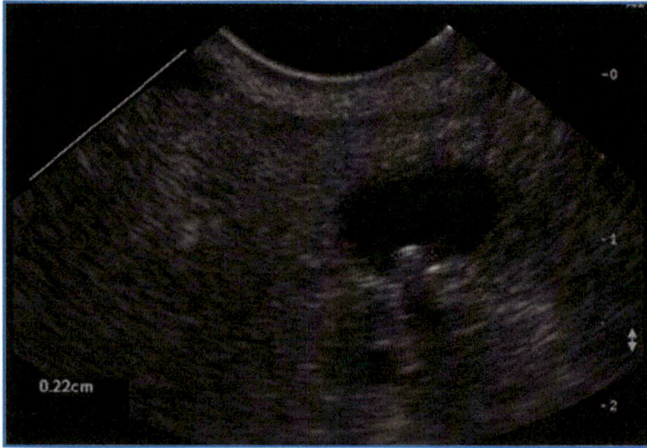

Fig. 7.2 Gallstone (*calipers*) in the main bile duct at EUS

Transabdominal US is the imaging method of choice in patients with acute abdomen due to its wide availability and portability. However, several limitations can be encountered in patients with acute pancreatitis mainly related to abdominal pain, which makes compressions with the probe impossible, and abundant overlying gas owing to a paralytic ileus. Very often a partial or inadequate transabdominal US visualization of the pancreas will result. Therefore, CT is still of paramount importance for the first evaluation of the disease. However, during the course of the disease, US may serve as an excellent imaging tool for short-term follow-up studies. Another potential advantage of US is the good visualization of the biliary system. Biliary stones are the most frequent causes of acute pancreatitis. US can easily detect stones in the gallbladder and in the biliary tract with high diagnostic accuracy (Fig. 7.1). This is very useful to triage patients requiring endoscopic retrograde cholangiopancreatography (ERCP) and sphincterotomy. However, the diagnosis of a bile duct stone with US is obviously influenced by operator skill. One German study demonstrated that experienced examiners achieve a significantly higher diagnostic accuracy for the detection of choledocholithiasis than less experienced investigators (83% versus 64%) [5]. Other studies showed that with endoscopic ultrasonography (EUS) (Fig. 7.2) and magnetic resonance cholangiopancreatography (MRCP) better results can be achieved [6-8]. However, these methods should be used only in patients with suspected choledocholithiasis but without detection of stones at transabdominal US. Finally, interventional procedures, such as aspiration and drainage of fluid collections, may be performed under US guidance.

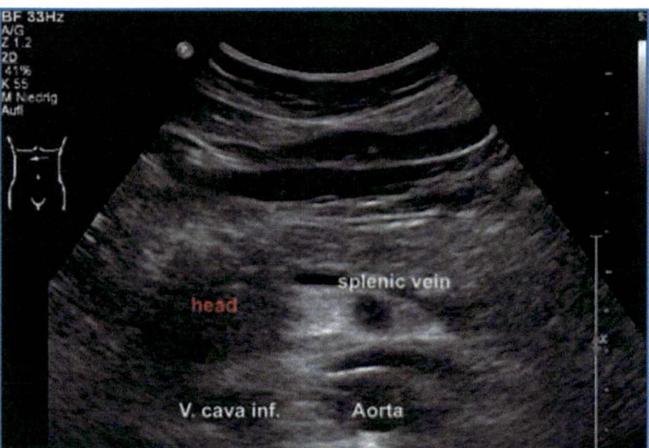

Fig. 7.3 Acute edematous pancreatitis located at the pancreatic head which appears enlarged and hypoechoic at transabdominal US

In early pancreatitis, the organ may be of normal size and echotexture. However, in most patients interstitial edema results in an enlargement of the gland and a subsequent hypoechoic appearance (Fig. 7.3). The acute inflammation can be focal or diffuse, depending on the distribution. Focal pancreatitis mostly occurs in the pancreatic head and presents as a hypoechoic mass that is sometimes difficult to differentiate from a tumor.

Complications of acute pancreatitis include acute fluid collections representing exudates, peripancreatic tissue necrosis or hemorrhage in various combinations, parenchymal necrosis, and vascular complications. Acute fluid collections are echopoor or echofree. They occur most commonly around the pancreas (Fig. 7.4) and usually spread into both the lesser sac and the anterior pararenal space up to the pericolic region. Furthermore, the enzyme-rich fluid can penetrate into

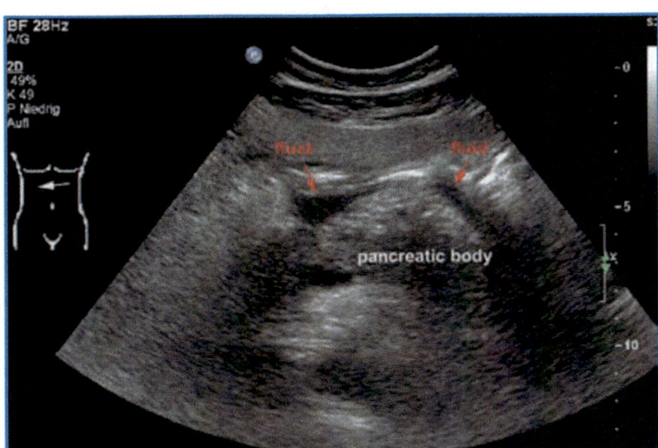

Fig. 7.4 Acute pancreatitis with enlargement of the pancreatic body and fluid collections around the pancreas at transabdominal US

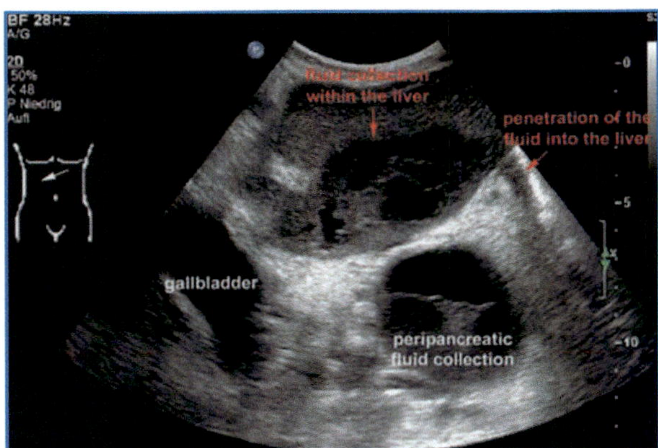

Fig. 7.5 Acute pancreatitis with peripancreatic fluid collection and involvement of the left liver lobe at transabdominal US

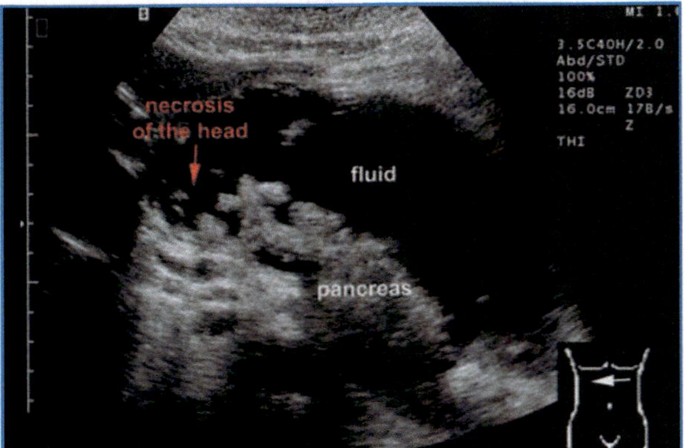

Fig. 7.6 Necrotizing pancreatitis at transabdominal US. The pancreatic head is destroyed and liquefied. The pancreatic body is enlarged and inhomogeneous. A peripancreatic fluid collection can also be appreciated

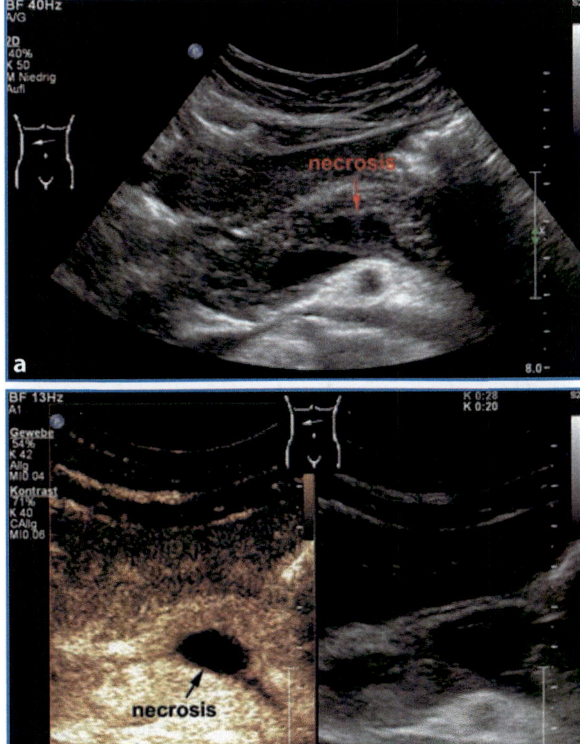

Fig. 7.7 a,b Necrotizing pancreatitis at transabdominal US. **a** Conventional US. Echopoor region (not liquefied necrosis) at the pancreatic body at B-mode US. A differentiation between necrosis and edema is impossible. **b** Contrast-enhanced US. The region shows no vascular structures and can therefore be characterized as necrotic

parenchymal organs, like the spleen or the liver (Fig. 7.5). In acute necrotizing pancreatitis, parts of the pancreas can be destroyed and liquefied (Fig. 7.6).

A major problem of conventional US is the detection of non-liquefied parenchymal necrosis because it cannot assess organ perfusion. Through the use of contrast media, however, even at US the vascular behavior of the pancreas can nowadays be examined. At CEUS necrotic areas of the pancreas show no vascular structures (Fig. 7.7). A paper published in 2006 showed that this method produces excellent results in the staging of acute pancreatitis severity [9]. This study demonstrated that the procedure is comparable to CT for the assessment of severe acute pancreatitis and can be recommended as a first-choice imaging procedure, especially when iodinated contrast medium injection is contraindi-

cated [9–12]. Ripollés et al. [13] reported that CEUS is comparable to CT in detecting pancreatic necrosis as well as predicting its clinical course and that therefore, when CT is contraindicated, CEUS may be a valid alternative. However, it has to be considered that in this study patients with incomplete US imaging of the pancreas were excluded. In light of the difficulties reported above regarding the exploration of the pancreas in patients with acute pancreatitis, one role of CEUS may be considered not in the first (staging) but in the further evaluation (follow-up) always required in the management of the disease. A positive outcome would be a significant reduction in the number of CT examinations performed. However, when CT is contraindicated, magnetic resonance imaging (MRI), with absolutely the same panoramic view of CT although less available and more expensive, can be used with good results [14, 15]. For instance, if the definition of a fluid collection proves difficult both at US and CT, it can be easily obtainable with MRI [14].

The most important complications of acute pancreatitis are infection of necrosis and vascular complications. Necrotic infection more frequently appears 15–20 days after the clinical onset of acute pancreatitis [16]. The probability of infection increases proportionately to the gravity of the acute pancreatitis at clinical and CT evaluation. Infection can be suspected in the presence of gas bubbles produced by anaerobic bacteria within the fluid collections. The detection of gas bubbles within the collections while difficult at US is instead immediate at CT. This is the reason why when infection of necrosis is first suspected CT must be performed again. Pancreatic abscess is a collection of suppurative fluid, surrounded by a fibrous capsule, adjacent to the pancreatic gland. An abscess secondary to acute pancreatitis probably starts off as infection of pancreatic necrosis. An abscess appears later than infection of the necrosis, usually after the fourth week [14]. Surgical necrosectomy or percutaneous debridement can be considered in treating infected pancreatic necrosis. Percutaneous drainage under imaging-guidance is highly efficient in the treatment of pancreatic abscess/infected pancreatic pseudocysts [14]. The mainly fluid content of the lesion explains the excellent clinical success of the procedure. Percutaneous drainage can be carried out under US or CT guidance, although CT is again preferable [14].

The most common vascular complications are thrombosis of the portal venous system, hemorrhage into a pseudocyst, arterial erosions and disruption, formation of collateral vessels or pseudoaneurysms, and rupture of a pseudoaneurysm (see also the paragraph about pseudocysts). In patients with a history of pancreatitis, the detection of a cystic lesion at US must be further evaluated with Doppler to exclude the presence of vascular complications [14, 17, 18]. The administration of microbubbles could potentially improve the diagnosis of vascular complications. However, CT evaluation remains mandatory for diagnostic confirmation and treatment planning. Angiography, playing no relevant role in the diagnostic phase, has to be immediately used for treating vascular lesions [14].

7.3 Chronic Pancreatitis

Irrespective of its etiology, chronic pancreatitis is described by fibrosis, destruction, and distortion of the pancreatic ducts with loss of parenchyma. The most common cause in Europe is alcohol abuse. Other causes include hereditary, tropical, autoimmune, and idiopathic pancreatitis. The diagnosis of chronic pancreatitis is based on clinical findings, laboratory evaluation of endocrine and exocrine pancreatic function, and imaging findings. Although early morphologic changes of chronic pancreatitis are difficult to recognize at imaging with different techniques, the findings of advanced disease are easily detected [19, 20]. ERCP has long been considered the diagnostic criterion standard in the diagnosis of chronic pancreatitis. However, today ERCP has been replaced by MRCP. MRI is nowadays a powerful noninvasive imaging modality for the study of chronic pancreatitis even in the early phase of the disease [15]. A complete MRI study for chronic pancreatitis includes imaging of the parenchyma before and after the administration of contrast material, and imaging of the duct before and after secretin stimulation to evaluate pancreatic exocrine function through the analysis of the pancreatic fluid output. EUS seems also to be highly sensitive in the detection of early morphologic changes [21]. Technologic advantages and new developments in US (compound and tissue harmonic imaging, high frequency probes, CEUS and elastography) have improved the value of US in the diagnosis of pancreatic diseases [22].

In the US study of chronic pancreatitis, alterations in the size of the pancreas may be seen in about 50% of patients affected by chronic pancreatitis. However, the finding of a gland with normal size does not exclude the diagnosis of chronic pancreatitis. Pancreatic atrophy and focal alterations in size can be easily identified (Fig. 7.8). However, these changes in pancreatic volume are signs of advanced stages of the disease [23]. The

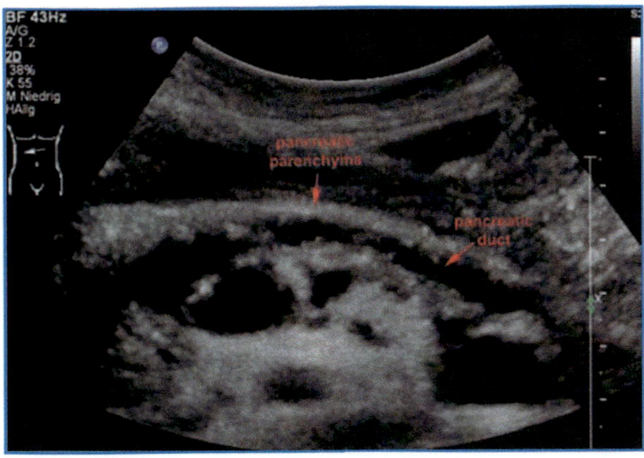

Fig. 7.8 Atrophy of the pancreatic parenchyma at transabdominal US in a patient with late-stage chronic pancreatitis. The pancreatic duct is dilated with very small intraductal plugs

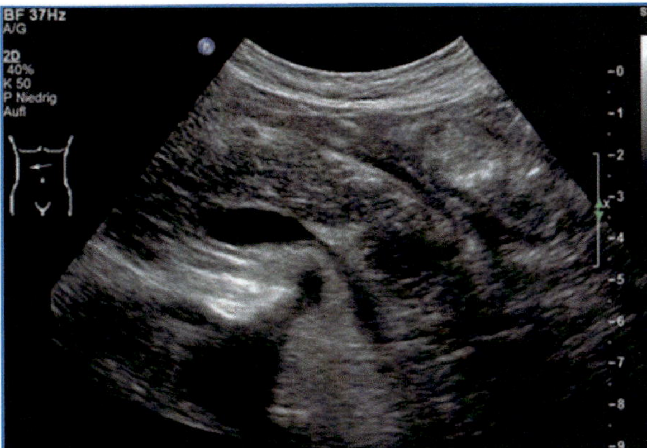

Fig. 7.9 Early-stage chronic pancreatitis at transabdominal US. The pancreatic parenchyma is inhomogeneous and coarse (*lobulated parenchyma*)

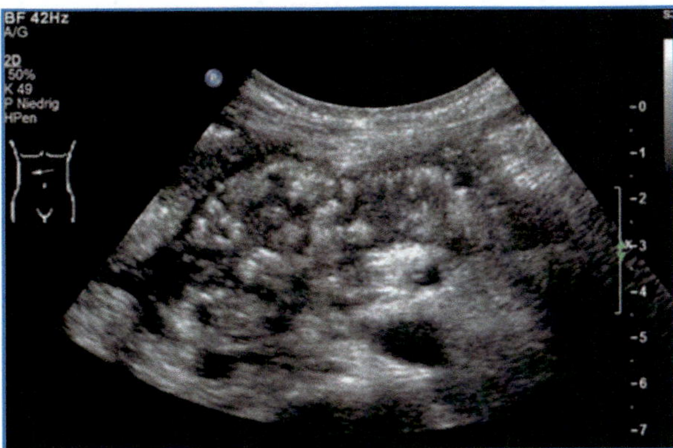

Fig. 7.10 Chronic pancreatitis at transabdominal US with an increased volume of the pancreatic gland and the presence of multiple calcifications

echogenicity of the pancreas may be increased in chronic pancreatitis due to fatty infiltration and fibrosis, although this sign is not absolutely specific. In fact, it can also be found in obese patients and the elderly. Parenchymal alteration is a more specific sign of chronic inflammation and represented by inhomogeneous and coarse *lobulated parenchyma* pattern due to the coexistence of hyperechoic and hypoechoic parts of fibrosis and inflammation, respectively (Fig. 7.9). These findings can be diagnosed presumably with the highest sensitivity at EUS [21, 23, 24].

The most important diagnostic sign of chronic pancreatitis is the presence of calcifications (Fig. 7.10) [25, 26]. These calcifications are calcium carbonate deposits. At US they appear as hyperechoic spots with posterior shading. Small calcifications may be hardly detectable. The diagnosis can be improved by the use of the so-called twinkling artifact (Fig. 7.11). Twinkling artifact is characterized by a rapidly fluctuating mixture of Doppler signals that occurs behind a strongly re-

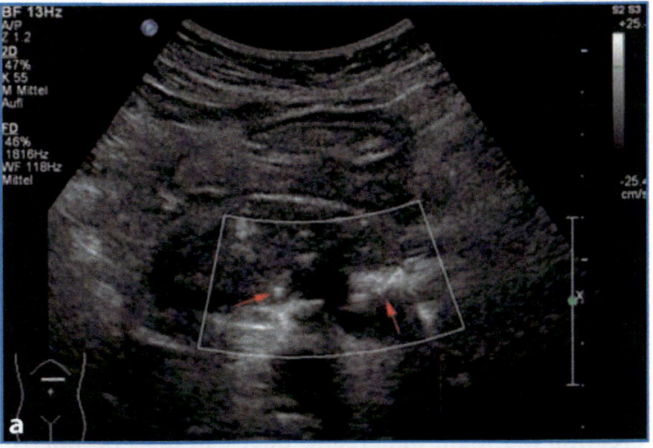

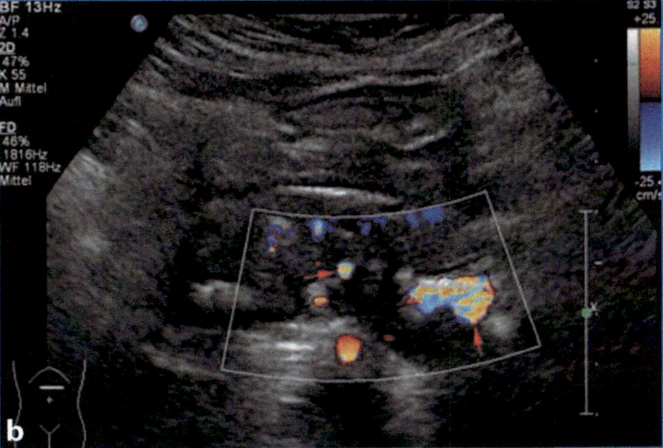

Fig. 7.11 a,b Chronic pancreatitis with small calcifications at percutaneous B-mode US (**a**, *arrows*) which generate typically twinkling artifacts at color-Doppler mode (**b**, *arrows*)

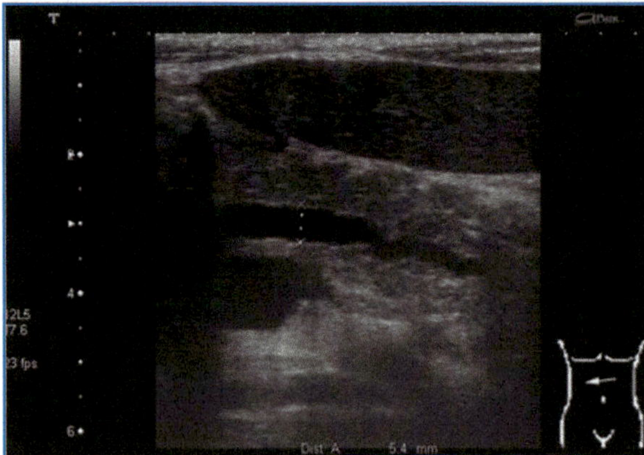

Fig. 7.12 Late-stage chronic pancreatitis at transabdominal US. The pancreatic duct is dilated (5 mm) and shows an irregular course. For better delineation the linear probe is used

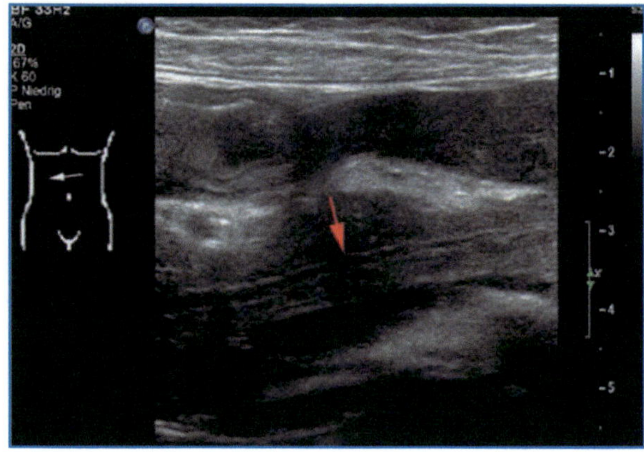

Fig. 7.13 Early-stage chronic pancreatitis at transabdominal US. The pancreatic duct (*arrow*) is not dilated but shows an irregular course. For better delineation the linear probe is used

flecting granular interface such as pancreatic calcifications [27]. The demonstration of pancreatic calcifications may be improved by the use of harmonic imaging and high resolution US, by using high US beam frequency, increasing US diagnostic accuracy [15]. Intraductal plugs with little or no calcium carbonate deposits appear at US as echoic spots almost without posterior shading (Fig. 7.8). The high spatial and contrast resolution of current US systems allow an accurate identification of pancreatic microcalcifications and microdeposits. Intraductal deposits such as plugs (Fig. 7.8) if not yet calcified can be better identified by means of the US than the CT study.

A further important sign of chronic pancreatitis is the dilatation of the main pancreatic duct of more than 3 mm [28, 29] (Fig. 7.12). However, in chronic pancreatitis the main pancreatic duct can also be not yet dilated but irregular in course (Fig. 7.13). Former studies have found that for the sonographic diagnosis of chronic pancreatitis pancreatic duct dilation is the most easily identified sign with a sensitivity of about 60%–70% and a specificity of about 80%–90% [28, 29].

Focal pancreatitis typically involves the pancreatic head [23]. The differentiation of mass-forming pancreatitis from ductal adenocarcinomas is notoriously problematic due to their similar patterns [12]. Mass-forming pancreatitis usually occurs in patients with a history of chronic pancreatitis and must be differentiated from pancreatic ductal adenocarcinoma. The differential diagnosis with a neoplastic disease may be difficult due to the very similar US features, presenting in most cases as a hypoechoic mass, and also because mass-

forming pancreatitis and pancreatic cancer may present with the same symptoms and signs [12]. The presence of small calcifications at US in the lesion may suggest its inflammatory nature, but this is low in specificity [12]. For diagnosis, biopsy is often mandatory. In many cases fine needle aspiration (FNA) or biopsy is in fact still necessary and can be US-guided either percutaneously or endoscopically.

CEUS can improve the differential diagnosis between mass-forming pancreatitis and pancreatic adenocarcinoma [30]. In particular, while ductal adenocarcinoma remains hypoechoic in all contrast-enhanced phases, due to its intense desmoplastic reaction with poor mean vascular density of the lesion, the inflammatory mass shows parenchymal enhancement in the early contrast-enhanced phase [12, 30]. The CEUS finding consistent with an inflammatory origin is therefore the presence of parenchymal enhancement similar to that of the adjacent pancreas during the dynamic study. The intensity of this parenchymal enhancement is related to the length of the underlying inflammatory process. It has been observed that, the more the inflammatory process is chronic and long-standing, the less intense is the intralesional parenchymal enhancement, probably in relation to the entity of the associated fibrosis. As opposed to this, in mass-forming pancreatitis of more recent onset the enhancement is usually more intense and prolonged [31-34].

Autoimmune pancreatitis is a rare cause of recurrent acute or chronic pancreatitis. It is characterized by periductal inflammation, caused by infiltration of lymphocytes and plasma cells, with evolution to fibrosis [35, 36]. In most cases, the echogenicity is reduced

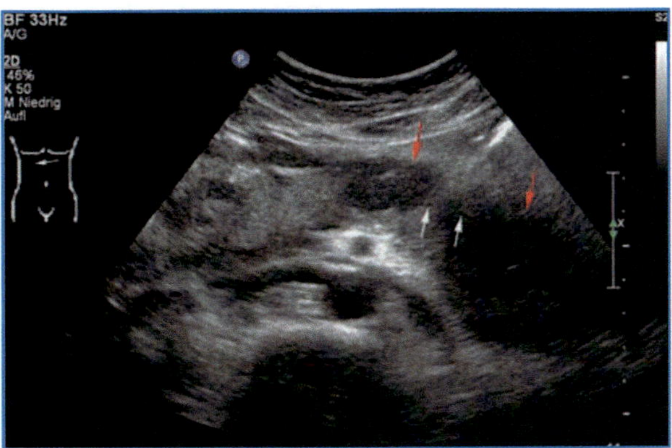

Fig. 7.14 Autoimmune pancreatitis at transabdominal ultrasound with focal enlargements of the pancreatic gland (*red arrows*) and compression of the pancreatic duct (*white arrows*)

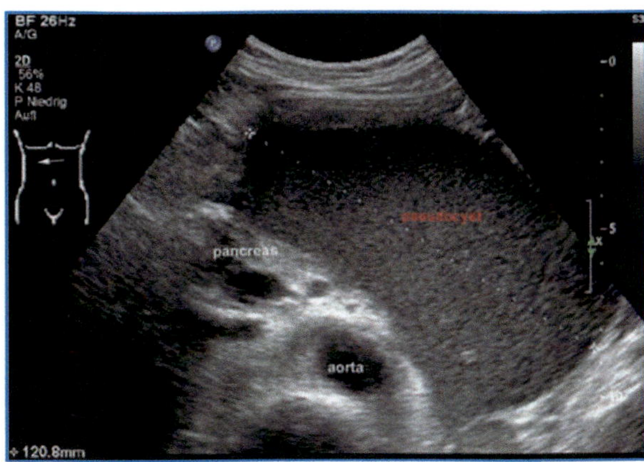

Fig. 7.15 Pancreatic pseudocyst at transabdominal US

(Fig. 7.14), the gland volume shows focal (Fig. 7.14) or diffuse (*sausage-like*) enlargement, and the pancreatic duct may be compressed by glandular parenchyma (Fig. 7.14). US findings are characteristic in the diffuse form when the entire gland is involved. In the focal form US features are less characteristic and very similar to those of mass-forming chronic pancreatitis. Focal autoimmune pancreatitis at the pancreatic head is often characterized by the dilation of the common bile duct alone [37]. The vascularization of autoimmune pancreatitis can be demonstrated at CEUS showing relatively intense parenchymal enhancement. CEUS of autoimmune pancreatitis shows fair and often from moderate to marked enhancement in the early contrast-enhanced phase, though inhomogeneous [37]. The CEUS findings may be especially useful in the study of focal forms of autoimmune chronic pancreatitis, in which differential diagnosis with ductal adenocarcinoma is a priority [30].

7.4 Pseudocysts

Pseudocyst of the pancreas is a fluid collection that contains pancreatic enzymes, surrounded by a fibrotic wall with no epithelial layer. They are caused by pancreatic ductal disruption following increased luminal pressure, either due to stenosis or calculi obstructing the ductal system, or as a result of parenchymal necrosis. Pseudocysts complicate the course of pancreatitis in 30% to 40% [38], appearing 3-6 weeks or longer following fluid collection organization [15].

At US a pseudocyst is seen as a sharply delineated and anechoic lesion with *distal acoustic enhancement*, and it is typically oval or round (Fig. 7.15). Sometimes it may have inclusions (debris), thus simulating a cystic tumor (e.g. cystadenoma or cystadenocarcinoma). Only if there is a history of acute or chronic pancreatitis or there are imaging signs of chronic pancreatitis can the diagnosis of pseudocysts be considered. Pseudocysts must be differentiated from pancreatic cystic tumors, especially mucinous cystadenoma, as they require completely different therapeutic approaches. CEUS can improve the differential diagnosis between pseudocysts and cystic tumors [39, 40]. Differential diagnosis between pseudocysts and cystic tumors of the pancreas is more reliable thanks to the evaluation of the vascularity of intralesional inclusions. Even if characterized by an inhomogeneous content at US, all the inclusions in pseudocysts are always completely avascular, becoming homogeneously anechoic during CEUS examination [40]. In fact, in contrast to CT and MRI the results of the CEUS study of a pseudocyst may be different. Harmonic microbubble-specific software filter all the background tissue signals during CEUS examination and this makes the examination accurate for distinguishing debris from tumoral vegetations. Therefore the accuracy of CEUS in the diagnosis of pseudocyst is high [39]. The wall of the pseudocysts may be more or less vascular at imaging and also at CEUS [39, 40].

Pseudocyst may be followed up if small in size and if not complicated and without involvement of adjacent structures. Otherwise drainage or surgical treatments have to be considered. The surgical approach is recommended if an open communication between the pseudocyst and the ductal system exists.

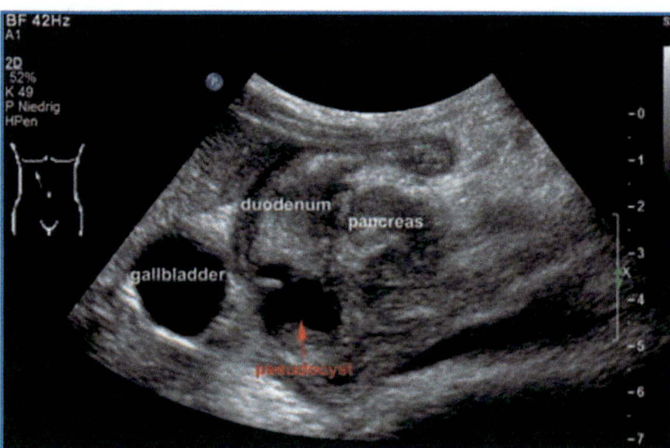

Fig. 7.16 Pancreatic pseudocyst within the wall of the duodenum at transabdominal US

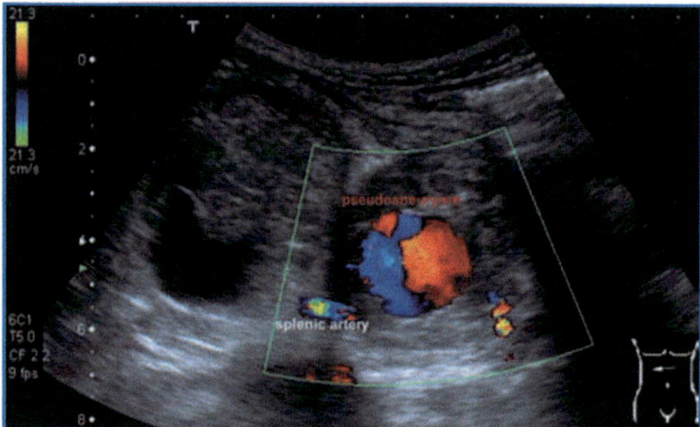

Fig. 7.17 Pseudoaneurysm of the splenic artery. With color-Doppler sonography blood flow can be appreciated within the pseudocyst

Pancreatic pseudocysts can involve adjacent organs [14] and the duodenum (Fig. 7.16), stomach and colon. Furthermore, fistulas between pseudocysts and the bile duct system have been reported [41].

The identification of small cystic formations in a thickened duodenal wall on the pancreatic side is however a specific finding for cystic dystrophy of the duodenal wall [42]. Cystic dystrophy of the duodenal wall and groove pancreatitis are in a border site (groove region) between the pancreas and duodenum, a site that can be correctly evaluated with EUS.

Bleeding is a further severe complication due to erosion and may occur into the pseudocyst or into the gastrointestinal tract or peritoneal cavity. When bleeding occurs into the pseudocyst, the cyst changes in echogenicity and may enlarge causing pain and pressure effects or blood may pass through the main pancreatic duct into the duodenum, which is known as *hemosuccus*

pancreaticus. An additional issue is whether bleeding is caused by erosion of a vessel wall or because of rupture of a pseudoaneurysm. The splenic artery appears to be the most common artery involved with major bleeding (Fig. 7.17). Helpful information can be obtained by Doppler US [43, 44].

References

1. Rickes S, Uhle C (2009) Advances in the diagnosis of acute pancreatitis. Postgrad Med J 85:208-212
2. Balthazar EJ (1989) CT diagnosis and staging of acute pancreatitis. Radiol Clin North Am 27:19-37
3. Uhl W, Warshaw A, Imrie C et al (2002) IAP Guidelines for the surgical management of acute pancreatitis. Pancreatology 2:565-573
4. Balthazar EJ, Freeny PC, van Sonnenberg E (1994) Imaging and intervention in acute pancreatitis. Radiology 193:297-306.
5. Rickes S, Treiber G, Mönkemüller K, et al (2006) Impact of operators experience on value of high-resolution transabdominal ultrasound in the diagnosis of choledocholithiasis: A prospective comparison using endoscopic retrograde cholangiography as gold standard. Scand J Gastroenterol 41:838-843
6. de Lédinghen V, Lecesne R, Raymond JM et al (1999) Diagnosis of choledocholithiasis: EUS or magnetic resonance cholangiography? A prospective controlled study. Gastrointest Endosc 49:26-31
7. Soto JA, Barish MA, Alvarez O, Medina S (2000) Detection of choledocholithiasis with MR cholangiography: Comparison of three dimensional fast spin-echo and single- and multisection half-Fourier rapid acquisition with relaxation enhancement sequences. Radiology 215:737–745
8. Moo JH, Cho YD, Cha SW et al (2005) The detection of bile duct stones in suspected biliary pancreatitis: comparison of MRCP, ERCP, and intraductal US. Am J Gastroenterol 100:1051-1057
9. Rickes S, Uhle C, Kahl S et al (2006) Echo-enhanced ultrasound: a new valid initial imaging approach for severe acute pancreatitis. Gut 55:74-78
10. Rickes S, Mönkemüller K, Malfertheiner P (2007) Acute severe pancreatitis: contrast-enhanced sonography. Abdom Imaging 32:362-364
11. Rickes S, Rauh P, Uhle C et al (2007) Contrast-enhanced sonography in pancreatic diseases. Eur J Radiol 64:183-188
12. D´Onofrio M, Zamboni G, Faccioli N et al (2007) Ultrasonography of the pancreas. 4. Contrast-inhanced imaging. Abdom Imaging 32:171-181
13. Ripollés T, Martínez MJ, López E et al (2010) Contrast-enhanced ultrasound in the staging of acute pancreatitis. Eur Radiol 20:2518-2523
14. Procacci C (2002) Non-traumatic abdominal emergencies: imaging and intervention in acute pancreatic conditions. Eur Radiol 12:2407–2434
15. Balthazar EJ (ed) (2009) Imaging of the pancreas. Acute and chronic pancreatitis. Springer, Berlin
16. Laws HL, Kent RB III (2000) Acute pancreatitis: management of complicating infection. Am Surg 66:145–152
17. Dörffel T, Wruck T, Rückert RI et al (2000) Vascular com-

plications in acute pancreatitis assessed by color duplex ultrasonography. Pancreas 21:126-33

18. Kinney TP, Freeman ML (2008) Recent advances and novel methods in pancreatic imaging. Minerva Gastroenterol Dietol 54:85-95

19. Choueiri NE, Alkaade S, Burton FR, Balci NC (2010) Advanced imaging of chronic pancreatitis. Curr Gastroenterol Rep 12:114-120

20. Aheed JS, Miller F (2007) Chronic pancreatitis: ultrasound, computed tomography, and magnetic resonance imaging features. Semin Ultrasound CT MR 28:384-394

21. Kahl S, Glasbrenner B, Leodolter A et al (2002) EUS in the diagnosis of early chronic pancreatitis: a prospective follow-up study. Gastrointest Endosc 55:507-511

22. Rickes S, Böhm J, Malfertheiner P (2006) SonoCT improves on conventional ultrasound in the visualization of the pancreatic and bile duct: A pilot study. J Gastroenterol Hepatol 21:552-555

23. Martinez-Noguera A, D´Onofrio M (2007) Ultrasonography of the pancreas. 1. Conventional imaging. Abdom Imaging 32:136-149

24. Bolondi L, Priori P, Gullo L et al (1987) Relationship between morphological changes detected by ultrasonography and pancreatic exocrine function in chronic pancreatitis. Pancreas 2:222-229

25. Homma T, Harada H, Koizumi M (1997) Diagnostic criteria for chronic pancreatitis by the Japan Pancreas Society. Pancreas 15:14-15

26. Ring EJ, Eaton SB, Ferrucci JT, Short WF (1973) Differential diagnosis of pancreatic calcification. Am J Roentgenol Radium Ther Nucl Med 117:446–452

27. Kim HC, Yang DM, Jin W et al (2010) Color Doppler twinkling artifacts in various conditions during abdominal and pelvic sonography. J Ultrasound Med 29:621-632

28. Niederau C, Grendell JH (1985) Diagnosis of chronic pancreatitis. Gastroenterology 88:1973–1995

29. Hessel ST, Siegelman SS, McNeil BJ et al (1982) A prospective evaluation of computer tomography and ultrasound of the pancreas. Radiology 143:129–133

30. D'Onofrio M, Zamboni G, Tognolini A et al (2006) Mass-forming pancreatitis: value of contrast-enhanced ultrasonography. World J Gastroenterol 12:4181-4184

31. Rickes S, Unkrodt K, Neye H et al (2002) Differentiation of pancreatic tumours by conventional ultrasound, unenhanced and echo-enhanced power Doppler sonography. Scand J Gastroenterol 37:1313-1320

32. Rickes S, Unkrodt K, Wermke W et al (2000) Evaluation of Doppler sonographic criteria for the differentiation of pancreatic tumours. Ultraschall in Med 20:253–258

33. Rickes S, Mönkemüller K, Malfertheiner P (2006) Contrast-enhanced ultrasound in the diagnosis of pancreatic tumors. J Pancreas 7:584-592

34. Rickes S, Unkrodt K, Ocran K et al (2003) Differentiation of neuroendocrine tumours from other pancreatic lesions by echo-enhanced power Doppler sonography and somatostatin receptor scintigraphy. Pancreas 26:76-81

35. Neuzillet C, Lepère C, El Hajjam M et al (2010) Autoimmune pancreatitis with atypical imaging findings that mimicked an endocrine tumor. World J Gastroenterol 21:2954-2958

36. Khan KJ (2010) Prevalence, diagnosis, and profile of autoimmune pancreatitis presenting with features of acute or chronic pancreatitis. Clin Gastroenterol Hepatol 8:639-640

37. Numata K, Ozawa Y, Kobayashi N et al (2004) Contrast enhanced sonography of autoimmune pancreatitis. Comparison with pathologic findings. J Ultrasound Med 23:199-206

38. Habashi S, Draganov PV (2009) Pancreatic pseudocyst. World J Gastroenterol 15:38-47

39. Rickes S, Wermke W (2004) Differentiation of cystic pancreatic neoplasms and pseudocysts by conventional and echo-enhanced ultrasound. J Gastroenterol Hepatol 19:761-766

40. D'Onofrio M, Barbi E, Dietrich C et al (2011) Pancreatic multicenter ultrasound study (PAMUS). Eur J Radiol doi:10.1016/j.ejrad.2011.01.053

41. Rickes S, Mönkemüller K, Peitz U et al (2006) Sonographic diagnosis and endoscopic therapy of a biliopancreatic fistula complicating a pancreatic pseudocyst. Scand J Gastroenterol 41:989-992

42. Procacci C, Graziani R, Zamboni G et al (1997) Cystic dystrophy of the duodenal wall: radiologic findings. Radiology 205:741–747

43. Rickes S, Kolfenbach S, Kahl S, Malfertheiner P (2004) Gastrointestinal bleeding and pancreatic pseudocysts. J Gastroenterol Hepatol 19:711

44. Rickes S, Mönkemüller K, Venerito M, Malfertheiner P (2006) Pseudoaneurysm of the splenic artery. Dig Surg 23:156–158

Solid Pancreatic Tumors

8

Christoph F. Dietrich, Michael Hocke, Anna Gallotti
and Mirko D'Onofrio

8.1 Introduction

Diagnostic imaging plays a crucial role in the study of pancreatic tumors, with the primary aims being their correct detection and characterization [1, 2]. A further accurate staging is of fundamental importance for treatment planning. Ultrasonography (US) is often the non-invasive imaging modality chosen for the first evaluation of the pancreas, as it is inexpensive, easy to perform and widely available [3]. The more precise and accurate the initial evaluation, the more appropriate the management of the patient will be. In recent decades, the introduction of new technologies has improved the image quality of conventional imaging with very high spatial and contrast resolution [4-6]. Adenocarcinoma is the most common primary malignancy of the pancreas, thus each single pancreatic solid mass detected at US has a high probability of being an adenocarcinoma. Otherwise not all the solid pancreatic masses detected at US are adenocarcinoma [7]. Therefore improving the US capability for the characterization and differential diagnosis will lead to both a faster diagnosis of ductal adenocarcinoma and a more accurate differential diagnosis in respect to other pancreatic tumor histotypes or non-neoplastic mass-forming conditions.

This chapter is focused on the actual possibility of detection and characterization, considering the most clinically relevant differential diagnoses, and staging of pancreatic ductal adenocarcinoma by means of US.

C.F. Dietrich (✉)
Department of Clinical Medicine
Caritas-Krankenhaus, Bad Mergentheim, Germany
e-mail: christoph.dietrich@ckbm.de

8.2 Pathology and Epidemiology

Ductal adenocarcinoma is the most common primary malignancy of the pancreas, accounting for 80% of malignant pancreatic tumors and almost three-fourths of all pancreatic cancers [8-10]. Macroscopically, pancreatic ductal adenocarcinoma is a white-yellow and firm mass owing to the presence of fibrosis and desmoplasia, with infiltration of the ductal epithelium [7]. Microscopically, it is composed of infiltrating glands surrounded by dense and reactive fibrous tissue [11]. The presence of intratumoral fibrosis and necrosis, typical for highly aggressive types with a reduction in the microvascular density and in perfusion, the presence of perineural invasion and distant metastases (commonly in the liver, lungs, peritoneum and adrenal glands) predict a worse survival [9, 10, 12-14].

In more than 95% of cases, regardless of the site of localization, pancreatic ductal adenocarcinoma is diagnosed at an advanced stage, with locally advanced or metastatic disease requiring palliative therapy [12-14]. Only 10 to 20% of patients are candidates for surgery [11]. The prognosis and the treatment approach are based on whether the tumor is resectable or non-resectable at presentation, which is mostly dependent on the time of diagnosis [2].

8.3 Adenocarcinoma

8.3.1 Detection

The detection of a pancreatic ductal adenocarcinoma at transabdominal US is basically related to both explo-

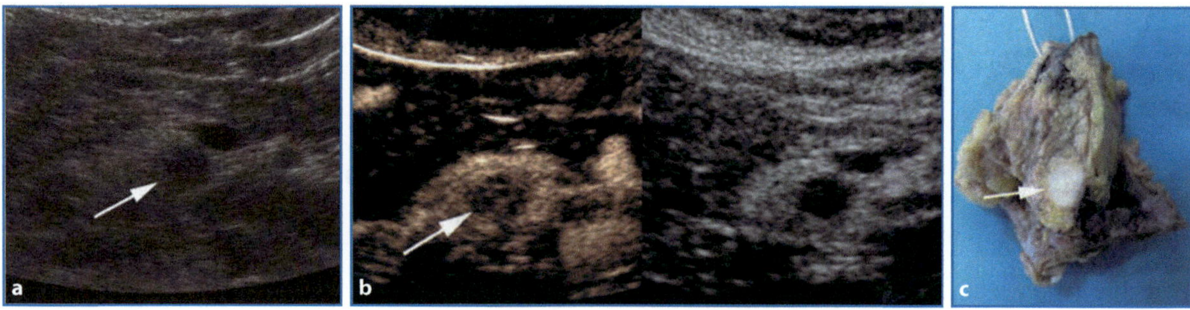

Fig. 8.1 a-c Small pancreatic adenocarcinoma. US (**a**) incidental detection of a small hypoechoic nodule (*arrow*) in the uncinate process of the pancreas appearing hypovascular (*arrow*) at CEUS (**b**) with final diagnosis of small ductal adenocarcinoma (*arrow*) at pathology (**c**)

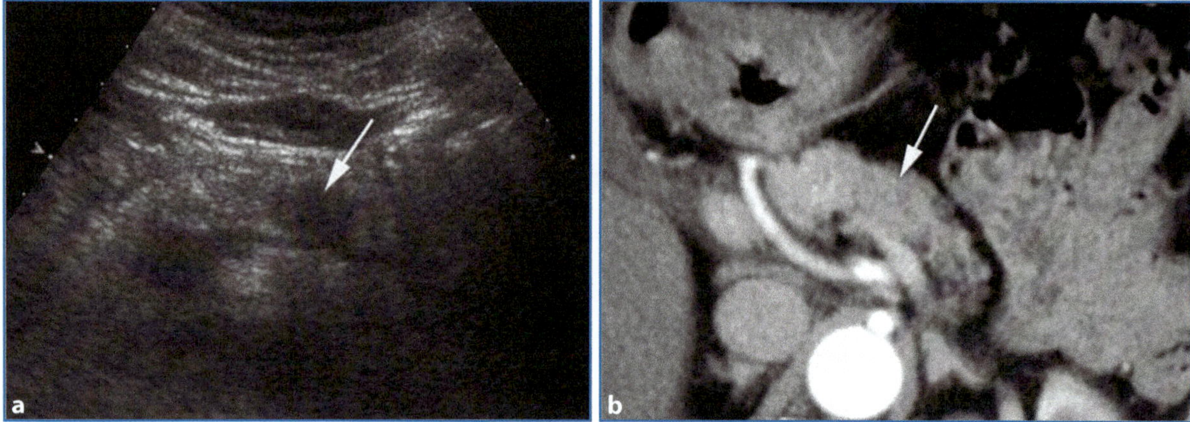

Fig. 8.2 a,b Small pancreatic adenocarcinoma. US (**a**) direct identification of a ductal adenocarcinoma of the pancreatic body appearing hypoechoic (*arrow*), but isoattenuating (*arrow*) at CT (**b**)

ration of the pancreatic region and conspicuity of the lesion in terms of size and echogenicity. Good visualization of the gland, which is difficult in the presence of tympanites or in obese patients, can be achieved by applying compression with the probe. Filling the stomach with water is not useful and makes compression more difficult. Moreover air bubbles are ingested together with the water generating artifacts. Patient position is also important. Changing the patient decubitus, such as on the left or right flank or in orthostasis, can provide a good visualization of the pancreatic region. These operations take time but very often a good result can be obtained [3, 15, 16]. On the other hand, a good conspicuity of the lesion is almost always instantaneous at US [1]. The high spatial resolution makes the US examination able to detect even very small pancreatic adenocarcinoma (Fig. 8.1). In fact, it has been argued that acoustic impedance of ductal adenocarcinoma is very low, with a significant difference between the lesion

and the pancreatic adjacent parenchyma always present [3]. This is the reason why the adenocarcinoma is usually markedly hypoechoic with respect to the pancreas (Fig. 8.2). Moreover this difference in impedance between the lesion and the adjacent parenchyma is sometimes greater than that observed at CT between beam attenuation in both pre- and post-contrast enhancement phases [3, 17, 18]. This could be experimentally proved by measuring and comparing the difference in echogenicity in respect to Hounsfield Units (HU) of the same lesion (Fig. 8.3) and explain some results already reported in the literature [17]. Pancreatic lesions are detectable at CT if a difference of 10-15 HU exists [18]. It has been reported that up to 11% of pancreatic adenocarcinoma at CT show no difference in attenuation compared to the surrounding pancreatic tissue, the so-called isoattenuating pancreatic adenocarcinoma [19-21]. Yoon et al. [20] reported that 27% of small (≤20 mm) pancreatic adenocarcinoma are isoattenuating at CT so not directly

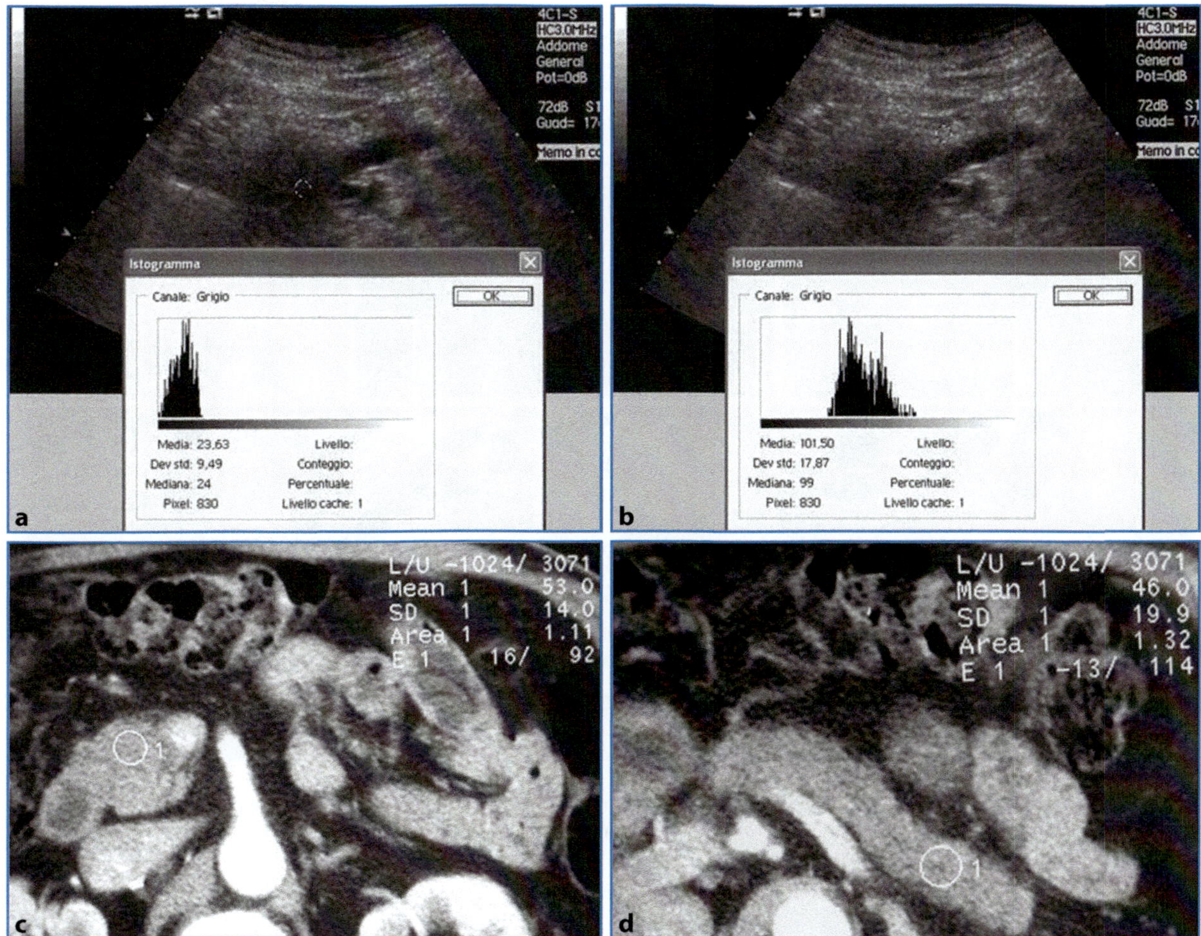

Fig. 8.3 a-d Pancreatic adenocarcinoma. **a,b** High difference in echogenicity between the pancreatic head lesion appearing hypoechoic (ROI in **a**) with respect to the pancreatic body (ROI in **b**). **c,d** Low difference in Hounsfield unit of the same lesion (ROI in **c**) with respect to the body-tail (ROI in **d**)

visible without the use of some secondary signs. But direct visualization (Fig. 8.2) is essential for the assessment of tumor dimensions and local staging. Moreover small well-differentiated pancreatic adenocarcinomas, which are associated with a better survival rate after resection, are isoattenuating in more than 50% of cases [20, 22]. Magnetic resonance imaging (MRI) and PET/CT, but also US (Figs. 8.2, 8.3) and contrast-enhanced ultrasound (CEUS) (Fig. 8.4), may be useful for detecting the lesion invisible at CT or if CT findings are inconclusive or when the patient is only suspected of having the lesion at CT [21]. In these cases in fact a *simple* US can cover the role of problem solving, in the same examination session, as the lesion can usually be immediately detected owing to its hypoechoic appearance and better conspicuity (Figs. 8.2-8.4) [17]. Hence

the integration of different imaging modalities is sometimes better for tumor detection yet in the first examination session to gain faster diagnosis [1].

The sensitivity and specificity of US in the detection of pancreatic adenocarcinoma varies in the medical literature, owing to the obvious impact of operator experience on the results. The mean sensitivity ranges from 72% to 98%, lower than that reported for CT, whereas specificity exceeds 90% [8, 17, 23, 24].

Regarding size, tumors smaller than 1 cm and limited to the ductal epithelium are considered early pancreatic duct adenocarcinoma [25, 26]. The imaging method with the highest possible resolution to visualize pancreatic tumors is endoscopic ultrasound (EUS), which takes advantage of the direct exploration of the gland [27-31]. Consequently all the described aspects of US detection of

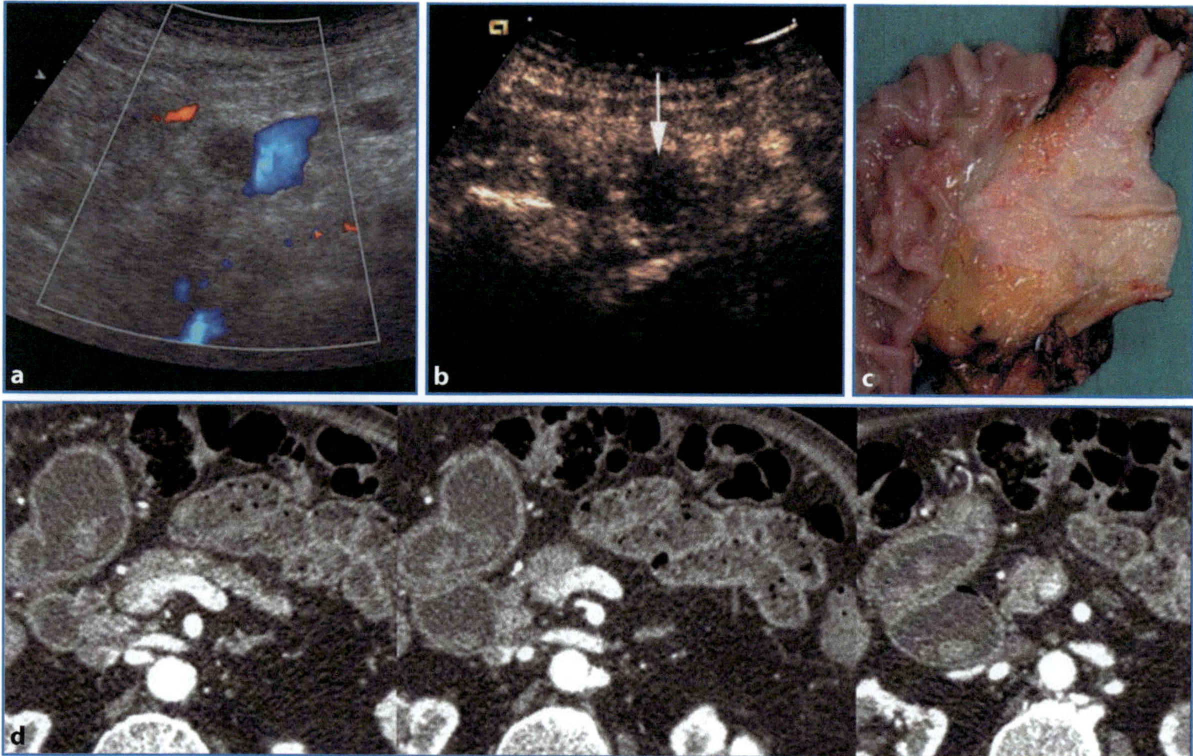

Fig. 8.4 a-d Pancreatic adenocarcinoma. US (**a**) direct identification of a ductal adenocarcinoma of the pancreatic neck appearing hypoechoic next to the superior mesenteric vein (*blue*) and hypoenhancing (*arrow*) at CEUS (**b**). Diagnosis of adenocarcinoma confirmed at pathology (**c**). The tumor is isoattenuating at CT (**d**)

pancreatic adenocarcinoma give better results. Tumors even smaller than 5 mm can be detected [8]. However, EUS cannot be used as a screening imaging method because of its mini-invasive approach. In addition, the procedure is complex to perform and different results have been reported in the literature, also in this case strongly correlated with the experience of the investigator [32, 33].

Even though the detection of pancreatic adenocarcinoma is a crucial point, most of the up to date diagnostic imaging methods show good sensitivity in an otherwise unchanged gland. The real problem for the differential diagnosis arises when the pancreatic tissue shows inflammatory changes. In comparative studies, the specificity of the major diagnostic tools are as low as 60-80%, not enough to guide clinical decisions [27]. Thus, the main efforts nowadays should focus on appropriate selection of the patient population at risk of developing pancreatic cancer requiring adequate diagnostic methods rather than increasing resolution of the imaging method.

At US, pancreatic adenocarcinoma almost always presents as a solid and markedly hypoechoic mass (Fig. 8.5) in comparison to the adjacent pancreatic parenchyma due to the very low US acoustic impedance of the tumor [3]. The main pancreatic duct is often infiltrated and dilated upstream. A tumor located in the pancreatic head also determines the dilation of the common bile duct (*double-duct sign*) [34, 35]. Thus, the identification of duct dilation with abrupt cutoff has to be considered a secondary sign suspicious of pancreatic cancer. Moreover due to the fact that the most common pancreatic tumor is the adenocarcinoma and most of them are localized in the head of the gland, a dilated pancreatic duct with abrupt cutoff is the most important sign for early detection even if the tumor itself cannot be visualized [36]. As a consequence, patients with unexplained dilatation of the pancreatic duct with abrupt cutoff should be referred to more specific imaging methods.

The newer US applications able to evaluate tissue stiffness could be used in the near future also to detect pancreatic lesions not visible at conventional US based on differences in acoustic impedance with respect to the adjacent parenchyma (Fig. 8.6).

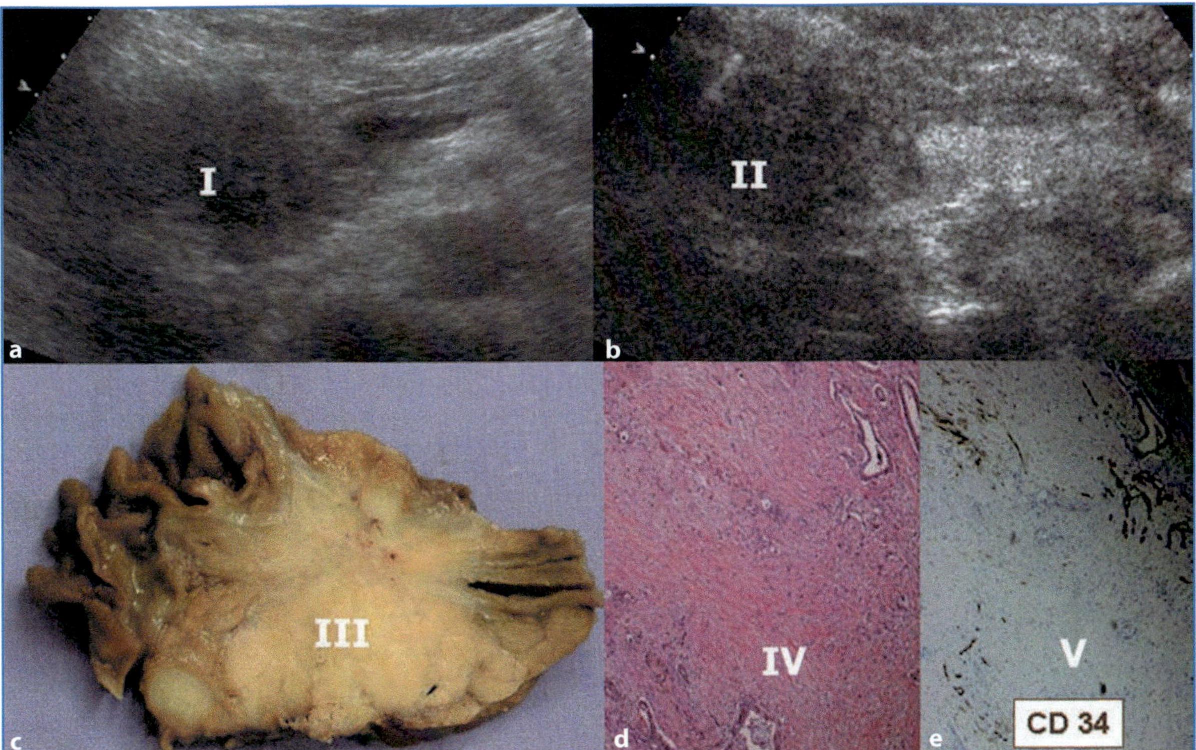

Fig. 8.5 a-e Pancreatic adenocarcinoma. US: hypoechoic pancreatic head mass (**a**). CEUS: hypovascular pancreatic head mass (**b**). Pathology: adenocarcinoma of the pancreas with marked desmoplasia (**c**), high fibrous changes (**d**) and low mean vascular density (**e**) at CD34 immunohistochemical staining

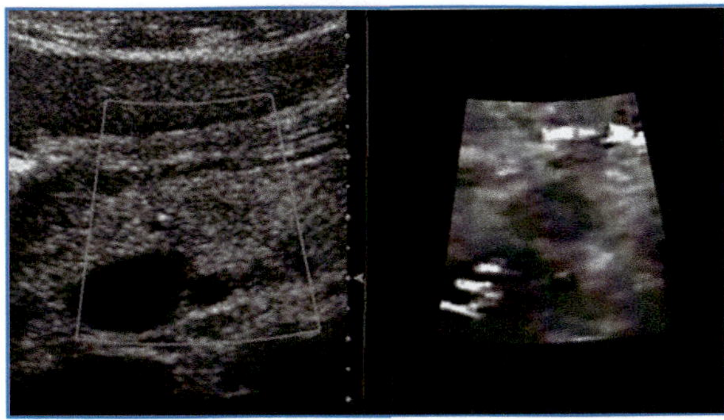

Fig. 8.6 Small focal pancreatic lesion. Isoechoic small pancreatic focal lesion detected at ARFI US imaging

8.3.2 Characterization and Differential Diagnosis

Pancreatic adenocarcinoma, as previously reported, typically presents at conventional US as a solid hypoechoic lesion with upstream dilation of the main pancreatic duct. The tumor is characterized by infiltrative margins and early diffusion of the tumor in the adjacent parenchyma and structures, justifying the often lack of clear-cut margins at US [1, 3]. As a result, sometimes the lesion can be difficult to identify or delineate. Harmonic US and compound techniques may improve the correct identification of the margins of the tumor [4]. The *double duct sign* can be observed in the presence of lesions located in the pancreatic head [34]. In highly aggressive form, necrosis and liquefaction are common, resulting from the difference between tumor growth rate and formation of new microvessels from neoangiogenesis [1]. The necrotic/liquid part of the tumor is mainly located centrally.

Real-time elastography [Hitachi Medical Systems, Tokyo, Japan] is a real-time technique able to improve the differential diagnosis between pancreatic lesions, displaying the mechanical hardness of examined tissues thus providing important additional information [31, 37, 38]. Basically, as a result of marked desmoplasia which is very often present in pancreatic adenocarci-

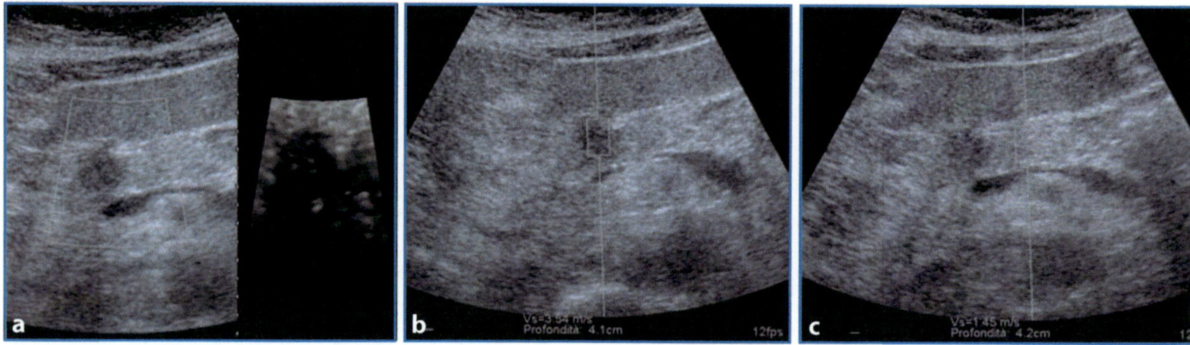

Fig. 8.7 a-c Small pancreatic adenocarcinoma. US incidental detection of a pancreatic small stiff (*black*) hypoechoic nodule at ARFI imaging (**a**) with high wave velocity value (Vs=3.54) at ARFI quantification (**b**) in respect to the normal adjacent pancreatic parenchyma (**c**)

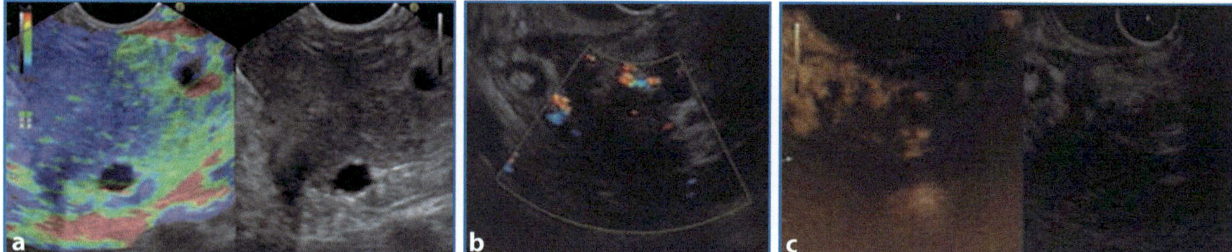

Fig. 8.8 a-c Dynamic study using high and low mechanical index (MI) CE-EUS and endoscopic elastography of pancreatic adenocarcinoma. **a** Elastography of a pancreatic carcinoma, the dense structure of the carcinoma is shown in blue codification of the elastography. **b** Only few vessels are visible using high MI CE-EUS in color-Doppler mode. **c** Poor enhancement of the lesion using low MI CE-EUS

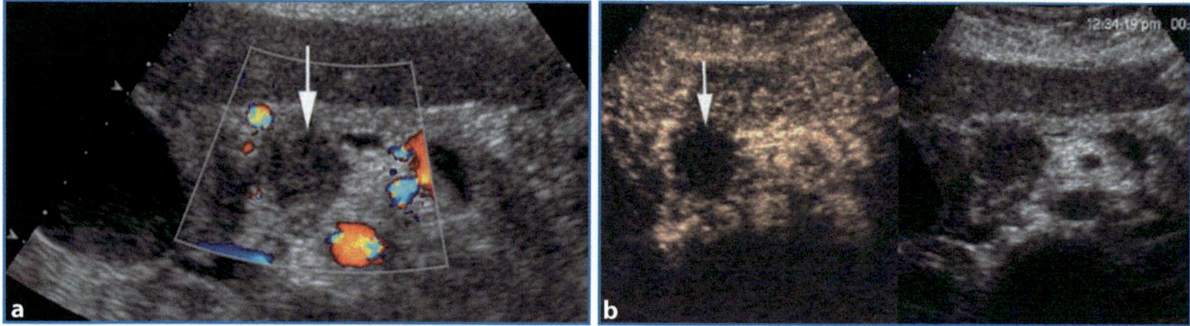

Fig. 8.9 a,b Pancreatic adenocarcinoma. Hypoechoic pancreatic head mass (*arrow*) without intralesional vascular signals at color-Doppler examination (**a**) appearing typically markedly hypovascular, hypoenhancing (*arrow*) at CEUS (**b**)

noma, the tumor appears stiff at transabdominal (Fig. 8.7) and endoscopic (Fig. 8.8) elastographic evaluation [1, 39, 40]. The quantitative analysis i.e. by means of Virtual touch tissue quantification (Siemens, Erlangen, Germany), makes the results more objective and reproducible. The wave velocity value measured inside a pancreatic ductal adenocarcinoma is higher (usually >3 m/s; Fig. 8.7) than that in the adjacent parenchyma (mean value in the healthy pancreas of 1.4 m/s) [1, 6].

At Doppler study, the detection of tumor vessels within the lesion often characterizes hypervascular masses (i.e. endocrine tumors), while no tumor vessels are usually observed within hypovascular ones, such as pancreatic ductal adenocarcinoma (Fig. 8.9) [5, 41].

Table 8.1 Accuracy of hypoenhancement as a sign of ductal adenocarcinoma

	Sensitivity [%]	Specificity [%]	PPV [%]	NPV [%]	Accuracy [%]
Hypoenhancemement as a sign of adenocarcinoma	90.0 (80.5-95.9)	100 (91.6-100)	100 (94.3-100)	85.7 (72.8-94.1)	93.8 (87.6-97.5)
Hyperenhancement as a sign of non-adenocarcinoma	100 (91.6-100)	90.0 (80.5-95.9)	85.7 (72.8-94.1)	100 (94.3-100)	93.8 (87.6-97.5)

The introduction of contrast agents has significantly strengthened US, increasing the accuracy of the first-line examination in the characterization of pancreatic tumors (especially pancreatic adenocarcinoma) [12, 42-45]. To discriminate between the most common focal pancreatic lesions, transabdominal and EUS studies with contrast agents achieve similar results [1, 46-48].

Ductal adenocarcinoma shows poor enhancement in all phases at transabdominal (Figs. 8.1, 8.5, 8.9) and contrast-enhanced EUS (CE-EUS) (Fig. 8.8). In fact the mean vascular density (MVD) is low and often inferior to the normal pancreatic parenchyma [12, 49, 50]. The marked desmoplasia (Fig. 8.5) and the low MVD of the lesion, together with the presence of necrosis or mucin justify the typical imaging features [12]. So at CEUS ductal adenocarcinoma typically presents as a hypoenhancing mass (Figs. 8.5, 8.9) compared to the adjacent parenchyma. This pattern is present in about 90% of cases [43, 51, 52]. As reported in the PA-MUS multicenter study (Pancreatic Multicenter Ultrasound Study) among the 987 adenocarcinomas included, 891 (90%) were hypovascular [52]. In a personal series of 112 solitary undetermined pancreatic masses, the hypoenhancemement as a sign of ductal adenocarcinoma showed a sensitivity of 90%, specificity of 100% and an accuracy of 93.8% (Table 8.1).

The MVD of pancreatic adenocarcinoma is influenced by different degrees of tumor differentiation. It has been shown that the enhancement pattern at CEUS correlates with tumor differentiation, aggressiveness and prognosis [12]. In particular, a markedly hypovascular pattern with avascular intratumoral areas identifies undifferentiated adenocarcinoma. And for this reason, this pattern of enhancement appears as a useful parameter for preoperative prognostic stratification. Moreover, CEUS can demonstrate changes in tumor vascularity during chemotherapy, raising the hope for a future application in clinical practice [49, 53].

Moreover, during CEUS examination tumor margins and size are better visible (Fig. 8.10), as well as the relations with peripancreatic arterial and venous vessels

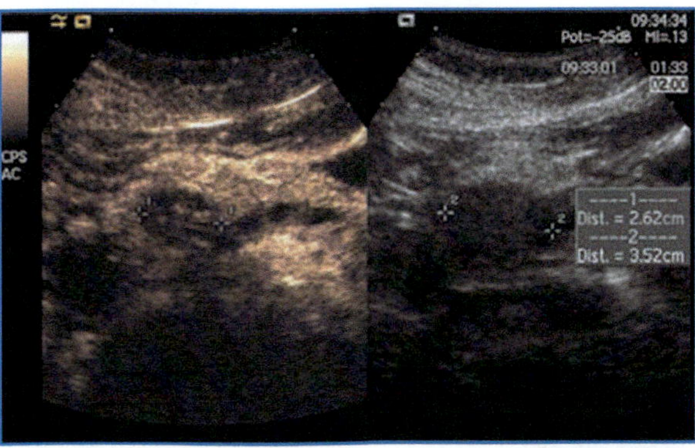

Fig. 8.10 Pancreatic adenocarcinoma. Pancreatic head mass hypoechoic at US (*right*) and hypoenhancing at CEUS (*left*) with different dimension (diameter 1 vs 2) at the two examinations

for local staging and presence of metastatic lesions for liver staging [1, 44, 45, 54, 55].

Compared to US, CEUS can also improve the differential diagnosis between mass-forming pancreatitis and pancreatic adenocarcinoma. In particular, while ductal adenocarcinoma remains hypoenhanced during all the dynamic phases, the inflammatory mass shows a parenchymal enhancement, as reported by published data from the Verona group [56]. The presence of a parenchymal enhancement somewhat similar to that of the adjacent pancreas during the dynamic study is therefore a CEUS finding consistent with an inflammatory origin. The intensity of this parenchymal enhancement is related to the length of the underlying inflammatory process [57]: the more chronic and long-standing the inflammatory process, the less intense the intralesional parenchymal enhancement. It is likely that this is related to the entity of the associated fibrosis. In contrast, in acute mass-forming pancreatitis the enhancement is usually more intense and prolonged [56].

It can be concluded that the use of CEUS can increase the differential diagnosis between pancreatic lesions by far and should be recommended in patients with a visualization of the gland at US. Contrast enhanced transabdominal and EUS are nowadays reported

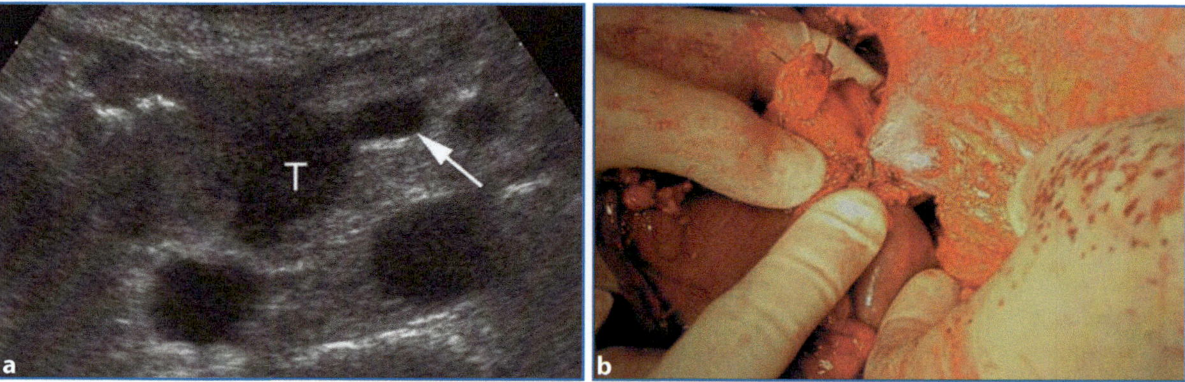

Fig. 8.11 a,b Local staging of pancreatic adenocarcinoma. **a** US local staging of a hypoechoic pancreatic head mass (*T*) infiltrating the superior mesenteric vein (*arrow*) with focal disappearance of the echoic interface between the tumor and the lumen of the vessel. **b** Intraoperative confirmation of a neoplastic tangential infiltration of the superior mesenteric vein

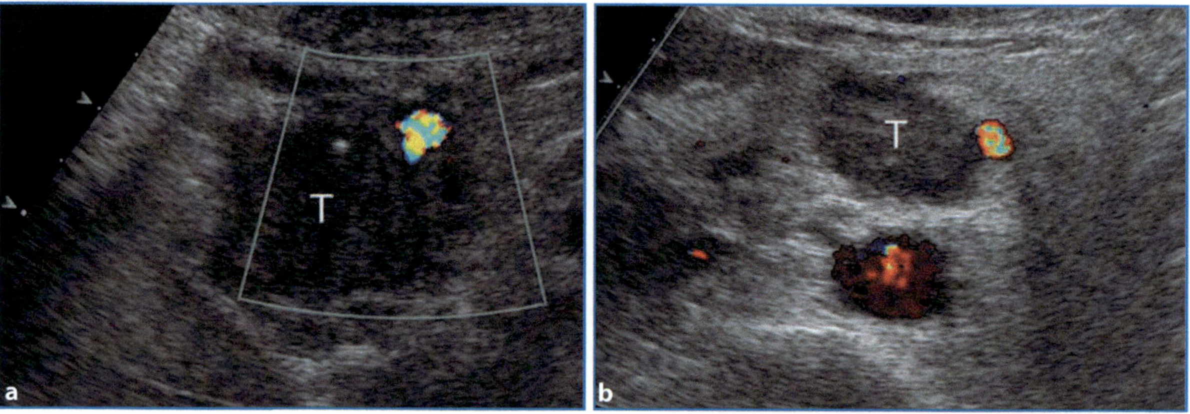

Fig. 8.12 a,b Local staging of pancreatic adenocarcinoma. **a** Color-Doppler US local staging of a hypoechoic pancreatic head mass (*T*) infiltrating the superior mesenteric vein (*colored*) with typical teardrop deformation. **b** Color-Doppler US local staging of a hypoechoic pancreatic head mass (*T*) infiltrating the superior mesenteric artery (*colored*)

in the literature as valuable imaging methods for the characterization of pancreatic lesions.

In summary, at CEUS examination pancreatic ductal adenocarcinoma usually presents as an ill-defined mass, showing poor enhancement in all dynamic phases. So a solid hypovascular pancreatic mass at CEUS has to be considered a ductal adenocarcinoma until proven otherwise.

8.3.3 Local and Liver Staging

The pancreatic study must include the evaluation of the adjacent vascular structures, mainly to distinguish between resectable and non-resectable lesions. The preserved echogenic fatty interface between tumor and vessels or a short contiguity between them suggest the resectability of the lesion, whereas the infiltration or compression or encasement imply unresectability, especially from an oncologic point of view [17, 58-61].

At conventional US, the vascular invasion is defined by a focal disappearance of the echogenic interface (Fig. 8.11) forming the vessel wall, or by a narrow lumen [1]. In cases of pancreatic head tumor, the simple evaluation of the site of potential resection for a duodenopancreatectomy can immediately indicate unresectability. In particular, if the dilated pancreatic duct stops at the same level as the superior mesenteric vein the pancreatic neck can be involved making pancreatic resection unsafe at this level.

To improve the visualization of tumor margins and

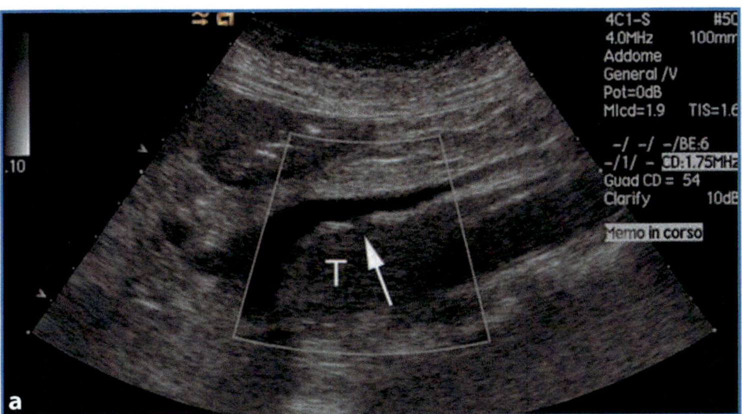
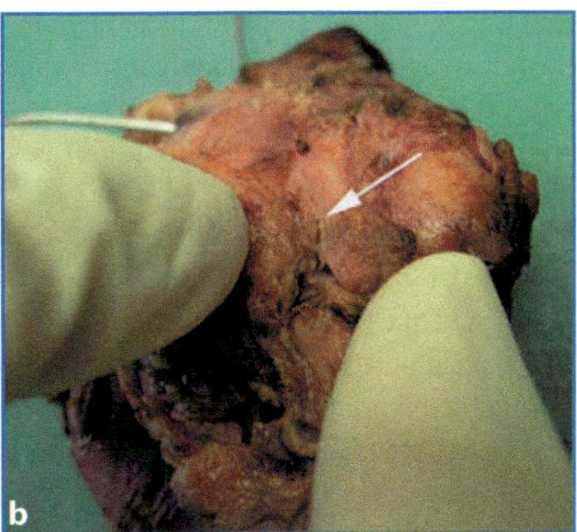

Fig. 8.13 a,b Local staging of pancreatic adenocarcinoma. a Doppler based US imaging of a hypoechoic head-uncinate process pancreatic mass (*T*) infiltrating the superior mesenteric vein with millimetric focal disappearance (*arrow*) of the echoic interface between the tumor and the lumen of the vessel. b Confirmation on the specimen of the focal tumoral infiltration resulting in a millimetric interruption (*arrow*) of the surface for the superior mesenteric vein

vessel walls, harmonic, compound and Doppler-based imaging can be used; the aim is not only to gain the best visualization of the tumor margins but also to gain a better evaluation of the relationship between them and major peripancreatic vessels (Fig. 8.12). At harmonic and compound imaging the conspicuity of the lesion is increased with a better delineation of the tumor, while some Doppler based imaging such as Clarify Vascular Enhancement (Acuson, Siemens) enhances the B-mode display with information derived from power-Doppler, clearly differentiating vascular anatomy from acoustic artifacts and surrounding tissue (Fig. 8.13) [59, 62].

At Doppler, localized aliasing and mosaic pattern are waveform changes due to increased flow velocities and turbulent blood flow at the site of a vascular stenosis, due to the presence of a pancreatic lesion involvement, which can be confirmed with duplex Doppler interrogation [60, 61]. Downstream from the infiltrated tract the flow velocity decreases, with the typical *parvus et tardus* waveform [17]. However, these hemodynamic changes usually occur in advanced tumors only, when vascular involvement is usually obvious at grey scale as well. Color-Doppler has contributed to assessing the involvement of the major peripancreatic arteries and of the portal venous system. The arterial infiltration of the tumor can involve the superior mesenteric, the splenic, celiac, hepatic and left renal arteries, in descending order of frequency. Venous involvement can affect the superior mesenteric, splenic, portal and left renal veins. In the presence of tumor encasement of the superior mesenteric vein, changes in blood flow velocity at Doppler study can be detected.

However, a normal waveform does not exclude infiltration of the superior mesenteric and portal veins [1].

Several studies have evaluated the role of color-Doppler in assessing the arterial involvement by pancreatic cancer, suggesting its accuracy greater than gray-scale US [5, 17, 58-60]. In fact, color-Doppler US allows recognition of vessels that are barely visible with grey scale US because of small caliber or deep location.

Combining grey scale and color-Doppler US, sensitivity, specificity, and overall accuracy of 79%, 89%, and 84% have been reported for the diagnosis of vascular involvement from pancreatic tumor [5]. When involvement of the portal vein is considered, sensitivity, specificity and overall accuracy of 74%, 95%, and 89% have been reported [60]. When in contrast only peripancreatic arteries are considered, sensitivity of 60%, specificity of 93% and overall accuracy of 87% were found [63]. Most false negative results occur in patients with limited venous involvement of the portal-mesenteric junction [5].

New technologies that use digitally encoding techniques to suppress tissue clutter and improve sensitivity for direct visualization of blood reflectors have been developed such as Bflow imaging (GE Medical Systems Co., Milwaukee, WI, USA) and eflow imaging (Aloka, Tokyo, Japan) [5]. The weak signals from blood echoes are enhanced and correlated with the corresponding signals of the adjacent frames to suppress non-moving tissues. The rest of the data processing is essentially the same as in conventional grey-scale imaging. In comparison with Doppler techniques these new US flow imaging modalities are not affected by aliasing and have the advantages of a significantly lower angle dependency and better spatial resolution with reduced overwriting [64]. As a consequence, evaluation of vessel profiles is markedly improved.

Usually tumor involvement of adjacent vessels established by means of US and Doppler study can be confirmed at CEUS. CEUS is reported to be very useful in establishing non-resectable patients already considered resectable on primary radiologic image material [65].

Moreover at CEUS, the evaluation of the whole liver is mandatory after pancreatic study [45, 55]. The late phase of enhancement, 120 s after bolus injection, is the best for the detection of metastatic liver lesions and each solid hypoechoic focal liver lesion detected during the late phase should be considered a metastasis until otherwise proven [45, 54, 55].

8.4   Neuroendocrine Tumor

Pancreatic neuroendocrine tumors or islet cell tumors arise from the neuroendocrine cells of the pancreas. These tumors are classified as functioning or non(hyper)functioning based on the presence or absence of symptoms related to hormone production. Insulinomas and gastrinomas are the most common functioning islet cell tumors and are usually small at the time of diagnosis [1, 66]. Insulinomas are usually benign and solitary lesions, while gastrinomas tend to be larger, malignant and multiple. Nonfunctioning tumors are frequently large at presentation and often malignant [67].

The diagnosis is usually based on clinical and biochemical work-up. Diagnostic imaging is needed to localize the tumor and to study the relations with vital structures for potential surgical resection. Abdominal US can detect only about 60% of isolated islet cell tumors. Better results in tumor detection are reported for EUS [67].

8.4.1   Functioning

Insulinomas are the most frequently found functioning neuroendocrine tumor of the pancreas (about 60% of all neuroendocrine tumors) and in the majority of cases are benign (85-99%) and solitary (93-98%) [3]. Preop-

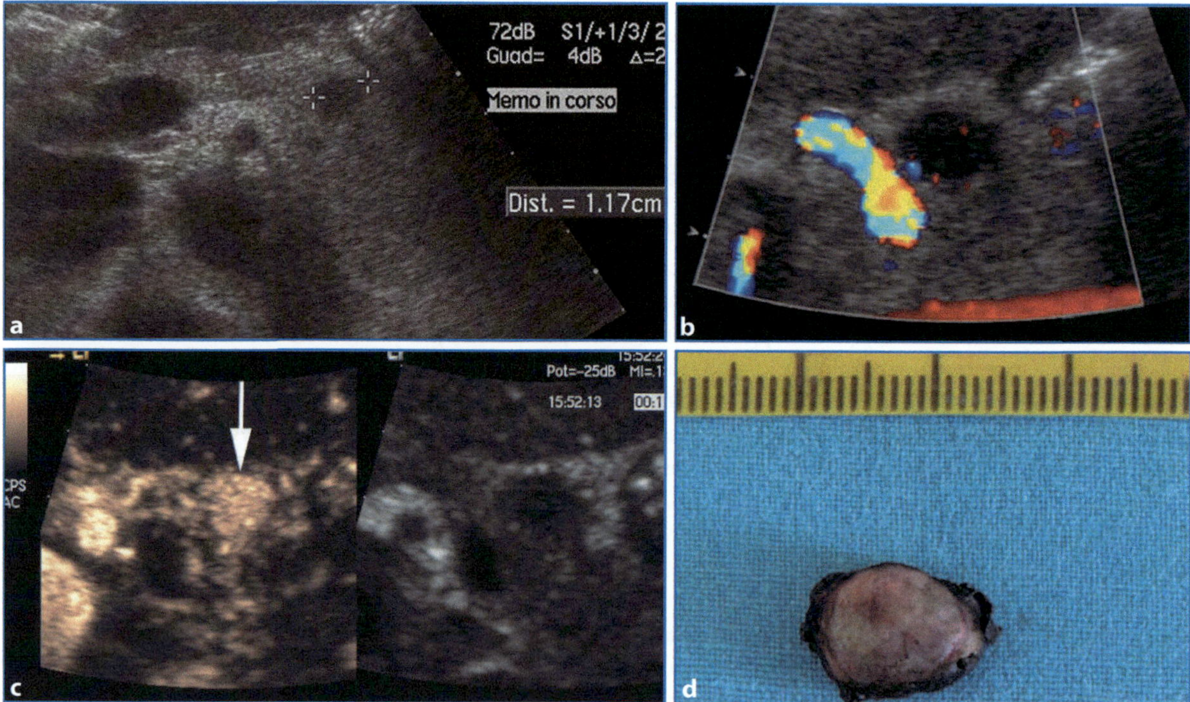

Fig. 8.14 a-d Pancreatic insulinoma. US (**a**) detection of a small hypoechoic nodule (*caliper*) with small intralesional vessels at color-Doppler evaluation (**b**). At CEUS (**c**) the nodule is hypervascular hypoenhancing (*arrow*) in the early dynamic phases. Resected specimen (**d**) with final diagnosis of insulinoma

erative US detection of insulinomas is sometimes difficult but possible. The US detection rate of insulinomas has steadily increased in recent years, thanks to the increase in spatial, lateral and contrast resolution provided by technologic developments [68]. The majority of insulinomas appear at US as hypoechoic nodules, usually capsulated, and hyperenhancing at CEUS (Fig. 8.14). Sometimes very small calcifications can be present, especially in the larger lesions [66, 67]. At the time of clinical presentation 50% of the tumors are smaller than 1.5 cm [68, 69]. When rarely malignant, they are generally greater than 3 cm and about a third of these have metastases at the time of diagnosis [3].

Gastrinomas are the second most frequently found functioning neuroendocrine tumors of the pancreas (about 20% of all neuroendocrine tumors) and differ from insulinomas by site, size and vascularity [1, 69, 70]. They occur within the gastrinoma triangle (junction of the cystic duct and common bile duct – junction of the second and third parts of duodenum – junction of the head and neck of the pancreas) of which only the pancreatic side can be correctly explored by US [3]. Identification of pancreatic gastrinomas can be easy considering their moderate size. Liver metastases are present in 60% of cases at the time of diagnosis [69].

The other functioning neuroendocrine tumors (VIPoma, glucagonoma and somatostatinoma) are rare; all together they account for about 20% of the functioning neuroendocrine tumors of the pancreas [67-69].

8.4.2 Non(hyper)functioning

Nonfunctioning islet cell tumors (NFETs) account for up to 33% of the neuroendocrine tumors of the pancreas ranging from 1 to 20 cm in diameter and showing a high malignancy rate, up to 90% [7]. They are, however, less aggressive than ductal adenocarcinoma. The clinical presentation of NFETs is nonspecific being due to the mass effect. In fact, these tumors, predominantly characterized by expansive growth, are clinically silent until adjacent viscera and structures are involved [67]. At US they appear well marginated and usually easy to detect thanks to their large size which justify their tendency to necrosis and hemorrhage giving them a typical nonhomogeneous appearance, sometimes with very small internal calcifications [4, 66, 71]. Larger nonfunctioning islet cell tumors show cystic degeneration or cystic change [69]. A well-organized relationship between neoplastic cells and neovessels travelling into the tumor stroma exists and

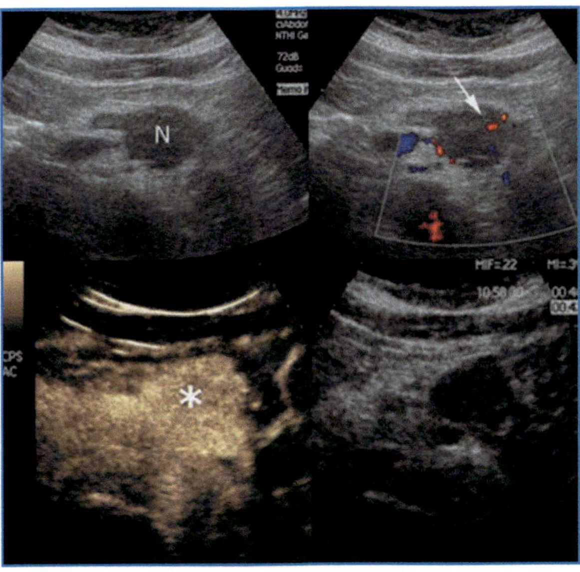

Fig. 8.15 Non hyperfunctionning neuroendocrine tumor. US: solid hypoechoic mass (*N*) of the pancreatic body. Color-Doppler US: small intralesional vessels (*arrow*). CEUS: hypervascular mass (*) of the pancreatic body

explains the hypervascular pattern [72]. For this reason the characterization depends on the demonstration of their hypervascularity [70-72]. Imaging differential diagnosis between NFETs and ductal adenocarcinoma is fundamental for therapeutic strategy and prognosis. At color- and power-Doppler US a *spotted pattern* can be demonstrated inside the endocrine tumors [5]. However, Doppler *silence* can be present in hypervascular endocrine tumors because of the small size of the lesion or of the tumor vascular network [1, 5]. At CEUS different enhancement patterns can be observed in relation to the size of the tumor and its vessels [42]. NFETs show a rapid intense enhancement in the early dynamic phases at transabdominal (Fig. 8.15) and endoscopic (Fig. 8.16) CEUS, with exclusion of the necrotic intralesional areas, and microbubble entrapment in the late phase [42, 70]. In moderate-size tumors a capillary blush enhancement can be present in the early phase, mirroring the most characteristic angiographic feature of these tumors [72]. Considering that the characterization of NFETs at imaging is mainly linked to their frequent hypervascularity, a high sensitivity in the detection of tumor macrocirculation and microcirculation is required [42, 71]. Last but not least, nonfunctioning neuroendocrine tumors can be hypovascular [70]. This is directly related to the amount of stroma inside the lesion which is dense and hyalinized. However,

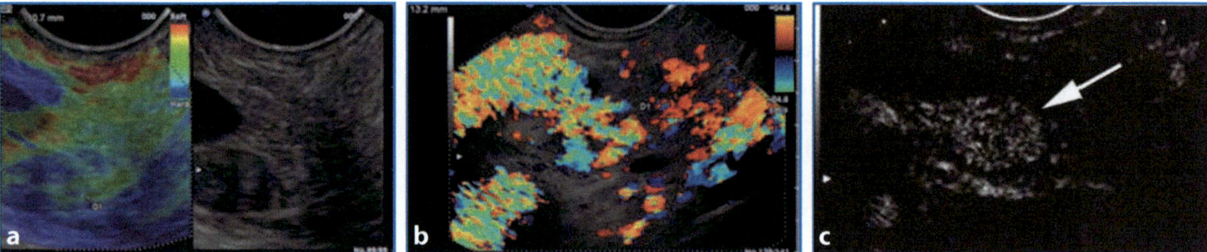

Fig. 8.16 a-c Dynamic study using high and low mechanical index (MI) contrast-enhanced endosonography and endoscopic elastography of neuroendocrine tumor. **a** Elastography of a neuroendocrine tumor: the tumor shows a dense structure in relation to the surrounding pancreas. **b** High MI CE-EUS: many microvessels are visible using color-Doppler mode. **c** Low MI CE-EUS: hypervascular appearance of the lesion (*arrow*) resulting hyperechoic

in some pancreatic neuroendocrine tumors appearing hypodense at dynamic CT, a clear enhancement is visible at CEUS [70]. The high capability of CEUS in demonstrating pancreatic tumor vascularity is a result of the high resolution power of the state-of-the-art US imaging, combined with the size and the distribution (blood pool) of the microbubbles [1, 30]. CEUS may improve identification and characterization of endocrine tumors allowing an accurate locoregional and hepatic staging as reported by Malagò et al. [72]. In the same paper, the authors reported good positive correlation between CEUS pattern and Ki67 index, which is considered the most reliable independent predictor of tumor malignancy. A prognostic stratification based on CEUS evaluation of whole tumor could therefore be considered.

8.5 Incidental Solid Pancreatic Lesion: Risk Factor and Management

At conventional US the detection of a solid hypoechoic mass in the pancreatic gland should be considered a ductal adenocarcinoma until proven otherwise, so requiring rapid and adequate management. However, US can occasionally still be not accurate in defining the solid or cystic nature of the lesion.

CEUS is a safe and feasible imaging method to better characterize pancreatic lesions immediately after US detection. At US the detection of a focal pancreatic lesion requires a first mandatory differentiation between its solid or cystic nature and CEUS is able to best solve this task (Fig. 8.17), thus playing a key role in the management of patients.

A solid lesion requires multidetector computed tomography (MDCT) confirmation, while a cystic lesion

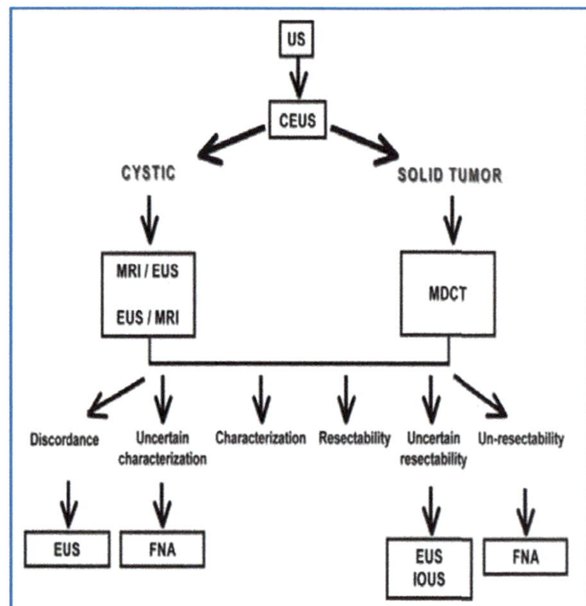

Fig. 8.17 CEUS in the work-up algorithm proposed for focal pancreatic tumors detected at conventional ultrasonography

should be investigated with MRI. Therefore, the injection of contrast agents can improve the accuracy of the first line investigation. Immediate diagnosis is very important especially when dealing with pancreatic ductal adenocarcinoma [1].

Pancreatic ductal adenocarcinoma typically shows poor enhancement during all the dynamic phases. Therefore, at CEUS the detection of a solid hypoechoic, hypovascular mass in the pancreatic gland has to be considered a ductal adenocarcinoma until proven otherwise. After immediate and mandatory CT staging, surgical treatment can be more rapidly applied.

8.6 Special Topics

8.6.1 Mean Vascular Density (MVD) of Solid Tumor and Microvessel

CEUS is the only imaging method able to provide a real-time evaluation of enhancement throughout all the dynamic phases [1]. Real-time evaluation of enhancement is possible by maintaining the same scanning frame rate of the previous conventional B-mode examination [42]. Dynamic observation of the contrast-enhanced phases (early arterial, arterial, pancreatic, portal/venous and late/sinusoidal phases) begins immediately after the injection of a second generation contrast medium.

Pancreatic solid lesions, even if poorly vascular or characterized by rapid-flow circulation, always show intratumoral micro- and macrovasculature. Taking advantage of a continuous observation of the contrast-enhanced phases, CEUS allows a real-time study of the tumor vascular network [1]. As a consequence, the study of tumor vasculature shows better results at CEUS than at CT [73]. Moreover, the correlation between CEUS pattern and MVD of pancreatic tumors can be so strong that a prognostic stratification, based on CEUS features, can be proposed both for ductal adenocarcinoma [11] and endocrine tumors [70]. In fact, association between MVD and tumor aggressiveness has been already proved: markedly hypovascular lesions, usually characterized by necrotic degeneration, turn out to be undifferentiated at pathology and having a worse prognosis [1].

To obtain a more objective evaluation of tumor perfusion at CEUS, a quantification analysis can nowadays be obtained directly on the US scanner (Fig. 8.18). The resulting color maps (Fig. 8.19) actually seem very similar to those obtained at perfusion CT.

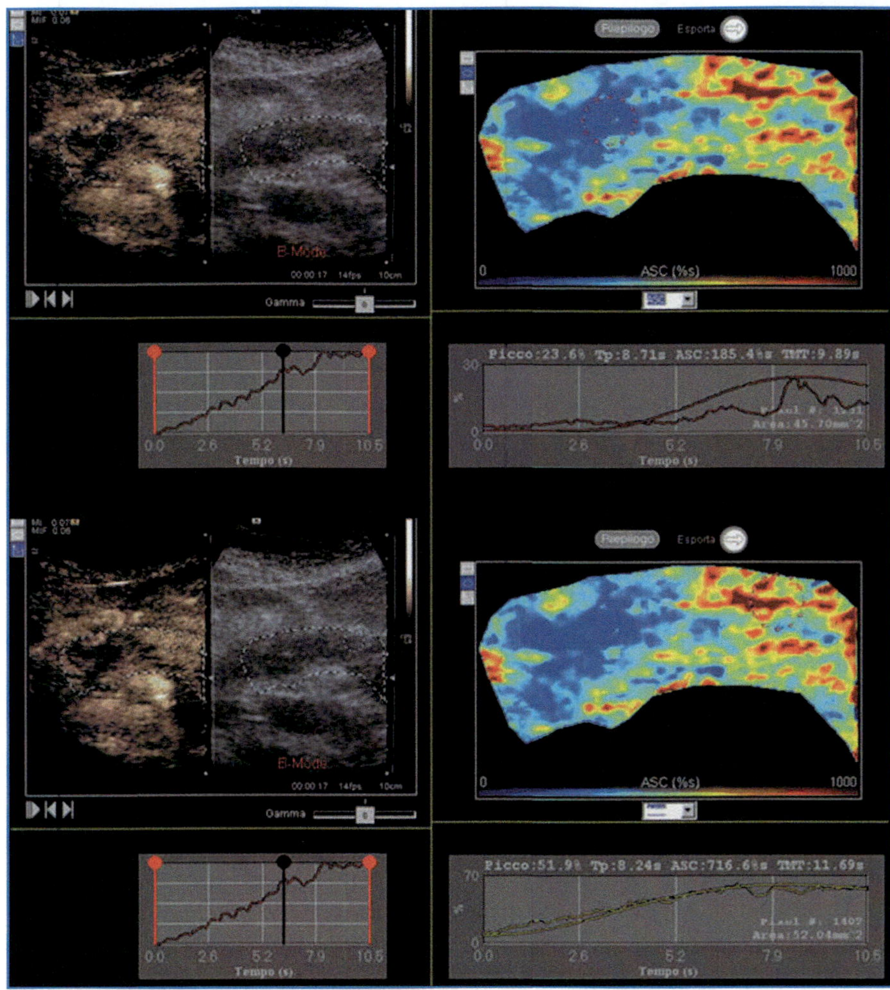

Fig. 8.18 Pancreatic adenocarcinoma: quantitative perfusion analysis at CEUS. The pancreatic tumor (blue colored on the maps) shows low enhancement (ROI placed in the tumor) in respect to the adjacent parenchyma (ROI placed in the pancreas), thus providing an objective characterization of the lesion based on the evaluation of tumor vascularity

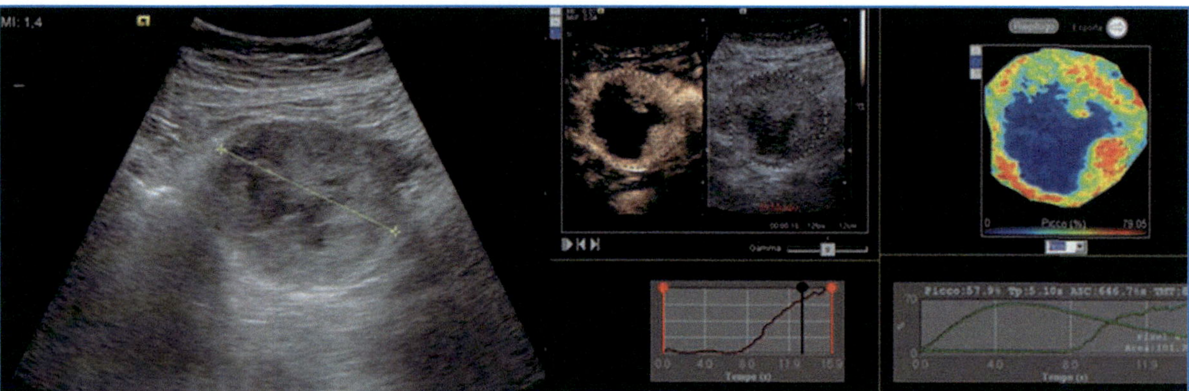

Fig. 8.19 Non-hyperfunctioning neuroendocrine tumor of the pancreas: quantitative perfusion analysis at CEUS. Pancreatic head mass with large necrotic avascular central area (*colored in blue on the map*); surrounded by viable neoplastic tissue irregular in thickness and vasculature (*colored in green and red on the map*). Enhancement quantification of the highest vascular portion of the tumor can be obtained by drafting a ROI in a selected area on the colored map

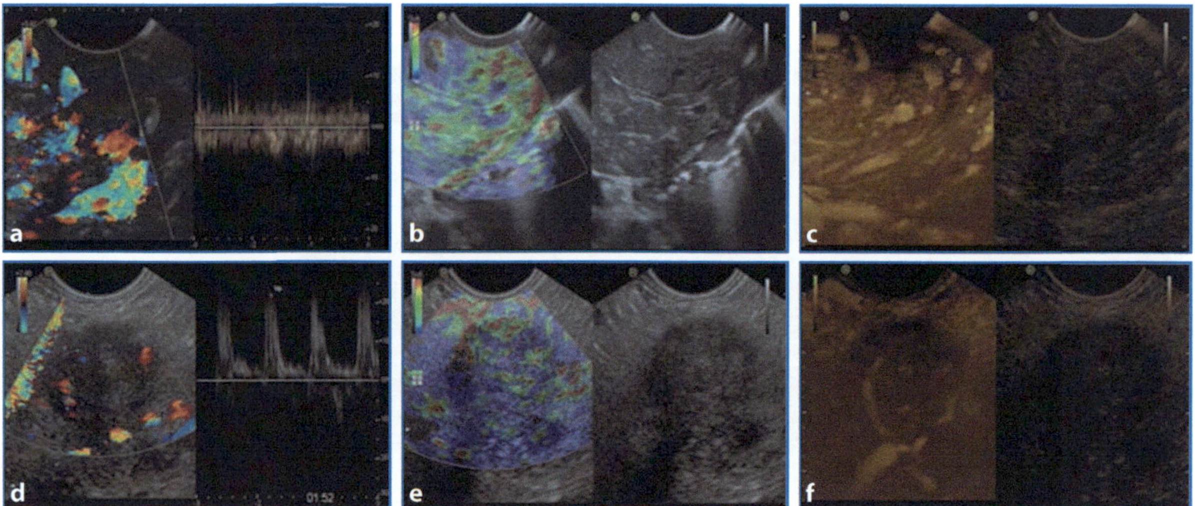

Fig. 8.20 a-f Differential diagnosis of pancreatic carcinoma and chronic pancreatitis. Chronic pancreatitis (**a-c**). CE-EUS in high MI Doppler mode with microvessel analysis (**a**), elastography (**b**) and CE-EUS in low MI mode (**c**): multiple vessels with venous signal in high MI mode, honeycomb pattern in elastography and contrast enhancing effect in low MI mode. Pancreatic adenocarcinoma (**d-f**). CE-EUS in high MI Doppler mode with microvessel analysis (**d**), elastography (**e**) and CE-EUS in low MI mode (**f**): only a few arterial vessels are visible using pulse waved Doppler mode, blue color meaning dense structure in elastography and non contrast enhancing effect in low MI mode

Microvessels in pancreatic tumor are generally hard to detect by unenhanced power or color-Doppler mode with the exception of lesion with neuroendocrine origin. However, US contrast enhancers can be used as signal improving agents in high mechanical color-Doppler mode especially during endoscopic study [47, 48]. Preliminary results were published by Bhutani et al. [74]. The advantage of EUS in comparison to all other diagnostic methods is the high resolution, allowing the description of the vessel system and the discrimination between arterial and venous vessels. This could open up new diagnostic possibilities. Chronic inflammatory pancreatic tissue can be differentiated from cancer tissue just by analyzing those microvessels [28, 75-77]. The typical finding of a chronic pancreatitis is a netlike rich vessel system with regular appearance and arterial and venous vessels side by side. On the other hand, the typical finding of pancreatic cancer is a rarefication of irregular

Table 8.2 Results of contrast enhanced endosonography regarding criteria of hyper- and hypovascularity as well as vessel structure and visibility of venous vessels

	Chronic pancreatitis	Pancreatic adenocarcinoma
Sum	73	121
Hypervascularity	55	28
Hypovascularity	18	93
Irregular vessels	21	97
Venous vessels	70	10

vessels and, using the contrast enhanced endoscopic Doppler mode, no visible venous vessels in the lesion. The visible difference between normal and cancerous vessels can be described by pathology as well [78]. However, no investigation about arterial or venous microvessels is ongoing due to the major difficulty in discriminating vessels in microscopic dimensions without immunostaining. The sensitivity and specificity of EUS in the discrimination of chronic pancreatitis could be improved to 91.7 and 95.9% using those criteria [48]. The results of our study are shown in Table 8.2.

The principle of the phenomenon consists of the invasive and compressive behavior of the pancreatic tumor. Therefore, the analysis of arterial and venous vessels by contrast enhanced Doppler US is a reliable method for discriminating chronic pancreatitis from pancreatic carcinoma (Fig. 8.20).

8.6.2 Pancreatic Intraepithelial Neoplasia (PanIN)

During the last few years due to the fatal prognosis of pancreatic carcinoma, great efforts have been made to investigate precursor lesions of invasive neoplasia. Pancreatic intraepithelial neoplasias (PanIN) have been recognized as precursor lesions of ductal adenocarcinoma, and are classified into different grades from PanIN-1 to PanIN-3 [79]. Molecular analyses have helped to define a progression model for pancreatic neoplasia. The most important step seems to be the occurrence of a PanIN-3 lesion which defines a high risk of malignant transformation [80].

PanIN-1A is a flat lesion with cylindrical epithelium with small round nuclei and plenty of supranuclear mucin. There is a broad overlap in histology to non-neoplastic lesions and neoplastic lesions without atypical epithelium.

PanIN-1B is an epithelial lesion with papillar and micropapillar structures and straight architecture, otherwise those lesions are comparable to the PanIN-1A lesions.

In PanIN-2 mucinous epithelial cells form flat lesions, but cell abnormalities are always present. The nuclei are enlarged and show signs of pseudo-stratifications. Mitosis is seldom.

PanIN-3 is a polypoid lesion in a papillary or micropapillary structure with signs of necrosis. The nuclei are often irregular and an increased mitosis rate is reported.

Whereas PanIN 1–2 lesions are invisible at EUS, there is a chance of visualizing PanIN-3 lesions due to the pancreatic duct irregularities (Fig. 8.21), which can be cytologically confirmed after fine needle aspiration [81].

As in PanINs, different types of intraductal papillary-mucinous neoplasms (IPMN) can be discriminated ranging from benign to invasive lesions. Becoming invasive, some of these tumors appear as ductal adenocarcinoma, others as colloid carcinoma with a much better prognosis [82, 83].

8.6.3 Autoimmune pancreatitis

The diagnosis of autoimmune pancreatitis (AIP) can be difficult in cases of tumor like lesions mimicking ductal adenocarcinoma of the pancreas. Real-time elas-

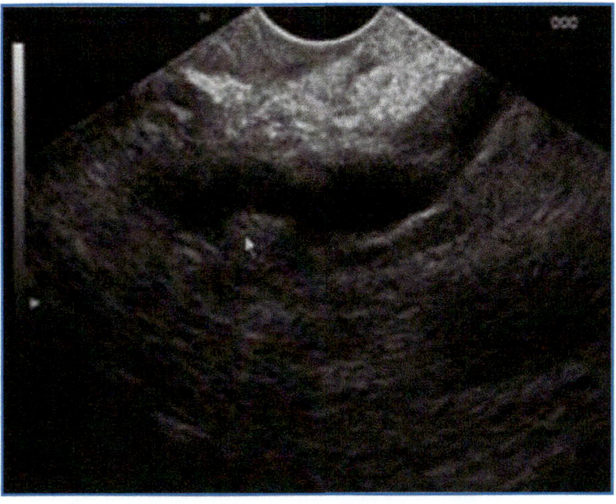

Fig. 8.21 PanIN-3. PanIN-3 lesion (*arrow*) visible in EUS

tography [84] is helpful in the differential diagnosis. Patients with AIP typically present with a unique pattern of mainly blue (stiff) colour signals not only in the tumour but also evenly spread over the surrounding pancreatic parenchyma. Using contrast enhanced ultrasound AIP is typically hyperenhancing [85, 86].

References

1. D'Onofrio M, Gallotti A, Pozzi Mucelli R (2010) Imaging techniques in pancreatic tumors. Expert Rev Med Devices 7:257-273
2. Sahani DV, Shan ZK, Catalano OA et al (2008) Radiology of pancreatic adenocarcinoma: current status of imaging. J Gastroenterol Hepatol 23:23-33. Review
3. Martinez-Noguera A, D'Onofrio M (2007) Ultrasonography of the pancreas. 1. Conventional imaging. Abdom Imaging 32:136-149
4. Hohl C, Schmidt T, Honnef D et al (2007) Ultrasonography of the pancreas. 2. Harmonic imaging. Abdom Imaging 32:150-160
5. Bertolotto M, D'Onofrio M, Martone E et al (2007) Ultrasonography of the pancreas. 3. Doppler imaging. Abdom Imaging 32(2):161-170
6. Gallotti A, D'Onofrio M, Pozzi Mucelli R (2010) Acoustic radiation force impulse (ARFI) technique in the ultrasound study with Virtual Touch tissue quantification of the superior abdomen. Radiol Med 115:889-897
7. Procacci C, Biasiutti C, Carbognin G et al (2001) Pancreatic neoplasms and tumor-like conditions. Eur Radiol 11[Suppl 2]:S167-S192
8. Schima W, Ba-Ssalamah A, Kölblinger C et al (2007) Pancreatic adenocarcinoma. Eur Radiol 17:638-649. Review
9. Cubilla AL, Fitzgerald PJ (1984) Tumors of the exocrine pancreas. 2nd Series Ed. Washington, DC: Armed Forces Institute of Pathology
10. O'Connor TP, Wade TP, Sunwoo YC et al (1992) Small cell undifferentiated carcinoma of the pancreas. Report of a patient with tumor marker studies. Cancer 70:1514-1519
11. Cameron JL (2001) Atlas of clinical oncology. Pancreatic Cancer. American Cancer Society. London, BC Decker Inc Hamilton
12. D'Onofrio M, Zamboni G, Malagò R et al (2009) Resectable pancreatic adenocarcinoma: is the enhancement pattern at contrast-enhanced ultrasonography a pre-operative prognostic factor? Ultrasound Med Biol 35:1929-1937
13. Nagakawa T, Mori K, Nakano T et al (1993) Perineural invasion of carcinoma of the pancreas and biliary tract. Br J Surg 80:619-621
14. Drapiewski JF (1994) Carcinoma of the pancreas: a study of neoplastic invasion of nerves and its possible clinical significance. Am J Clin Pathol 14:549-556
15. Martínez-Noguera A, Montserrat E, Torrubia S et al (2001) Ultrasound of the pancreas: update and controversies. Eur Radiol 11:1594-1606
16. Abu-Yousef MM, El-Zein Y (2000) Improved US visualization of the pancreatic tail with simethicone, water, and patient rotation. Radiology 217:780-785
17. Minniti S, Bruno C, Biasiutti C et al (2003) Sonography versus helical CT in identification and staging of pancreatic ductal adenocarcinoma. J Clin Ultrasound 31:175-182
18. Baron RL (1994) Understanding and optimizing use of contrast material for CT of the liver. Am J Roentgenol 163:323-331
19. Prokesch RW, Chow LC, Beaulieu CF et al (2002) Isoattenuating pancreatic adenocarcinoma at multi-detector row CT: secondary signs. Radiology 224:764-768
20. Yoon SH, Lee JM, Cho JY et al (2011= Small (<=20 mm) pancreatic adenocarcinomas: analysis of enhancement patterns and secondary signs with multiphasic multidetector CT. Radiology 259:442-452
21. Kim JH, Park SH, Yu ES et al (2010) Visually isoattenuating pancreatic adenocarcinoma at dynamic-enhanced CT: frequency, clinical and pathologic characteristics, and diagnosis at imaging examinations. Radiology 257:87-96
22. Barugola G, Partelli S, Marcucci S et al (2009) Resectable pancreatic cancer: who really benefits from resection? Ann Surg Oncol 16:3316-3322
23. Niederau C, Grendell JH (1992) Diagnosis of pancreatic carcinoma. Imaging techniques and tumor markers. Pancreas 7:66-86. Review
24. Karlson BM, Ekbom A, Lindgren PG et al (1999) Abdominal US for diagnosis of pancreatic tumor: prospective cohort analysis. Radiology 213:107-111
25. Rosewicz S, Wiedenman B (1997) Pancreatic carcinoma. Lancet 349:485-489
26. Ichikawa T, Haradome H, Hachiya J et al (1997) Pancreatic ductal adenocarcinoma: preoperative assessment with helical CT versus dynamic MR imaging. Radiology 202:655-662
27. Chaya CT, Bhutani MS (2007) Ultrasonography of the pancreas. 6. Endoscopic imaging Abdom Imaging 32:191-199
28. Brand B, Pfaff T, Binmoeller KF et al (2000) Endoscopic ultrasound for differential diagnosis of focal pancreatic lesions, confirmed by surgery. Scand J Gastroenterol 35:1221-1228
29. Dietrich CF, Jenssen C, Allescher HD et al (2008) Differential diagnosis of pancreatic lesions using endoscopic ultrasound. Z Gastroenterol 46:601-617
30. Becker D, Strobel D, Bernatik T et al (2001) Echo-enhanced color- and power-Doppler EUS for the discrimination between focal pancreatitis and pancreatic carcinoma. Gastrointest Endosc 53:784-789
31. Hirche TO, Ignee A, Barreiros AP et al (2008) Indications and limitations of endoscopic ultrasound elastography for evaluation of focal pancreatic lesions. Endoscopy 40:910-917
32. Muller MF, Meyenberger C, Bertschinger P et al (1994) Pancreatic tumors: evaluation with endoscopic US, CT, and MR imaging. Radiology 190:745-751
33. Mesihovic R, Vanis N, Husic-Selimovic A et al (2005) Evaluation of the diagnostic accuracy of the endoscopic ultrasonography results in the patients examined in a period of three years. Med Arh 2005;59:299-302
34. Menges M, Lerch MM, Zeitz M (2000) The double duct sign in patients with malignant and benign pancreatic lesions. Gastrointest Endosc 52:74-77
35. Dearden JC, Ayaru L, Wong V et al (2004) The double duct sign. Lancet 364:302
36. Tanaka S, Nakao M, Ioka T et al (2010) Slight dilatation of the main pancreatic duct and presence of pancreatic cysts as

predictive signs of pancreatic cancer: a prospective study. Radiology 254:965-972

37. Nightingale K, Soo MS, Nightingale R et al (2002) Acoustic radiation force impulse imaging, in vivo demonstration of clinical feasibility. Ultrasound Med Biol 28:227-235

38. Garra BS (2007) Imaging and estimation of tissue elasticity by ultrasound. Ultrasound Q 23:255-268

39. Giovannini M, Botelberge T, Bories E et al (2009) Endoscopic ultrasound elastography for evaluation of lymph nodes and pancreatic masses: a multicenter study. World J Gastroenterol 15:1587-1593

40. Saftoiu A, Vilmann P, Gorunescu F et al (2011) European EUS Elastography Multicentric Study Group. Accuracy of endoscopic ultrasound elastography used for differential diagnosis of focal pancreatic masses: a multicenter study. Endoscopy 43:596-603

41. Angeli E, Venturini M, Vanzulli A et al (1997) Color-Doppler imaging in the assessment of vascular involvement by pancreatic carcinoma. Am J Roentgenol 168:193-197

42. D'Onofrio M, Zamboni G, Faccioli N et al (2007) Ultrasonography of the pancreas. 4. Contrast-enhanced imaging. Abdom imaging 32:171-181

43. D'Onofrio, Martone E, Malagò R et al (2007) Contrast-enhanced ultrasonography of the pancreas. JOP 8[Suppl 1]:71-76

44. Faccioli N, D'Onofrio M, Zamboni G et al (2008) Resectable pancreatic adenocarcinoma, depiction of tumoral margins at contrast-enhanced ultrasonography. Pancreas 37:265-268

45. Claudon M, Cosgrove D, Albrecht T et al (2008) Guidelines and good clinical practice recommendations for contrast enhanced ultrasound (CEUS) - update 2008. Ultraschall Med 29:28-44

46. Dietrich CF, Braden B, Hocke M et al (2008) Improved characterisation of solitary solid pancreatic tumours using contrast enhanced transabdominal ultrasound. J Cancer Res Clin Oncol 134:635-643

47. Dietrich CF, Ignee A, Braden B et al (2008) Improved differentiation of pancreatic tumors using contrast-enhanced endoscopic ultrasound. Clin Gastroenterol Hepatol 6:590-597

48. Hocke M, Schmidt C, Zimmer B et al (2008) Contrast enhanced endosonography for improving differential diagnosis between chronic pancreatitis and pancreatic cancer. Dtsch Med Wochenschr 133:1888-1892

49. Numata K, Ozawa Y, Kobayashi N et al (2005) Contrast-enhanced sonography of pancreatic carcinoma, correlation with pathological findings. J Gastroenterol 40:631-640

50. Kloppel G, Schluter E (1999) Pathology of the pancreas. In: Baert AL, Delorme G, Van Hoe L (eds) Radiology of the Pancreas (2nd edn). Springer Verlag, Germany pp. 69-100

51. Kitano M, Kudo M, Maekawa K et al (2004) Dynamic imaging of pancreatic diseases by contrast enhanced coded phase inversion harmonic ultrasonography. Gut 53:854-859

52. D'Onofrio M, Barbi E, Dietrich CF et al (2011) Pancreatic multicenter ultrasound study (PAMUS). Eur J Radiol doi:10.1016/j.ejrad.2011.01.053

53. Tawada K, Yamaguchi T, Kobayashi A et al (2009) Changes in tumor vascularity depicted by contrast-enhanced ultrasonography as a predictor of chemotherapeutic effect in patients with unresectable pancreatic cancer. Pancreas 38:30-35

54. D'Onofrio M, Martone E, Faccioli N et al (2006) Focal liver lesions, sinusoidal phase of CEUS. Abdom Imaging 31:529-536

55. Piscaglia F, Nolsøe C, Dietrich CF et al (2011) The EFSUMB Guidelines and Recommendations on the Clinical Practice of Contrast Enhanced Ultrasound (CEUS): Update 2011 on non-hepatic applications. Ultraschall Med 2011 (epub in advance)

56. D'Onofrio M, Zamboni G, Tognolini A et al (2006) Mass-forming pancreatitis: value of contrast-enhanced ultrasonography. World J Gastroenterol 12:4181-4184

57. D'Onofrio M, Malago R, Martone E et al (2005) Pancreatic pathology. In: Quaia E (ed) Contrast media in ultrasonography. Berlin, Heidelberg: Springer Verlag pp. 335-347

58. Koito K, Namieno T, Nagakawa T et al (2001) Pancreas, imaging diagnosis with color/power-Doppler ultrasonography, endoscopic ultrasonography, and intraductal ultrasonography. Eur J Radiol 38:94-104

59. Yassa NA, Yang J, Stein S et al (1997) Gray-scale and color flow sonography of pancreatic ductal adenocarcinoma. J Clin Ultrasound 25:473-480

60. Ueno N, Tomiyama T, Tano S et al (1997) Color-Doppler ultrasonography in the diagnosis of portal vein invasion in patients with pancreatic cancer. J Ultrasound Med 16:825-830

61. Lu DSK, Reber HA, Krasny RM et al (1997) Local staging of pancreatic cancer, criteria for unresectability of major vessels as revealed by pancreatic-phase, thin-section helical CT. Am J Roentgenol 168:1439-1443

62. Hohl C, Schmidt T, Haage P et al (2004) Phase-inversion tissue harmonic imaging compared with conventional B-mode ultrasound in the evaluation of pancreatic lesions. Eur Radiol 14:1109-1117

63. Tomiyama T, Ueno N, Tano S et al (1996) Assessment of arterial invasion in pancreatic cancer using color-Doppler ultrasonography. Am J Gastroenterol 91:1410-1416

64. Umemura A, Yamada K (2001) B-mode flow imaging of the carotid artery. Stroke 32:2055-2057

65. Grossjohann HS, Rappeport ED, Jensen C et al (2010) Usefulness of contrast-enhanced transabdominal ultrasound for tumor classification and tumor staging in the pancreatic head. Scand J Gastroenterol 45:917-924

66. Dixon E, Pasieka JL (2007) Functioning and nonfunctioning neuroendocrine tumors of the pancreas. Curr Opin Oncol 19:30-35

67. Tamm EP, Kim EE, Chaan S (2007) Imaging of neuroendocrine tumors. Hematol Oncol Clin N Am 21:409-432

68. Lee LS (2010) Diagnosis of pancreatic neuroendocrine tumors and the role of endoscopic ultrasound. Gastroenterol Hepatol (NY) 6:520-522

69. Ros PR, Mortele KJ (2001) Imaging features of pancreatic neoplasms. JBR-BTR 84:239-249

70. D'Onofrio M, Mansueto GC, Falconi M et al (2004) Neuroendocrine pancreatic tumor: value of contrast enhanced ultrasonography. Abdom Imaging 29:246-258

71. Procacci C, Carbognin G, Accordini S et al (2001) Non-functioning endocrine tumors of the pancreas: possibilities of spiral CT characterization. Eur Radiol 11:1175-1183

72. Malagò R, D'Onofrio M, Zamboni GA et al (2009) Contrast-enhanced sonography of nonfunctioning pancreatic neuroendocrine tumors. Am J Roentgenol 192:424-430

73. D'Onofrio M, Malagò R, Zamboni G et al (2005) Contrast-enhanced ultrasonography better identifies pancreatic tumor vascularization than helical CT. Pancreatology 5:398-402

74. Bhutani MS, Hoffman BJ, van Velse A et al (1997) Contrast-enhanced endoscopic ultrasonography with galactose microparticles: SHU508 A (Levovist). Endoscopy 29:635-639

75. Rickes S, Malfertheiner P (2006) Echo-enhanced ultrasound—a new imaging modality for the differentiation of pancreatic lesions. Int J Colorectal Dis 21:269-275

76. Hocke M, Schulze E, Gottschalk P, Topalidis T, Dietrich CF (2006) The use of contrast enhanced endoscopic ultrasound in discrimination between focal pancreatitis and pancreatic cancer. World J Gastroenterol (WJG) 212:246-250

77. Hocke M, Ignee A, Topalidis T, Stallmach A, Dietrich CF (2007) Contrast enhanced endosonographic Doppler spectrum analysis is helpful in discrimination between focal chronic pancreatitis and pancreatic cancer. Pancreas 286-288

78. Ueda T, Oda T, Kinoshita T et al (2002) Neovascularization in pancreatic ductal adenocarcinoma: Microvessel count analysis, comparison with non-cancerous regions and other types of carcinomas. Oncol Rep 9:239-245

79. Koorstra JBM, Feldmann G, Habbe N et al (2008) Morphogenesis of pancreatic cancer: role of pancreatic intraepithelial neoplasia (PanINs). Langenbecks Arch Surg 393:561-570

80. Feldmann G, Beaty R, Hruban RH et al (2007) Molecular genetics of pancreatic intraepithelial neoplasia. J Hepatobiliary Pancreat Surg 14:224-232. Review

81. Canto MI (2007) Strategies for screening for pancreatic adenocarcinoma in high-risk patients. Semin Oncol 34:295-302

82. Haugk B (2010) Pancreatic intraepithelial neoplasia-can we detect early pancreatic cancer? Histopathology 57:503-14. Review

83. Recavarren C, Labow DM, Liang J et al (2011) Histologic characteristics of pancreatic intraepithelial neoplasia associated with different pancreatic lesions. Hum Pathol 42:18-24

84. Dietrich CF, Hirche TO, Ott M, Ignee A (2009) Real-time tissue elastography in the diagnosis of autoimmune pancreatitis. Endoscopy 41:718-720

85. Hocke M, Ignee A, Dietrich CF (2011) Contrast-enhanced endoscopic ultrasound in the diagnosis of autoimmune pancreatitis. Endoscopy 43:163-165

86. Dietrich CF (2011) Elastography Applications. Endo heute 24:177–212

Cystic Pancreatic Tumors

9

Mirko D'Onofrio, Paolo Giorgio Arcidiacono and Massimo Falconi

9.1 Introduction

Cystic lesions of the pancreas are increasingly being recognized due to the widespread use of cross-sectional imaging, and include a large variety of lesions with different etiology and biology, each requiring a different management strategy [1-5]. The exclusion of a pseudocyst, generally found in patients with a history of acute or chronic pancreatitis, is the first aim of the primary approach to a pancreatic cyst. The evaluation of a pancreatic cystic tumor should be directed toward differentiation between benign and malignant behavior [6].

Epithelial tumors of the exocrine pancreas, primarily represented by serous and mucinous lesions, make up the majority followed by other tumors potentially presenting with cystic changes, such as pseudopapillary tumor, neuroendocrine tumor and ductal adenocarcinoma [3].

The imaging modalities routinely used to characterize different cystic tumors of the pancreas are magnetic resonance imaging (MRI) and endoscopic ultrasound (EUS). Ultrasonography (US), together with harmonic US, Doppler study and nowadays elastosonography, are usually the first step in the diagnostic algorithm of pancreatic tumors, considering that US is still used as the first imaging modality for the initial evaluation of the pancreas especially in European and Asian countries [7]. The introduction of microbubble contrast agents has certainly improved the characterization of pancreatic tumors, first allowing definitive differentiation between solid and cystic lesions. Contrast-enhanced ultrasound (CEUS) can also immediately characterize solid and cystic pancreatic tumors through the real-time evaluation of the contrast enhancement [8]. In particular at CEUS, even if the lesion is characterized by a heterogeneous content at pre-contrast study, a pseudocyst shows avascular materials. On the other hand, cystic tumors of the pancreas are complex cystic lesions usually characterized by internal enhanced vegetations, such as septa and mural nodules [7-10]. CEUS has significantly improved the accuracy of the first-line examinations and may influence confidently the choice of the second-line investigations. The detection of a solid mass requires multidetector computed tomography (MDCT) confirmation, while a cystic lesion should be studied with an MRI examination. Therefore, while the pancreatic solid lesion characterized as ductal adenocarcinoma at CEUS requires an MDCT study as soon as possible to obtain a faster diagnosis, confirmation and staging, the pancreatic cystic lesions should be studied with MRI and magnetic resonance cholangiopancreatography (MRCP). MRI with MRCP in fact still remains the imaging modality of choice as it provides excellent contrast resolution and allows an accurate evaluation of the pancreatic ductal system [3, 11-16]. However, in recent years MDCT with its post-processing reconstructions has been reported to have a similar accuracy to MRI in detecting and characterizing cystic lesions of the pancreas [4, 17-19]. EUS is widely accepted as a significant test for the diagnosis of cystic pancreatic lesions (CPLs). EUS permits close, high resolution imaging of CPL morphology that may not be readily visualized by CT or

M. D'Onofrio (✉)
Department of Radiology
G.B. Rossi University Hospital, Verona, Italy
e-mail: mirko.donofrio@univr.it

MRI. Diagnostic accuracy of EUS imaging alone for detecting malignant or premalignant lesions is reported to be 82-96% [20-24].

Earlier literature described several EUS features of pancreatic cysts associated with increased malignancy risk, including thick wall, protruding tumor, presence of nodule or mass and thick septations [20, 21]. More recent studies, however, have uncovered the shortcomings of relying on EUS alone in differentiating benign from malignant CPLs. In the study by Ahmad et al. [23], blinded expert endosonographers reviewed 31 EUS videos of pathologically confirmed pancreatic cystic neoplasms and noted cystic features, type, and malignancy potential. The interobserver agreement was moderately good in detecting the solid component, but only fair for defining the diagnosis of neoplastic versus non-neoplastic lesions, and the overall accuracy rates ranged from 40% to 93%. A large multicenter prospective US study found that the accuracy of EUS imaging features alone for the diagnosis of mucinous lesions was only 51% [25].

Given the above limitation, EUS morphology alone is generally considered inadequate for further characterization of CPLs. However, EUS also allows for fine needle aspiration (FNA), which has been shown to be an effective and safe sampling method of CPLs [24]. Its safety has been confirmed by multiple studies and complication rates in recent literature were found to be around 1% or less [26-29]. The US transducer on the distal tip of the echoendoscope permits needle advancement into the lesion under real-time guidance. A variety of commercially available FNA needles is available and range in size between 19 and 25 gauge. It is recommended that Doppler is used to examine the projected path of the needle to avoid puncturing intervening blood vessels, while trying to minimize the amount of normal pancreatic tissue that has to be traversed. Once the gastric or duodenal wall is punctured and the needle enters the cyst, the stylet is withdrawn and suction is applied. If possible, complete cyst aspiration using only one biopsy is recommended.

The presence of on-site cytopathology for rapid interpretation is recommended and has been shown to improve the diagnostic yield [30].

The use of FNA for cytology and fluid analysis has been extensively evaluated. The specificity of EUS-FNA cytology for the diagnosis of CPLs is excellent and exceeds 90% in most published studies. On the other hand, the sensitivity of EUS-FNA remains widely variable with most studies reporting a sensitivity of about 50% [24, 25, 31-33].

Tumor markers in the fluid of pancreatic cysts which have been evaluated in various studies include: carcinoembryonic antigen (CEA), CA 19-9, CA 72-4, and CA 125. The most commonly evaluated marker is CEA, and this is generally found in high levels in mucinous lesions, but is lower in pseudocysts and non mucinous tumors. The largest prospective study to date determined that a cut-off of cyst fluid CEA of 192 ng/mL provided a sensitivity of 73% and specificity of 84% for differentiating mucinous from nonmucinous CPLs in 112 patients who underwent surgery [25]. No other combination of factors, including cytology, morphology, and CEA levels was found to be more accurate than CEA levels alone.

In recent years, there has been increased interest in identifying specific genetic markers associated with higher risk of malignancy in CPLs. Certain DNA analysis of genetic markers of cyst fluid have become available and could help differentiate mucinous from nonmucinous lesions.

Considering differences between countries and institutions and recognizing that first non-invasive and then mini-invasive or invasive diagnostic procedures should be used, cystic tumors uncertain at imaging require sampling under EUS guidance or need to directly undergo surgical resection because of the high risk-to-benefit ratio, especially in cases of mucinous lesions [34-36]. In this chapter, the main features of the most representative cystic tumors of the pancreas studied with different imaging modalities, but beginning with US, are reviewed.

9.2 Pathology and Epidemiology

In past literature, cystic tumors of the pancreas were reported to account for about 20% of all pancreatic tumors representing 10-15% of the cystic lesions of the pancreas [3, 6] and pseudocystic lesions were considered the most frequent pancreatic cystic lesions [37-39]. These are no longer valid statements due to the increasing number of incidental cysts discovered at imaging.

Due to the advances in imaging techniques, the detection of pancreatic cystic lesions in asymptomatic patients has significantly increased. The management of these incidental findings, also reported in the literature as *disease of technology*, is becoming an important argument of discussion [40, 41]. The diagnoses of intraductal papillary mucinous neoplasm (IPMN) as well as serous cystadenoma are increasing in number, having an effect on the epidemiology and distribution of cystic pancreatic lesions. From this experience, it is becoming clear that the prevalence of pseudocysts among cystic lesions of the pancreas is lower than previously thought [15]. As a result, the occurrence of pseudocystic lesions in series from referral centers for pancreatic diseases reported in the literature is absolutely low from 5.5% to 13.7% [42, 43].

The epidemiology of cystic pancreatic lesions comes from the new estimated relative frequency of the most common histotypes: pseudocyst (30%); mucinous (30%); serous (20%); others (20%) [44].

9.3 Serous Cystadenoma

Serous cystadenoma (SCA) is a pancreatic cystic tumor generally detected in 50-70 year-old females (sex-ratio: 2:1), usually located in the pancreatic head as a solitary lesion. SCA can be multifocal in patients with Von-Hippel Lindau disease [3]. SCA has a typical multilocular *honeycomb* architecture due to the presence of multiple microcysts (<20 mm), thin wall and thin multiple septa orientated towards the center [6]. SCA has a lobulated *cloud-like* morphology (Fig. 9.1), clearly demonstrable at US [45]. The cystic content appears homogeneously anechoic at US (Fig. 9.1), hypodense at CT and homogeneously hypointense on T1-weighted images at MRI examination. The T2-weighted images clearly demonstrate the microcystic pattern (Fig. 9.1) with the microcystic boundaries appearing hypointense on a typically highly hyperintense cystic fluid [7]. The US findings that make a cystic lesion comparable with SCA are: multilocular mainly microcystic architecture, thin septa and wall, lobulated morphology (Fig. 9.1). For these reasons in the presence of a cystic lesion with US findings comparable with SCA, the final report must address the need of an MRI with MRCP. SCA does not communicate with the ductal system of the pancreas (Fig. 9.2) and this

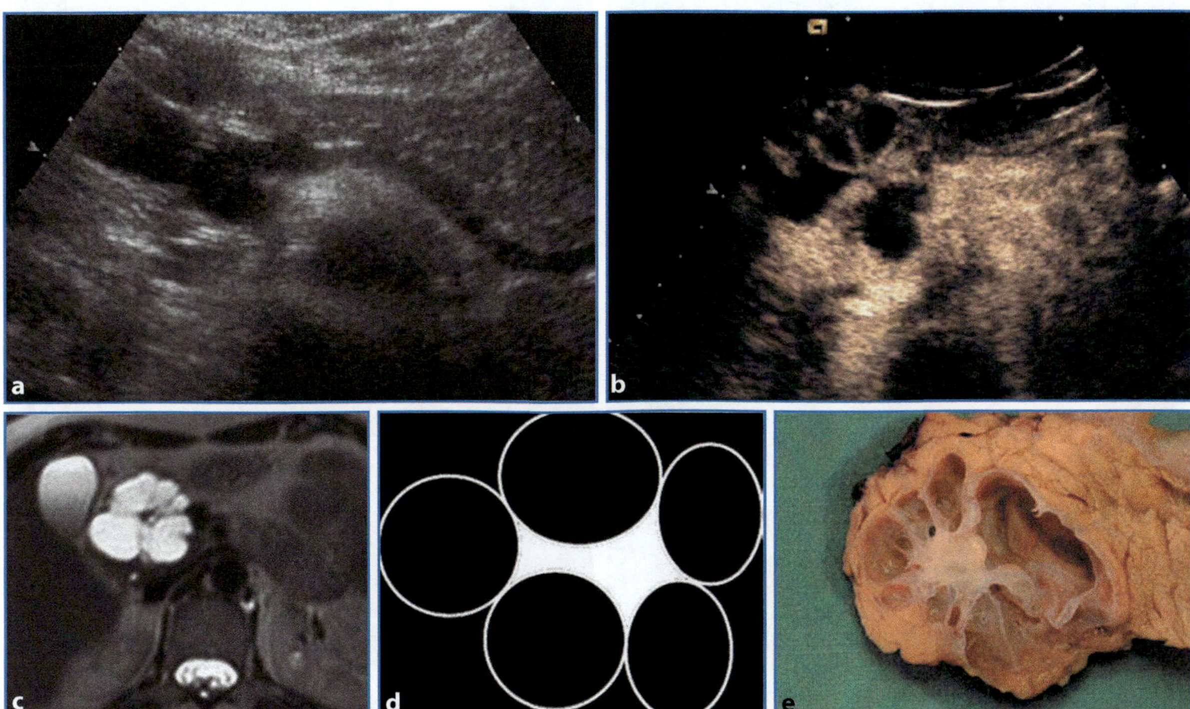

Fig. 9.1 a-e Serous cystadenoma. US (**a**) appearance of serous cystadenoma in the head of the pancreas with typical lobulated *cloud-like* morphology and vascularized centrally oriented septa at CEUS (**b**). Microcystic pattern on T2-weighted images at MRI (**c**). Lobulated *cloud-like* morphology: pattern (**d**). Specimen (**e**) resected owing to lesion dimensions causing initial main pancreatic duct compression

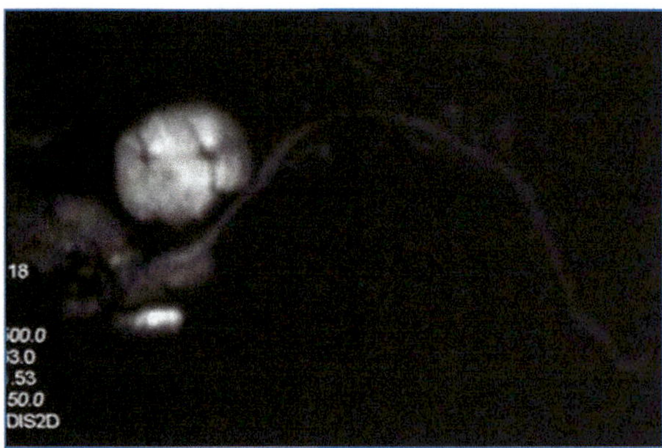

Fig. 9.2 Serous cystadenoma. Magnetic resonance colangiopancreatography (MRCP) perfectly showing a microcystic serous cystadenoma with complete absence of communication with the main pancreatic duct

is well demonstrated on MRCP [3, 11]. This finding, absolutely not demonstrable with US, remains crucial for the differential diagnosis in respect to IPMN of the branch duct that may present with a very similar appearance.

At US elastography, the serous content of SCA acts as simple fluid similar to a simple cyst [46]. As a result, stratification or a mosaic pattern may be present. Non-numerical values are reported in the quantitative US elastographic study of SCA made by means of acoustic radiation force impulse (ARFI) imaging (Fig. 9.3). Cystic lesions with different fluid contents could give different wave propagation speeds. In particular, it has been reported that while in pancreatic cystic lesions with simple fluid content such as serous cystadenomas almost always XXXX/0 (non-numeri-

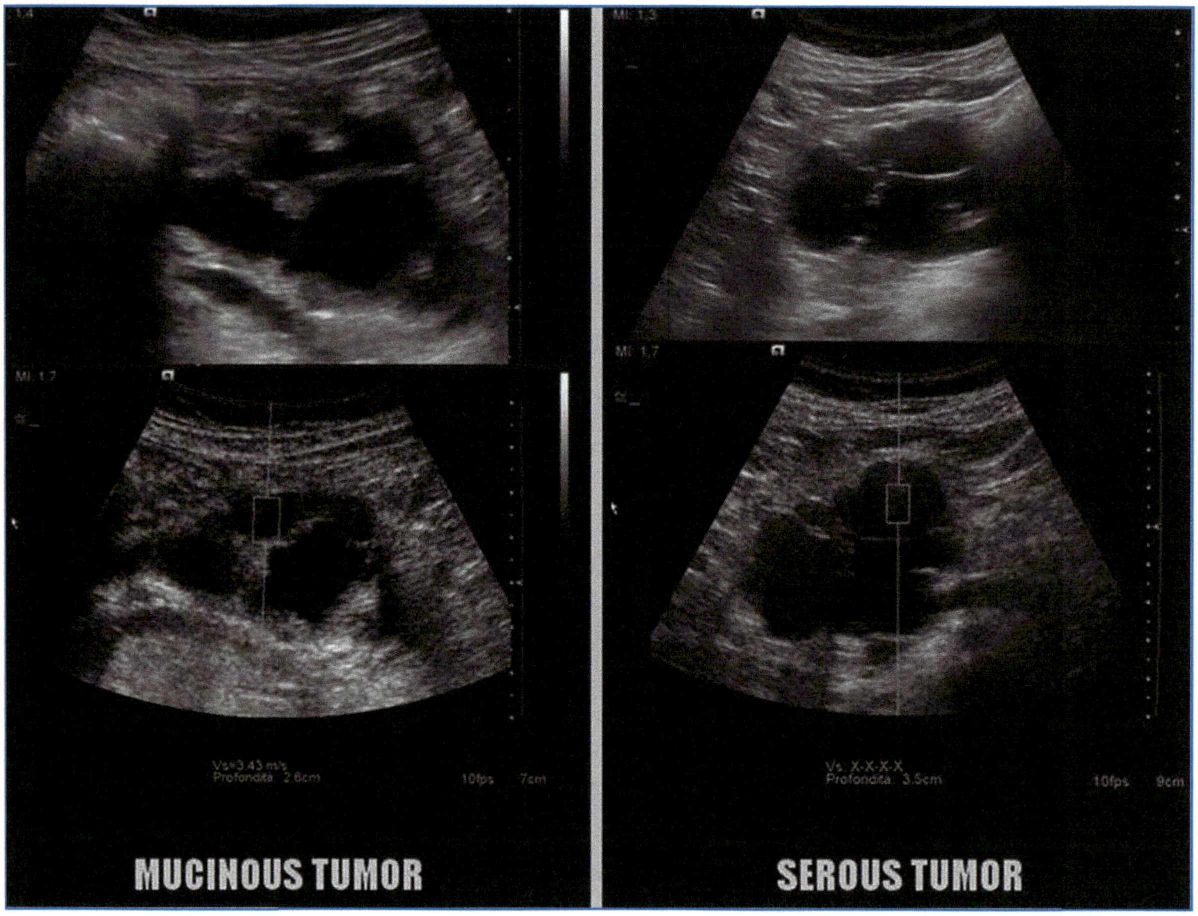

Fig. 9.3 ARFI US of cystic pancreatic tumors. *Left panel*: intraductal papillary mucinous neoplasm (IPMN) showing numeric value at virtual touch tissue quantification with the ROI (*small box*) placed in the fluid portion. *Right panel*: serous cystadenoma showing non-numerical value (XXXX or 0 in the new release) at virtual touch tissue quantification with the ROI (*small box*) placed in the fluid portion. Note that the two lesions present similar features at conventional US

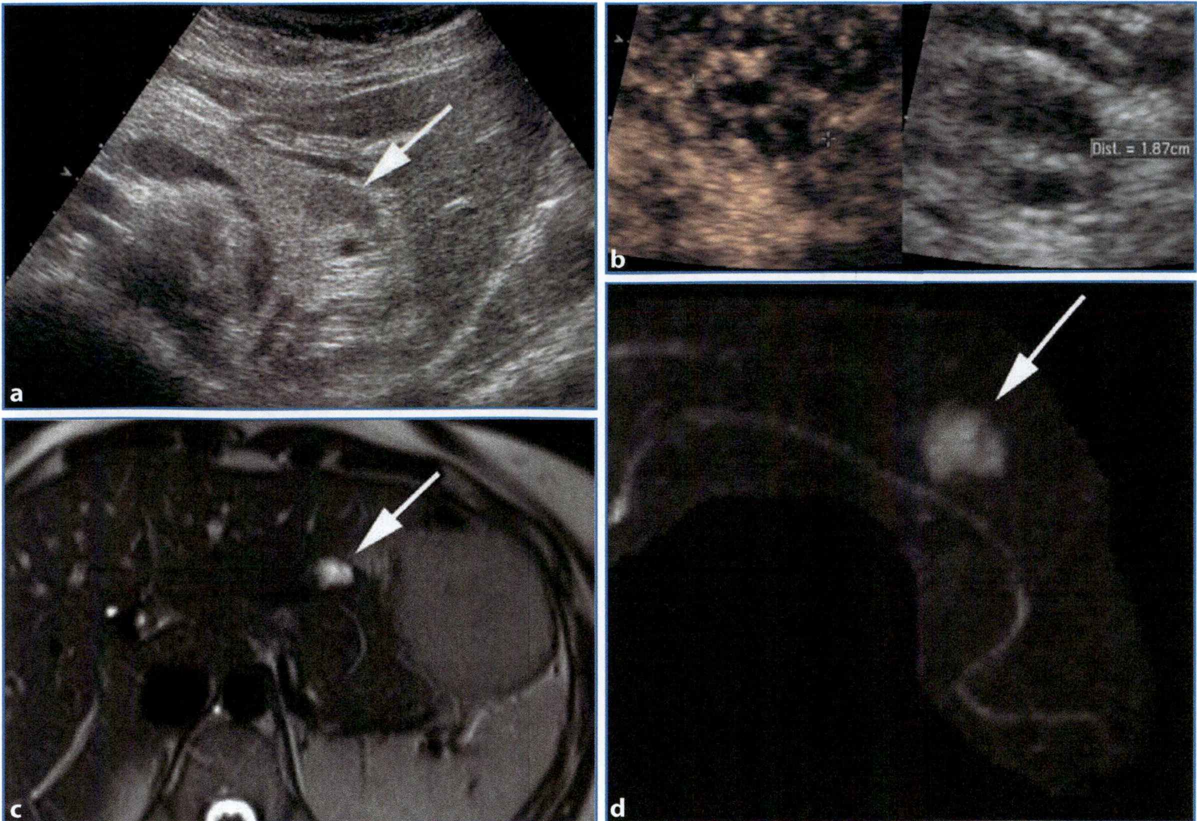

Fig. 9.4 a-d Serous cystadenoma. Pseudo-solid hypoechoic aspect of the lesion (*arrow*) at US (**a**) showing tiny microcysts at CEUS (**b**) confirmed at MRI (**c**) with diagnosis of microcystic serous cystadenoma (*arrow* in **c** and **d**) at T2-weighted image non communicating with the ductal system at MRCP (**d**)

cal) values are expected, in more complex fluids the evidence of numerical value is more frequent (Fig. 9.3). In vivo this could be due to a mucinous content, such as in mucinous tumors [47, 48]. The ARFI imaging seems able to potentially characterize the pancreatic cystic lesions through a new revolutionary approach: a non-invasive analysis of the fluid content (Fig. 9.3). The innovation is related to the fact that the study of pancreatic cystic lesions at imaging is nowadays still based only on the morphologic and architectural analysis, classifying the lesions by evaluating their shape, wall thickness, presence of septa, parietal nodules, calcifications and communication with the main pancreatic duct [3-13]. The ARFI US quantification seems to be able to non-invasively study the fluid content of pancreatic cystic lesions, thus potentially improving lesion characterization. At CEUS the enhancement of the internal septa is observed (Fig. 9.1), and sometimes a better identification of the mi-

crocystic feature (Fig. 9.4) is documented [5, 49]. In 15% of cases a central scar hypoechoic/hypodense/hypointense on T1-weighted images is observed [3, 45]. The scar is fibrovascular and a vessel can be visualized at Doppler study (Fig. 9.5). At US and CT examinations, calcifications potentially present are well detected. At imaging examinations, the extremely microcystic type (5%) may mimic a solid (Figs. 9.6, 9.7) lesion [5, 45] resembling an endocrine tumor of the pancreas after the administration of contrast agent (Fig. 9.8), owing to the homogeneous hyperenhancement of the extremely compacted internal septa [50]. Also in these cases, non-numerical values can be obtained at ARFI quantification, suggesting the nonsolid nature of the lesion [51]. The true cystic nature of the lesion can be easily demonstrated at MRI with a typical hyperintense signal on T2-weighted images (Figs. 9.6-9.8). This is the reason why a lesion with US features typical or suggestive of SCA has to be

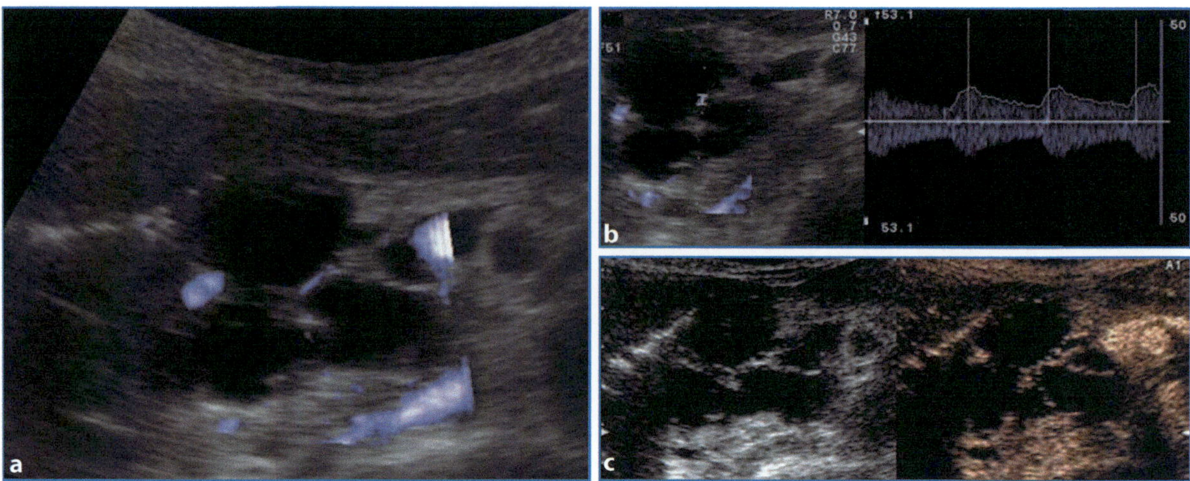

Fig. 9.5 a-c Serous cystadenoma. Pancreatic head microcystic lesion with tiny vessels at Doppler (**a,b**) along the septa appearing vascularized at CEUS (**c**)

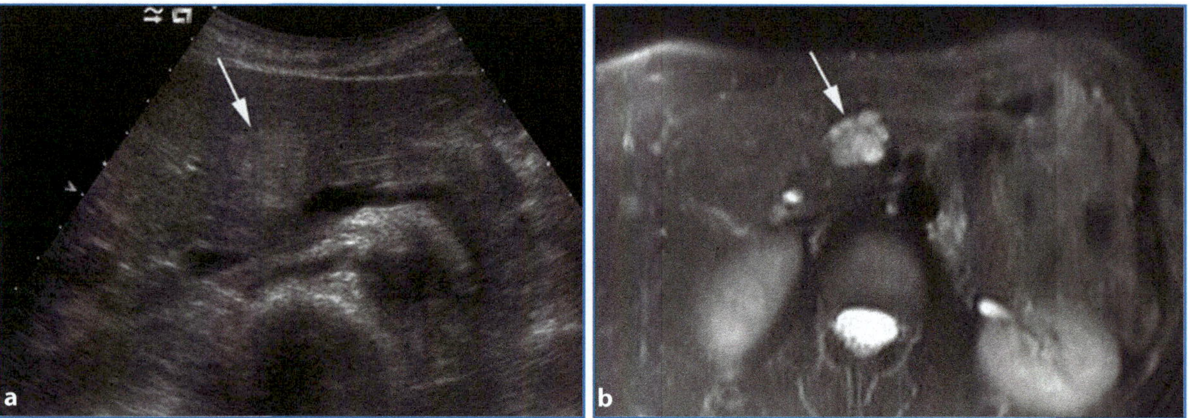

Fig. 9.6 a,b Serous cystadenoma. Pseudo-solid hyperechoic aspect of the lesion (*arrow*) at US (**a**) showing typical microcystic pattern (*arrow*) at MRI (**b**)

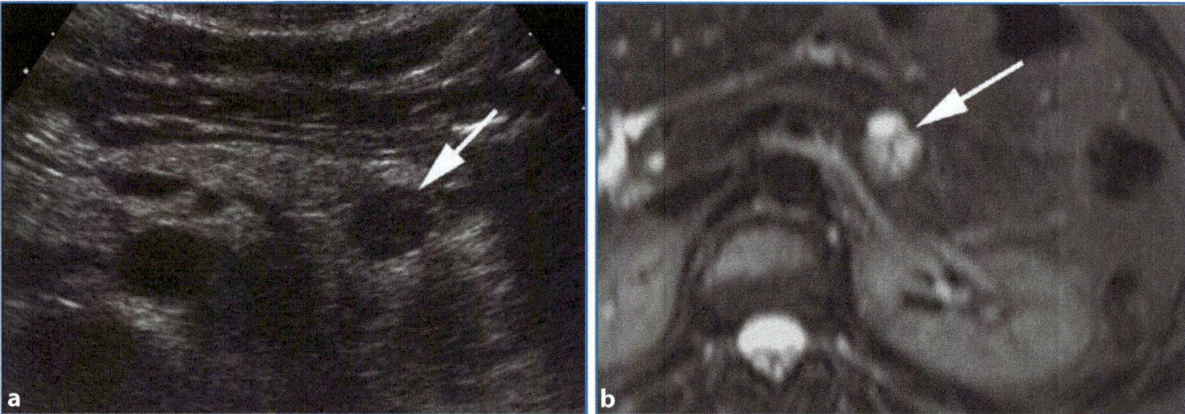

Fig. 9.7 a,b Serous cystadenoma. Pseudo-solid hypoechoic aspect of the lesion (*arrow*) at US (**a**) showing typical microcystic pattern (*arrow*) at T2-weighted image MRI (**b**)

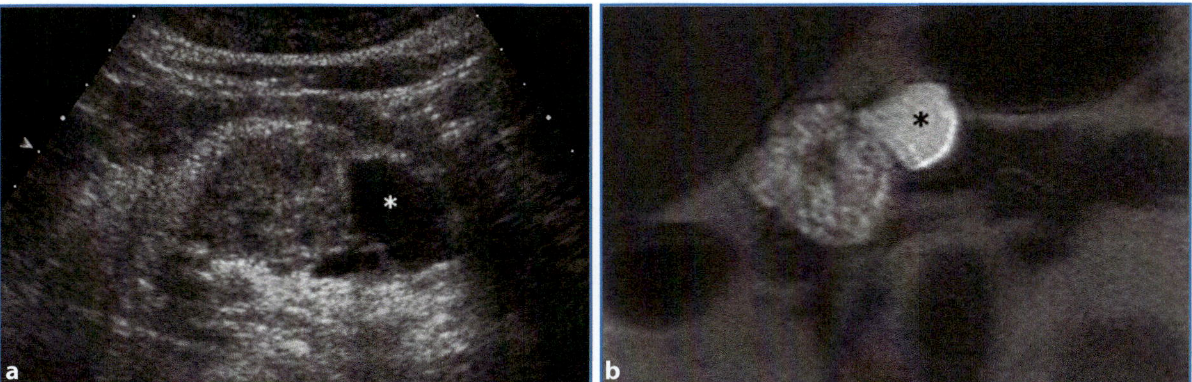

Fig. 9.8 a-c Serous cystadenoma. Pseudo-solid hypoechoic aspect of the lesion (*arrow*) at US (**a**) resulting hypervascular, hyperenhancing (*arrow*) at CEUS (**b**) showing typical microcystic pattern (*arrow*) at T2-weighted MRI (**c**)

Fig. 9.9 a,b Serous cystadenoma. Mixed type serous cystadenoma with pseudo-solid aspect of the main lesion at US (**a**) and macrocyst peripherically located (*asterisk*) and appearing with typical microcystic pattern at T2-weighted MRI (**b**) with macrocyst peripherically located (*asterisk*)

studied with MRI and MRCP which can easily confirm the diagnosis of SCA by excluding the communication with the ductal system of the pancreas. The macrocystic type (25%) comprises the mixed type (Fig. 9.9) with large (>20 mm) cysts and the unilocular type (Fig. 9.10), which is difficult to differentiate at imaging from a mucinous cystadenoma [52], and therefore FNA of these lesions is recommended [41, 53]. Finally the largest tumors can compress the ductal system, with consequent upstream dilatation.

The diagnostic yield of EUS-FNA for SCA is usually poor due to the small size of the cystic compartments and the relatively vascular intercystic septa (Fig. 9.11). Due to the distinctive EUS appearance of microcystic SCA, cyst sampling is generally not needed. If necessary, EUS-FNA of SCA should target the largest cystic compartments for fluid analysis. The fluid obtained is often thin, nonviscous and colorless. Cellularity is very low, and if any, cuboidal epithelial cells have been described on aspirate that stain positive for glycogen but not mucin [54]. CEA levels are low, usually less than 20 ng/mL.

SCA is a benign tumor of the pancreas, confirmed at pathology by sampling a glycogen-rich serous fluid, without atypia in the cell wall. However, this benign lesion requires follow-up, usually by US or MRI, while surgical treatment has to be considered only in symptomatic patients with a lesion generally larger than 4 cm in size [41]. In fact, progressive growth has been reported in the majority of incidental lesions without communication with the main pancreatic duct and larger than 3 cm in size [55]. Moreover, lesions characterized by micro-macrocystic or macrocystic pattern show a more significant growth compared to microcystic lesions [55].

9.4 Mucinous Cystadenoma

Mucinous cystadenoma (MCA) is a pancreatic cystic tumor with female sex predilection (sex ratio 9:1), generally occurring at a mean age of 50-60 years [3].

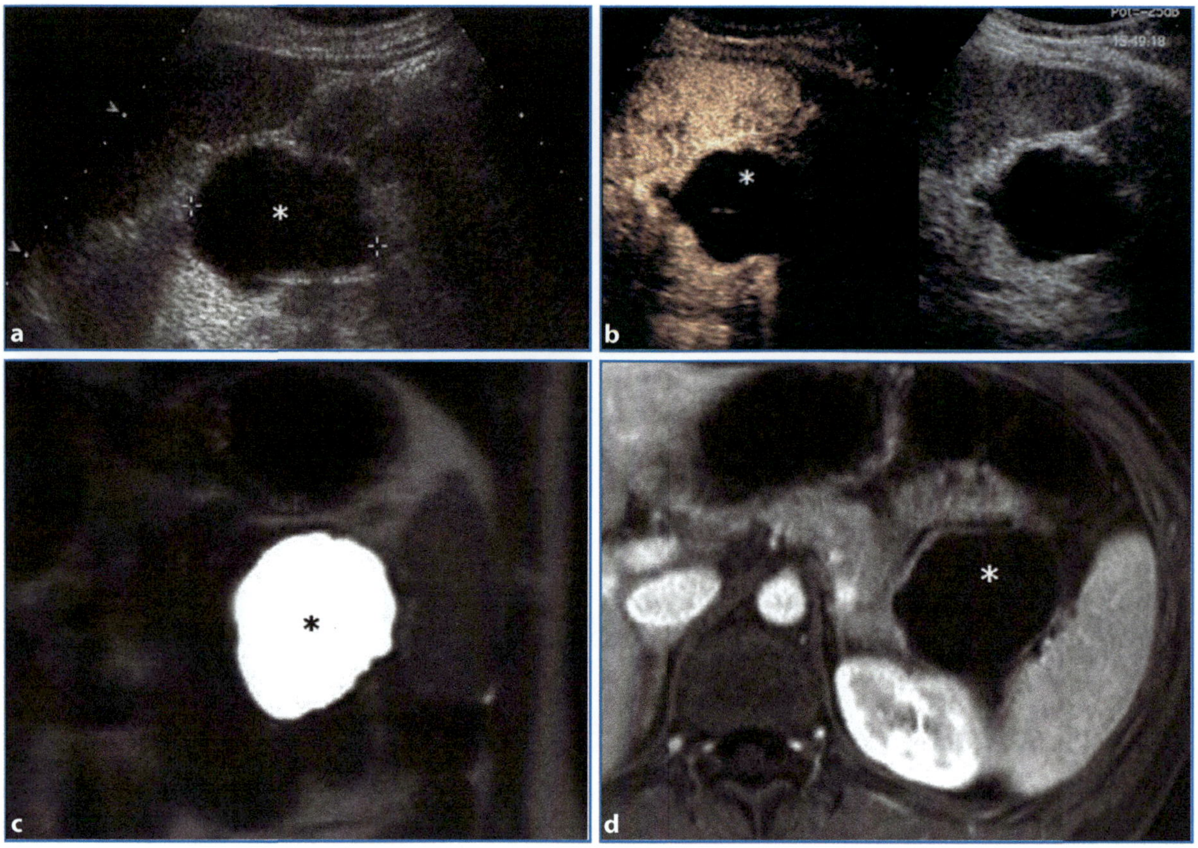

Fig. 9.10 a-d Serous cystadenoma. Macrocystic serous cystadenoma of the pancreatic tail with rounded unilocular cystic mass (*caliper and asterisk*) at US (**a**), CEUS (**b**), T2-weighted image MRI (**c**) and dynamic MRI (**d**) led to the wrong diagnosis of mucinous neoplasm. Tiny intralesional septum enhancement can be seen at CEUS

MCA is a benign mucin-producing lesion with a proven high malignant potential [56, 57]. Therefore, in respect to serous cystadenoma, MCA requires sur-

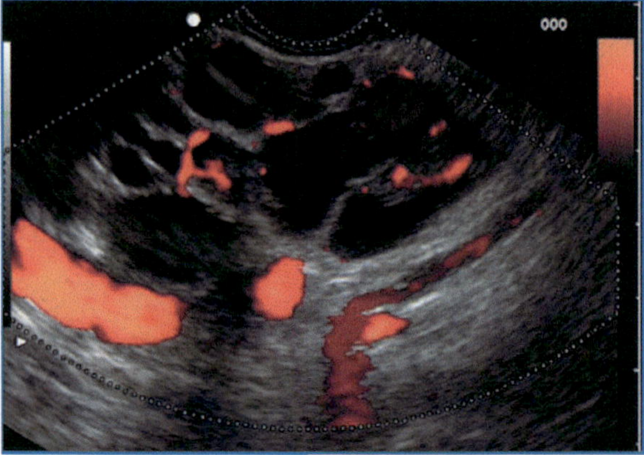

Fig. 9.11 Serous cystadenoma. EUS image of mixed macrocystic type serous cystadenoma with vascular intracystic septa

gical resection. As a consequence, the differential diagnosis between mucinous and nonmucinous (serous) cystic lesions of the pancreas is fundamental for management and treatment planning. The majority appears as a single lesion located in the body-tail of the pancreas, without communication with the main pancreatic duct, generally regular in caliber [6, 11]. MCA usually presents as a macrocystic lesion with rounded *ball-like* morphology (Fig. 9.12), irregular septa, thick wall and complex content that can be particle, viscous and dense owing to mucin and hemorrhage. This content very often makes the lesion heterogeneously hypoechoic at US, hypodense at CT and slightly hyperintense on T2-weighted images at MRI examination [7]. On T1-weighted images, the signal intensity can vary from hypointensity to hyperintensity, depending on the mucin concentration [2, 3, 6]. MRCP clearly demonstrates the lack of communication with the pancreatic ductal system. Unlike SCA, the intrale-

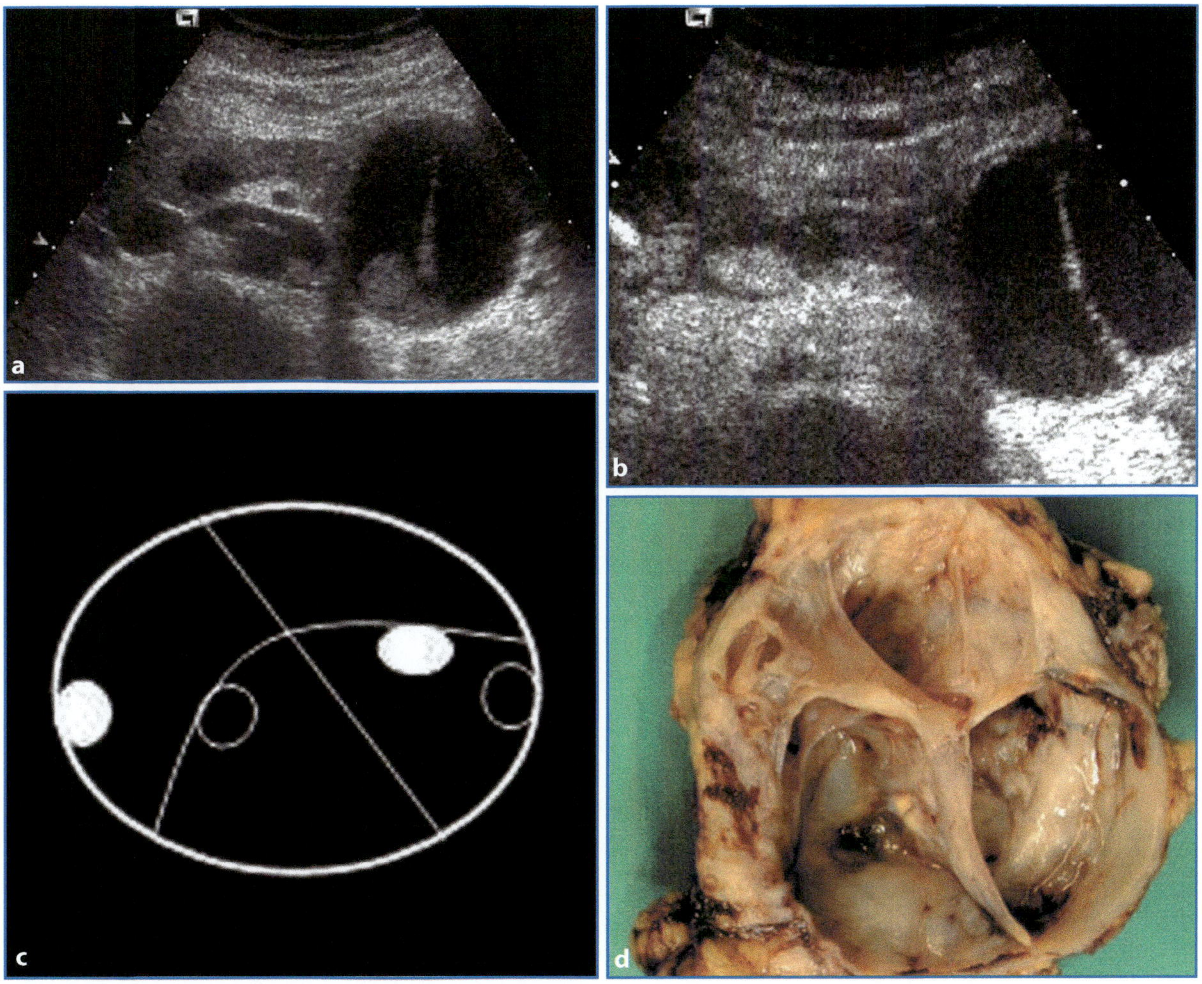

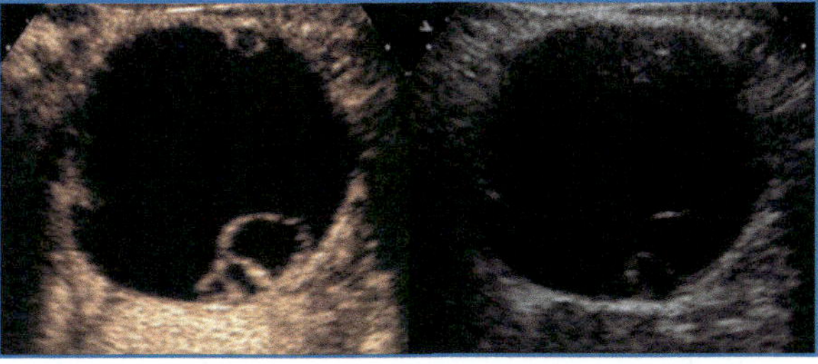

Fig. 9.12 a-d Mucinous cystadenoma. US (**a**) appearance of mucinous cystadenoma of the pancreatic tail with typical rounded "ball-like" morphology and vascular thick septa at CEUS (**b**). Rounded "ball-like" morphology: pattern (**c**). CEUS perfectly correlates with the specimen (**d**)

sional septa with disorganized distribution are peripherally located very often describing a *bridge* along the cystic wall (Figs. 9.13, 9.14) with a *pseudonodular* appearance. Unlike SCA, peripheral calcification along the thick wall have been reported in about 10-25% of patients [6, 37, 45, 58]. Rarely, MCA, especially when small in dimensions, can present as a grossly round and unilocular lesion. At imaging, the differential diagnosis between MCA and pseudocyst may be difficult and is still mainly based on the demonstration of the enhancement of internal vegetations [5, 6, 49, 59, 60]. This feature can be documented on different imaging modalities after the administration of contrast material. Some lesions at imaging appear grossly round and unilocular without

septa only because of the capability of the methods used. Therefore, some lesions can be perfectly unilocular without septa at CT but septa can be demon-

Fig. 9.13 Mucinous cystadenoma. CEUS perfectly demonstrates the vasculature of intralesional septa with disorganized distribution and peripherically located describing a *bridge* along the cystic wall

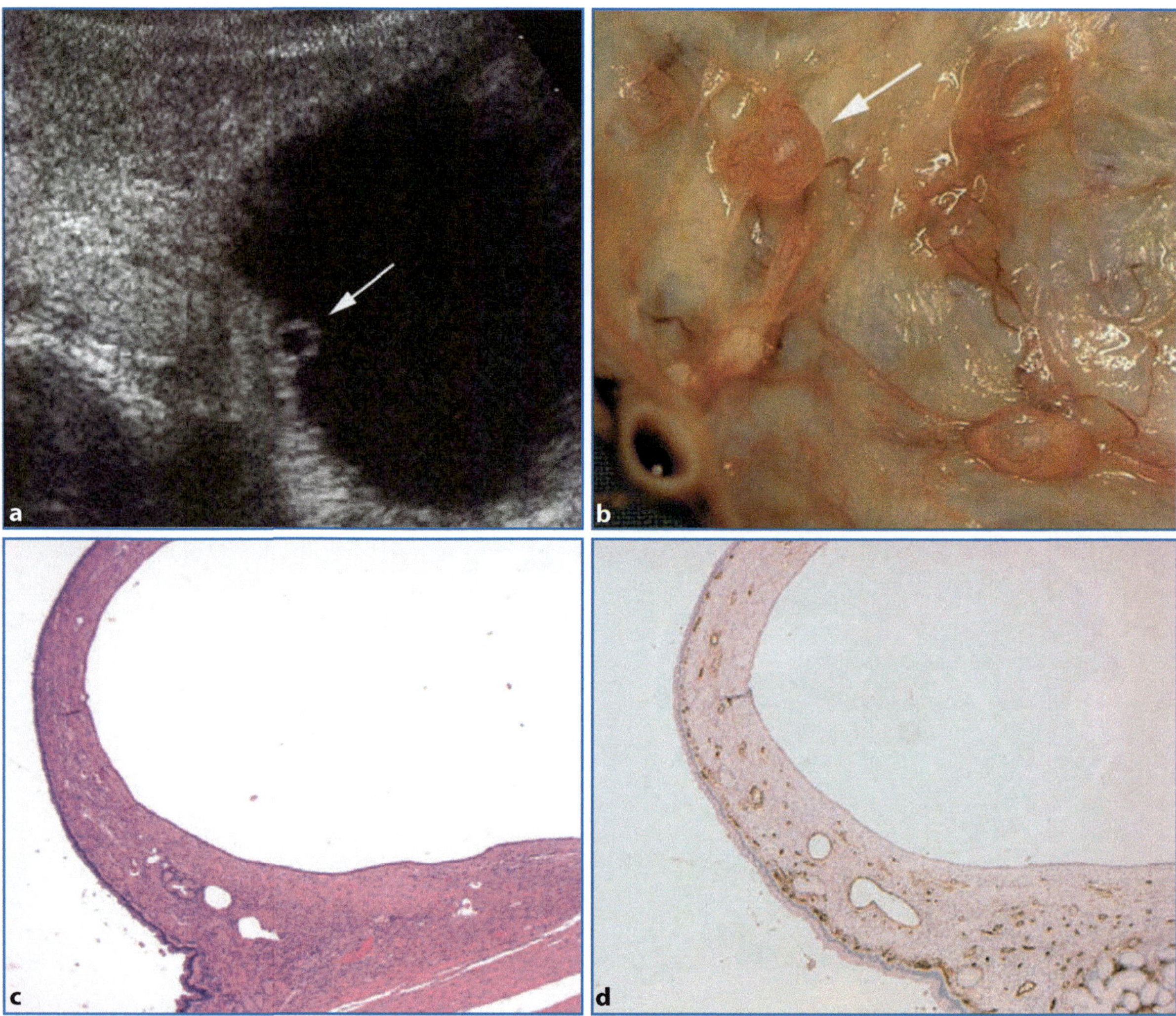

Fig. 9.14 a-d Mucinous cystadenoma. CEUS perfectly demonstrates the vasculature of a very small intralesional septum (*arrow*) describing a *bridge* along the cystic wall. The small septum is confirmed at pathology (*arrow*). Final diagnosis was mucinous neoplasm (**c**). CD 34 immunohistochemical stain confirms the presence of small capillary vessels within the septum (**d**)

strated at CEUS (Fig. 9.15) transabdominally or endoscopically performed [54, 60]. Owing to its special technical features (the dynamic evaluation of perfusion by using a blood pool contrast agent), sometimes CEUS can better demonstrate the enhancement than other imaging examinations, showing single microbubbles passing through the septa with a perfect correlation with the resected specimen (Fig. 9.16). During CEUS, microbubble-specific software on the sonographic console deletes all the background signal intensity so that the operator sees only the signal intensity produced by the contrast agent passing in vessels under the sonographic probe while the non-vascularized (unenhanced) tissue remains invisible [5]. This property can be readily exploited in the evaluation of the wall and architecture of cystic pancreatic lesions. The viable vascularized portions of cystic pancreatic tumors become progressively echogenic during CEUS as the contrast material passes into the capillary vessels of the septa (Figs. 9.12-9.15) or nodules (Fig. 9.16) inside the cysts [7]. Conversely, intralesional blood clots and debris, which are easily detectable on baseline sonograms, are completely invisible (Fig. 9.17) during CEUS [8, 9, 49, 60]. For this reason, CEUS is reported to improve the characterization of pseudocysts [8, 9, 49, 61]. Moreover,

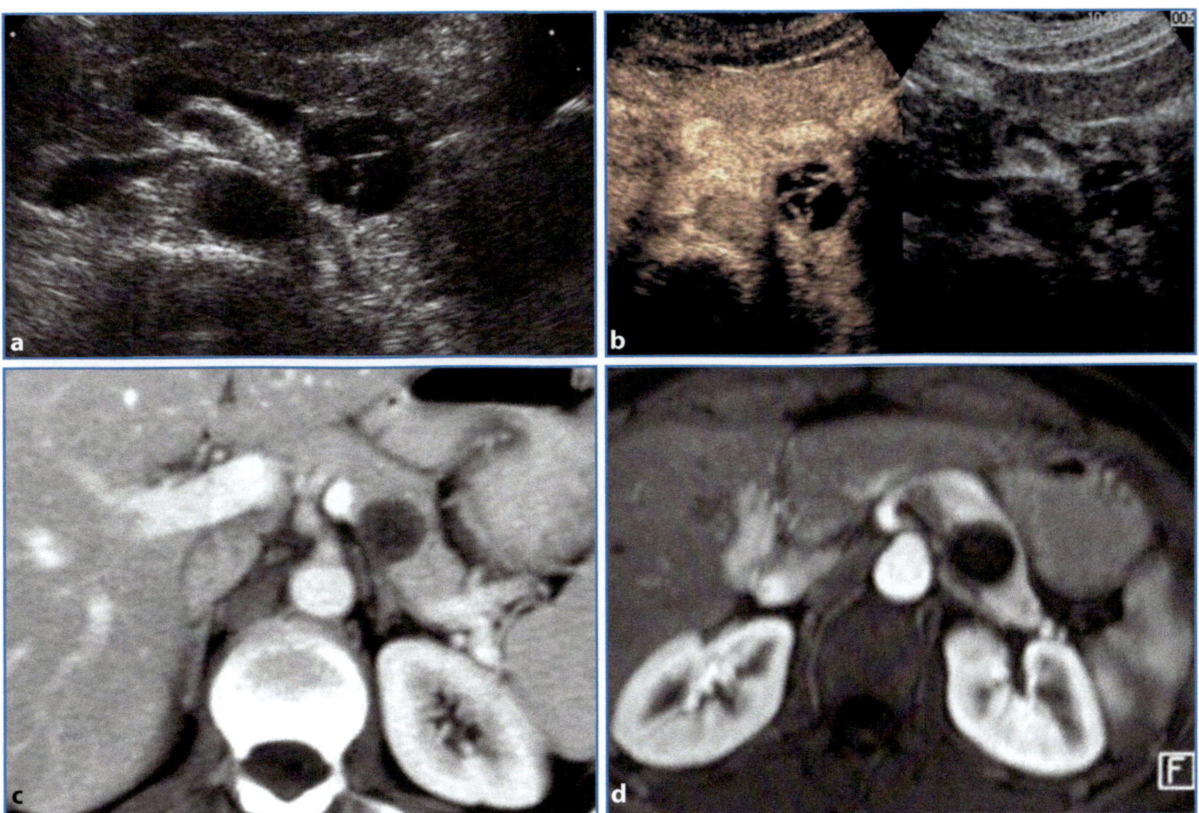

Fig. 9.15 a-d Small mucinous cystadenoma. Evident difference between US (**a**) with CEUS (**b**) in respect to both CT (**c**) and MRI (**d**) regarding the detection and the demonstration of vasculature of intralesional septa

owing to the deletion of the background tissue and of all the echogenic intracystic content (i.e. mucinous content or clots and debris), the detection rate of septa and nodules on CEUS is absolutely superior compared to transabdominal US, thus improving the characterization of cystic tumors [8, 62, 63]. In fact during unenhanced US, the viscosity of mucin within a lesion results in increased content echogenicity, which can obscure the internal wall [5, 45, 63]. Even with respect to MRI the results can sometimes be better considering that septa and nodules may be seen only on T2-weighted MR images and not on contrast-enhanced MRI, thus explaining possible false-positive results [10]. As a result, CEUS is reported to be an accurate method for the characterization of cystic lesions. Cystic tumor was correctly diagnosed at CEUS with an accuracy of 97.1% in the multicenter pancreatic US study [8].

The presence of enhanced mural nodules is strictly related to malignancy and the diagnosis of cystadenocarcinoma has to be suggested [56, 57]. In fact, the risk of malignant degeneration seems to increase with respect to the number of irregular thick septa and mural nodules. Since the change from adenoma to adenocarcinoma is progressive, surgical resection is therefore the accepted management for MCA even if asymptomatic [56-58, 64].

Clearly, the presence of evident features of malignancy, such as vascular involvement, regional lymph node enlargement or liver metastases, defines the malignant degeneration of MCA into mucinous cystadenocarcinoma [60, 65].

As reported above, ARFI seems to be able to non-invasively study the fluid content of pancreatic cystic lesions, potentially improving lesion characterization (Fig. 9.3). In particular, in contrast to serous lesions (Fig. 9.18), numerical values (Fig. 9.19) can be more often obtained during the study [48]. As reported, the useful information is the recurring presence of a numerical value which reflects the complex nature of the fluid, viscous, corpuscular and dense (Fig. 9.19) in respect to serous fluid. ARFI can be applied in the

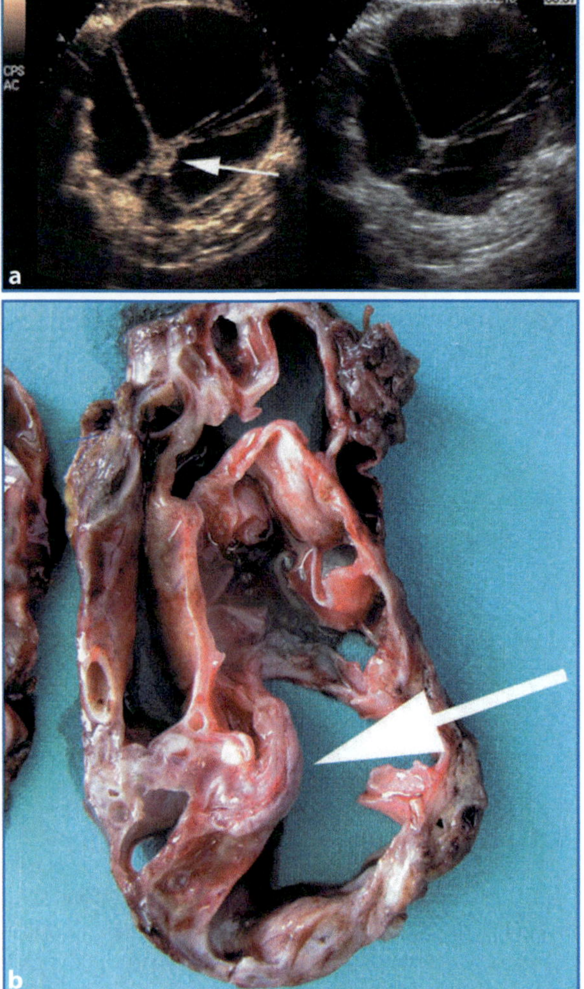

Fig. 9.16 a,b Mucinous cystic neoplasm. Perfect correlation between CEUS (**a**) with septa and nodule (*arrow*) enhancement and the resected specimen (**b**) confirming the presence of septa and nodule (*arrow*)

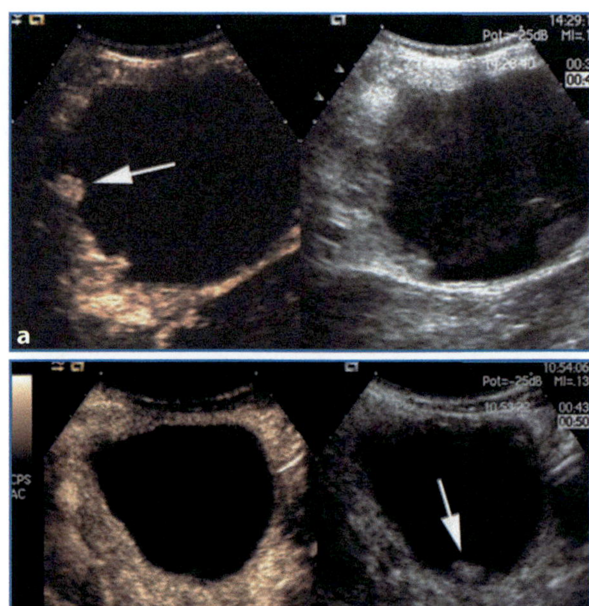

Fig. 9.17 a,b Differential diagnosis. **a** Mucinous neoplasm: at CEUS nodular (*arrow*) enhancement of the wall. **b** Pseudocyst: at CEUS no enhancement of debris and clot (*arrow*)

analysis of fluids and is potentially able to differentiate more complex (mucinous) from simple (serous) content in studying pancreatic cystic lesions [46, 47, 49]. In particular, the observed high sensitivity and positive predictive values in respect to a low specificity of this method could confer to ARFI, if confirmed in further larger studies, a potential role in the screening of mucinous content (Fig. 9.20) in cystic pancreatic lesions [46].

The extremely high spatial resolution makes EUS the best imaging modality for detecting very thin septa and small nodules in cystic pancreatic tumors. However, to confirm that intralesional vegetations are true neoplastic, vasculature has to be proven (Fig. 9.21). In addition, real-time sono-elastography (RTSE) is useful for a better characterization of lesions and increased accuracy of differential diagnosis [27]. RTSE is a technique which allows the calculation and visualization of tissue strain and hardness based on the average tissue strain in a selected region of interest. The technique allows the real-time visualization of the calculated strain values, displayed in a transparent layout over the gray-scale images, in a manner similar to color Doppler imaging [66]. In this way, this technique can selectively guide EUS fine needle aspiration where elastography suggests a hard mass (Figs. 9.22, 9.23) the vasculature of which can be proven by injecting contrast media (Fig. 9.23) and thus precisely identifying the viable portions of the tumor before sampling.

If there is any visible nodule to biopsy, EUS-FNA cytology could reveal columnar epithelial cells in up to half of the patients in association with extracellular mucin. Mucin is frequently identified on EUS-FNA of mucinous cystic neoplasm and cystic fluid is typically clear but often viscous with elevated CEA levels and low amylase [54]. However, there is not a direct

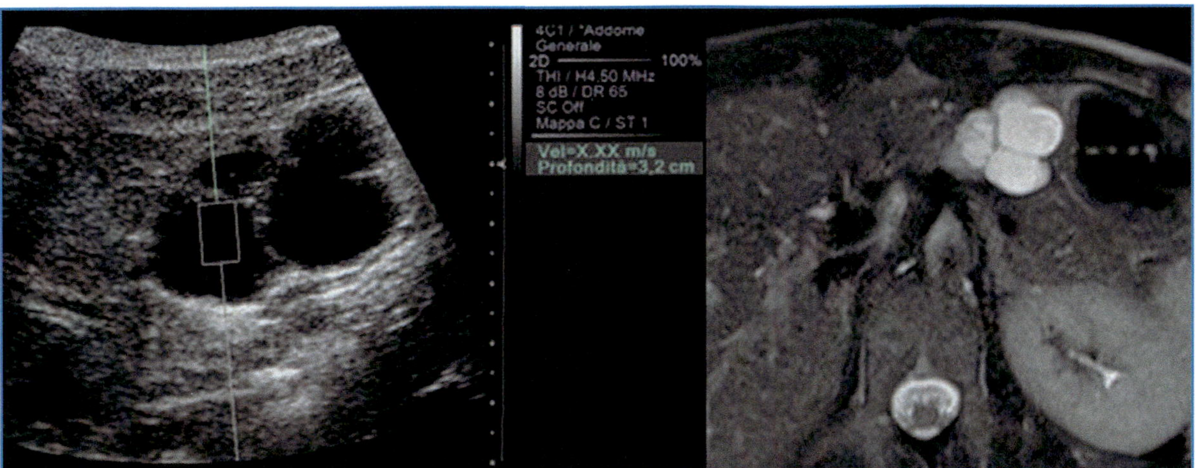

Fig. 9.18 Serous cystadenoma. Non-numerical values are obtained at ARFI US with virtual touch tissue quantification (*left panel*). MRI (*right panel*) confirms the diagnosis of serous cystadenoma

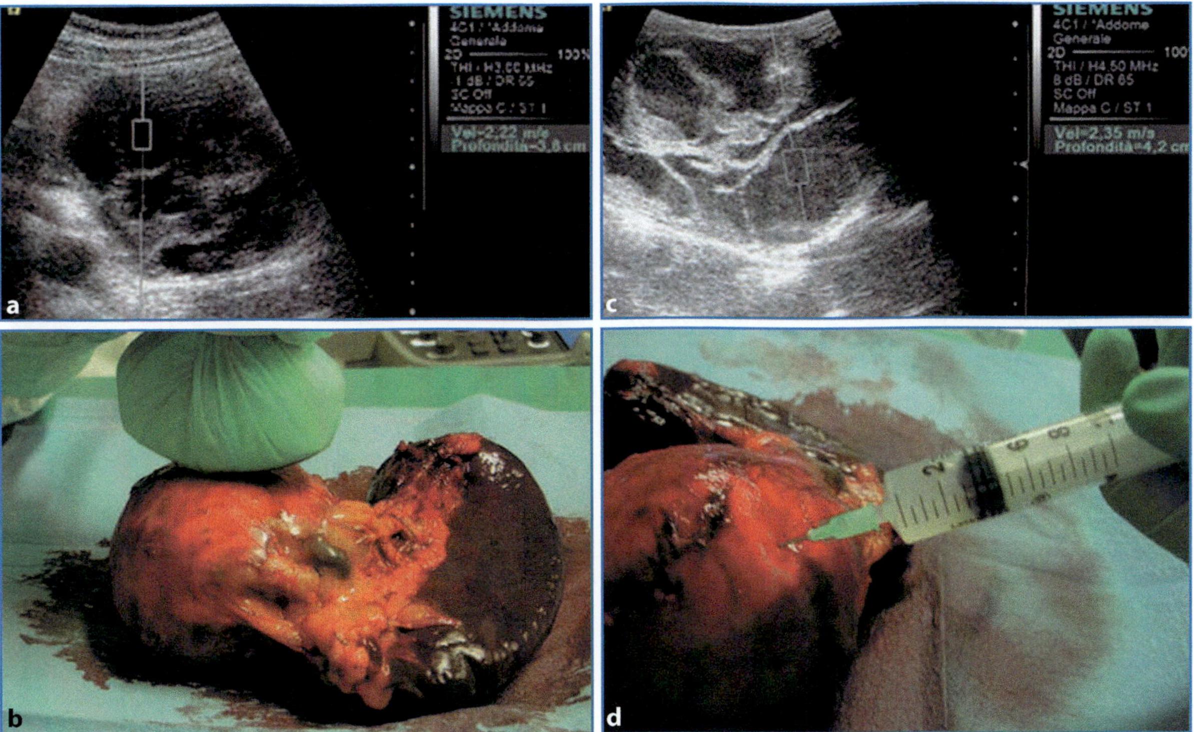

Fig. 9.19 a-d Mucinous neoplasm. At ARFI US with virtual touch tissue quantification (**a**) numerical values are obtained in the fluid. The possibility of obtaining numerical values is confirmed by applying virtual touch tissue quantification directly on the specimen (**b**) obtaining numerical values again (**c**). Aspiration confirms the presence of viscous particled (**d**) intralesional fluid

correlation between the risk of malignancy and the concentration of CEA. MCA with concordant and typical findings at noninvasive imaging (US, CEUS and MRI) should undergo resection without fluid analysis [7].

9.5 Mucinous Cystadenocarcinoma

Mucinous cystoadenocarcinoma represents the malignant neoplastic transformation of mucinous cys-

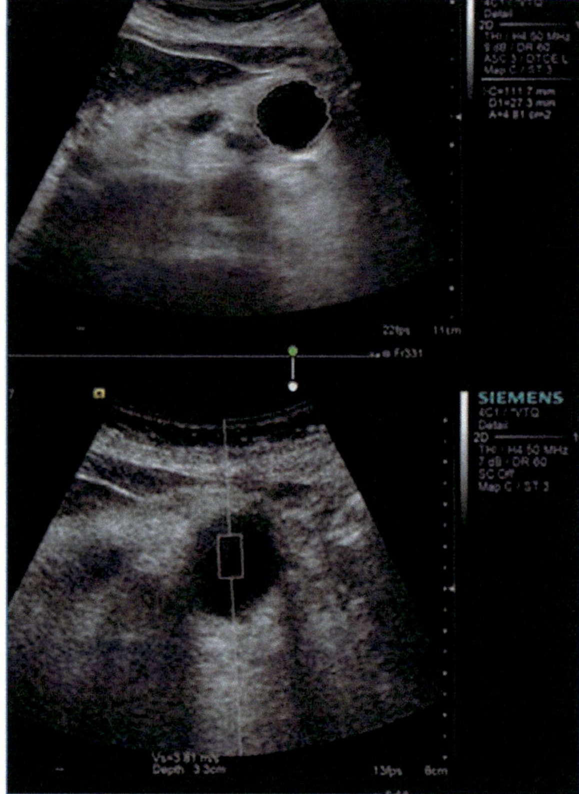

Fig. 9.20 Mucinous cystadenoma. Incidental simple small cystic pancreatic lesion with numerical values at ARFI with virtual touch tissue quantification and final diagnosis of mucinous cystadenoma

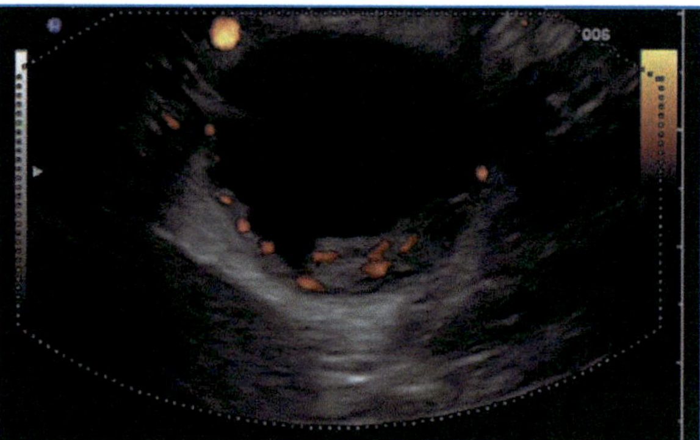

Fig. 9.21 Mucinous neoplasm. EUS image of a mucinous cystic lesion with evidence of wall thickening with solid component that appeared vascularized at Doppler imaging

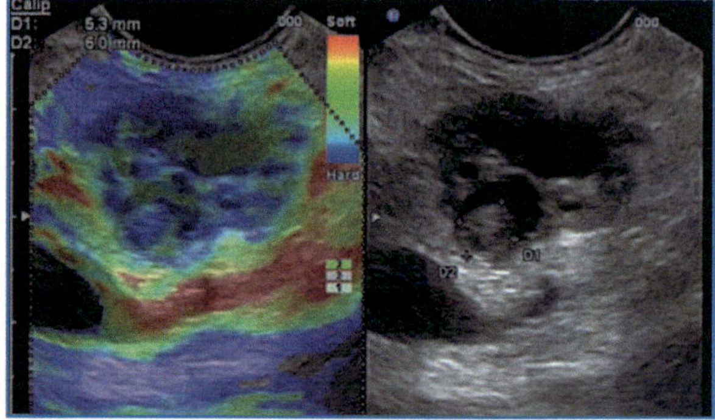

Fig. 9.22 Mucinous neoplasm. EUS elastographic image of a mucinous cystic lesion showing the hardness of a 6 mm mural nodule

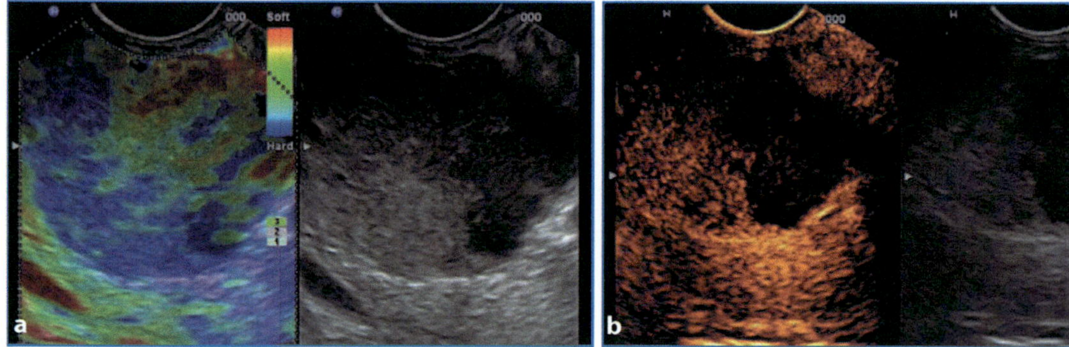

Fig. 9.23 a,b Mucinous neoplasm. **a** EUS elastographic image of a mucinous cystic lesion showing hard tissue (*blue*) with a soft area (*green*). **b** EUS image of a mucinous cystadenocarcinoma after contrast medium injection enhancing tumor vasculature

toadenoma and is characterized by thicker wall and septa, disomogeneous content and a greater number of nodules (Fig. 9.24). The significant cell proliferation is responsible for invasion, lymph nodes involvement and liver metastases [56-58]. CEUS is able to accurately demonstrate the enhancement of neoplastic vegetations [60,65]. Moreover quantitative perfusion analysis of the enhancement (Fig. 9.25) is nowadays possible, revealing higher perfusion values in the site of neoplastic degeneration (Fig. 9.25).

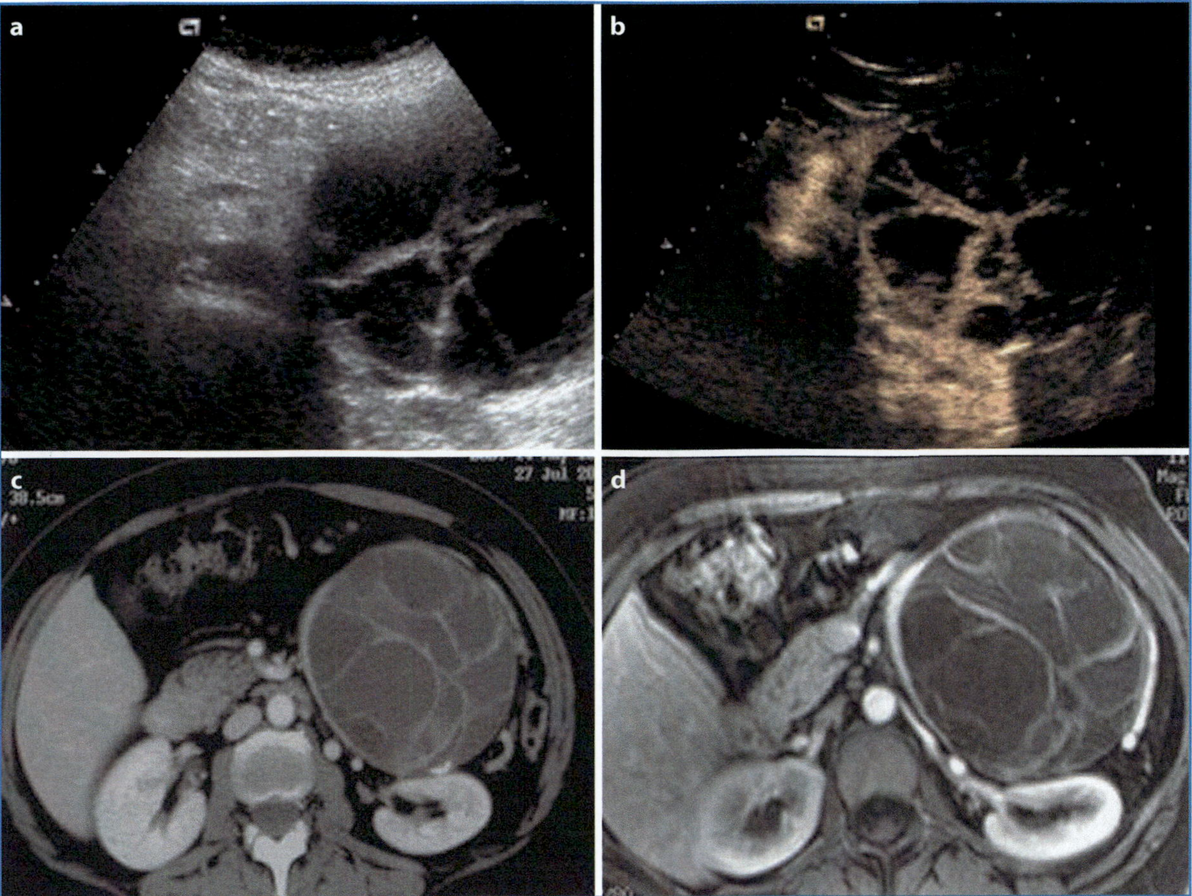

Fig. 9.24 a-d Mucinous cystadenocarcinoma. Huge cystic pancreatic mass with thick wall, thick septa and nodules enhancement. Perfect correlation between US (**a**) with CEUS (**b**), CT (**c**) and MRI (**d**)

9.6 Intraductal Papillary Mucinous Neoplasm (IPMN)

Intraductal papillary mucinous neoplasm (IPMN) is a group of exocrine mucin-producing tumors. A common occurrence in males with a mean age of 60 years old has been reported in the literature [6, 13]. However, improvements in image quality have led to the frequent incidental detection of pancreatic cystic lesions classified as IPMNs [41]. Three types of IPMNs have been described [6, 37, 67]: the main duct type, with a segmental or diffuse dilatation of the main pancreatic duct, without any abrupt cut-off [68]; the branch duct type, presenting as unilocular or multilocular cystic lesions, uni- or multi-focal, with grapelike clusters (pleomorphic cystic shape) [13]; and the mixed type, involving both the main duct and its side-branches

[69]. The demonstration of the involvement or the communication with the main pancreatic duct is needed for an appropriate diagnosis [3] (Fig. 9.6). MRI with MRCP is nowadays the imaging modality of choice for a correct diagnosis [3, 7, 13, 68], having replaced the invasive endoscopic retrograde cholangiopancreatography (ERCP), generally used for therapeutic approaches. Moreover, unlike ERCP, the ductogram provided by MRCP is not dependent upon pressure to fill all of the fluid (mucous)-filled side branches, allowing an accurate characterization of IPMN type and extent [11-14, 68, 70-73]. Dynamic evaluation before and after the intravenous secretin administration could be useful to better demonstrate the communication of the pancreatic cystic lesions with the ductal system. However, in recent years the application of secretin stimulation in the study of IPMNs has been routinely avoided. MRI with MRCP still remains a useful imag-

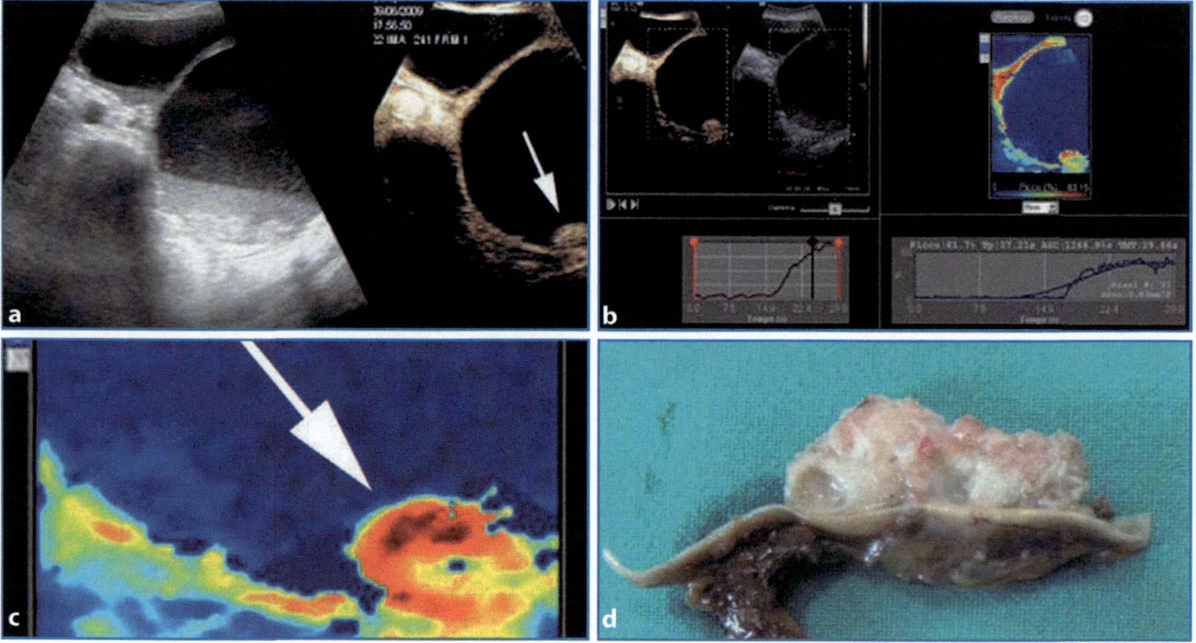

Fig. 9.25 a-d Mucinous cystadenocarcinoma. Huge cystic pancreatic mass with thick wall, thick septum and nodule (*arrow*) enhancing at CEUS (**a**). At enhancement quantification analysis (**b,c**) the highest values (*red*) are registered at the level of the septum and the nodule (*arrow*) confirmed at pathology (**d**)

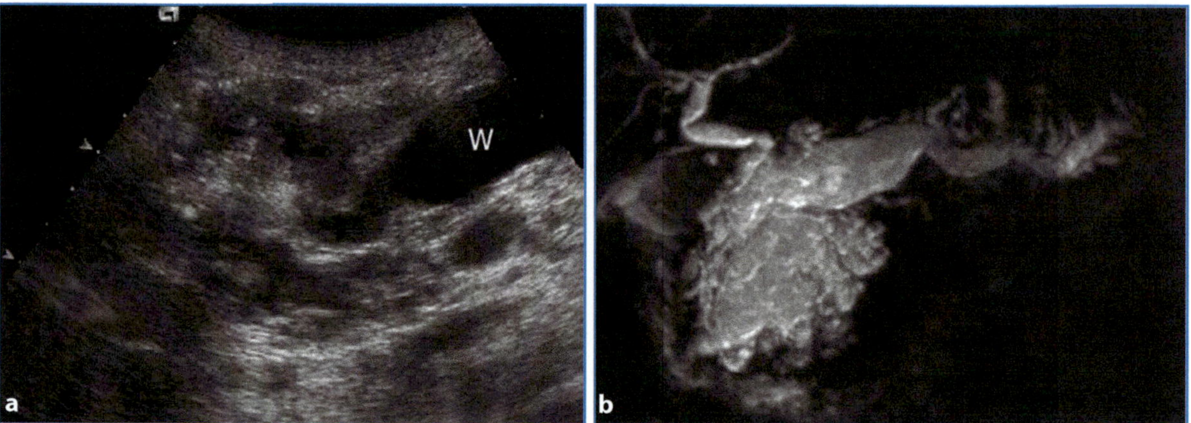

Fig. 9.26 a,b IPMN. Dilation of the main pancreatic duct (*W*) and large complex pancreatic head mass with mixed pattern at US (**a**) but with mainly cystic appearance at MRCP (**b**) and clear communication with the main pancreatic duct

ing modality for the study of IPMN able to noninvasively provide the diagnosis (communication with the ductal system) and correctly evaluate the disease (number of lesions). IPMN in fact derives from a degeneration of the ductal epithelium and can be considered an epiphenomenon of a whole ductal system disease also attested by the very often diffuse involvement (multifocal IPMN of the side branches).

In more recent papers, thin-section helical CT examination with high-quality post-processing reconstructions has been reported to have similar accuracy to MRI in detecting involvement or communication with the main pancreatic duct [4]. IPMNs consist of a variety of lesions, highly variable in type and extent, with different biological behavior, pathologically ranging from adenoma to invasive carcinoma passing from

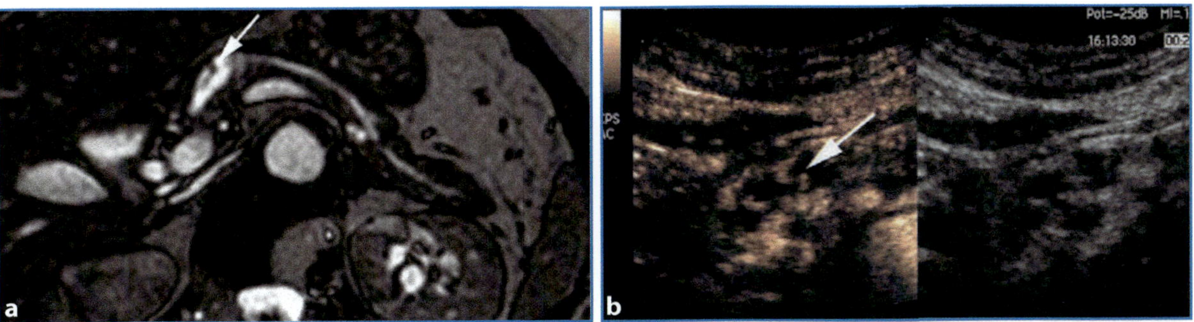

Fig. 9.27 a,b IPMN. MRI (**a**) shows segmental ductal dilation at the level of the neck of the pancreas containing very small vegetation (*arrow*) with vasculature identified at CEUS (**b**) appearing enhancing (*arrow*) during dynamic phases

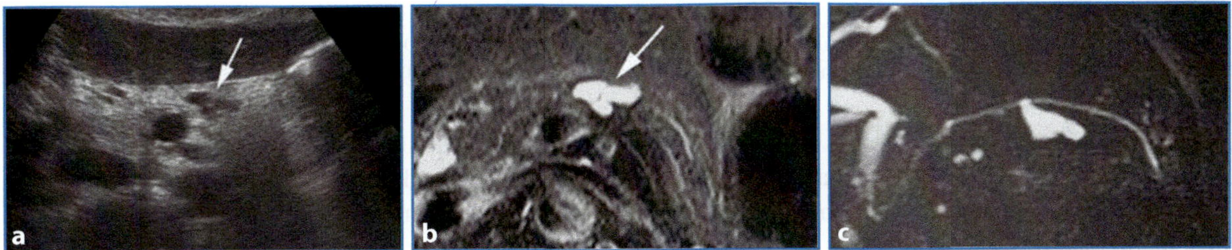

Fig. 9.28 a-c IPMN. Incidental finding at US (**a**) detecting a mixed small pancreatic body lesion (*arrow*). The lesion is clearly cystic (*arrow*) at MRI T2-weighted image (**b**) and the communication with the ductal system at MRCP (**c**) is well documented

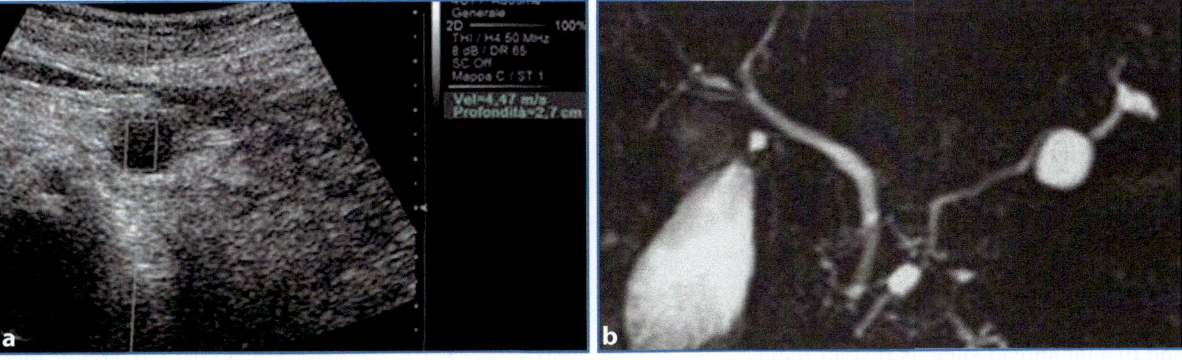

Fig. 9.29 a,b IPMN. Incidental finding at US (**a**) detecting a small cystic lesion in the pancreatic body with positive results at ARFI virtual touch tissue quantification. The suspected diagnosis of IPMN of the branch-duct is confirmed at MRCP (**b**), but more than one lesion is clearly visible

borderline lesions with different grades of atypia and noninvasive carcinoma [74-76]. Different pathologic degrees not necessarily reflect different imaging features. Therefore, a clear imaging differentiation between lesions with different pathologic behavior seems impracticable. However, several papers in the literature describe the imaging features usually observed in malignant tumors [68, 76-83]. The segmental or diffuse involvement of the main pancreatic duct, both in the main type and mixed type, defines lesions with higher risk of malignancy. In particular, a main duct with a diameter larger than 10 mm is highly suggestive of malignancy [4, 68, 76-83]. Other reported features of malignancy consist of the presence of peripheral or septal calcification, better detected on MDCT, the presence of enhanced mural nodules, enhanced solid mass in the dilated main duct or within the cystic lesions, thick septa, and enhanced ductal wall [4, 68,

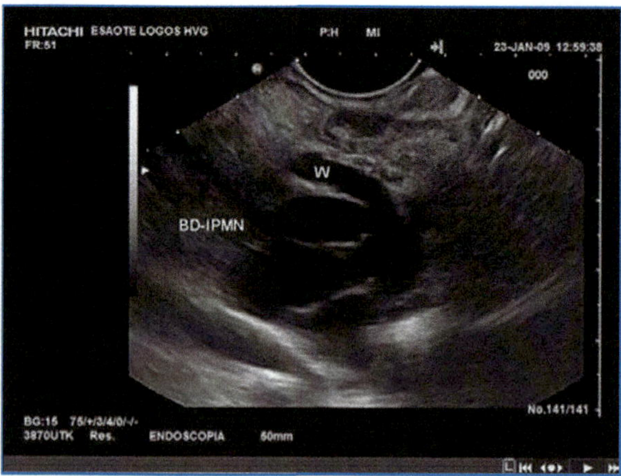

Fig. 9.30 IPMN. EUS image of a branch-duct intraductal papillary mucinous neoplasm (*BD-IPMN*) in communication with the Wirsung (*W*)

76-83]. At US, IPMN usually appears as a complex indefinite mass (Fig. 9.26) with dilation of the main pancreatic duct if involved [45, 84, 85]. As reported above for other cystic tumors of the pancreas, the enhancement of internal vegetations sometimes can be better demonstrated at CEUS than on other imaging modalities (Fig. 9.27). The real-time evaluation and the high spatial resolution allow the detection of single microbubbles passing through the septa and parietal nodules [59, 83]. However, US evaluation fails in two important aims: the demonstration of the communication with the pancreatic ductal system essential for the final diagnosis (Fig. 9.28) and the evaluation of the number of lesions (Fig. 9.29) essential for a correct evaluation of the disease.

At imaging, signs of local invasion, such as vascular encasement, peripancreatic lymph nodes enlargement and distant spread such as distant metastases are obvious features of malignancy [3-5, 37, 60, 69, 83]. In contrast, monitoring might be possible for those lesions smaller than 2.5 cm that spare the main pancreatic duct, without solid components [14, 41]. The international consensus guidelines recommend resection for all main-duct IMPNs and careful observation for asymptomatic branch-duct IPMNs measuring less than 3 cm in the absence of solid components or main-duct dilation [86]. On the other hand, cystic lesions only with a mean diameter equal to or larger than 30 mm are not uniformly considered with features of malignancy [4, 70, 87-92]. EUS again still provides the highest spatial resolution imaging of the pancreas with

an extremely accurate evaluation of the morphologic features of cystic tumors (Fig. 9.30). On EUS, any intraductal mass, mural nodule or projections noted within the main duct or off a cyst wall should be sampled by FNA [54]. If no visible lesions are noted, the main or branch duct can be punctured for cytology and tumor markers. Cytology usually reveals thick mucin and fragments of papillary mucinous epithelium can be seen on FNA. Since the results of EUS guided FNA cytology have been variable, many groups focused the attention at the application of molecular techniques to cyst fluid obtained by EUS-FNA. IPMNs are believed to follow a transformation process similar to the adenoma-carcinoma sequence in colon cancer, where lesions progress from hyperplasia to dysplasia and carcinoma [93]. K-ras gene mutation has been well studied and appears to occur early in the transformation sequence. In a multicenter prospective study, Khalid et al. evaluated the role of DNA analysis in 124 patients undergoing EUS-FNA with malignant cytology or later confirmed by surgical pathology. This study found that very high amounts of mutated DNA and mutational sequence of K-ras followed by allelic loss was very specific for malignant cyst [94]. The role of cyst fluid DNA analysis in clinical practice, however, remains to be determined.

Some authors have also studied the immunohistochemical analysis of aspirated cyst fluid. Mucins (MUCs), high-molecular-weight glycoproteins, are generally known to protect surface epithelia but often display deregulated expression in malignant cells. In 2004, a new classification of IPMN in four subtypes, on the basis of histologic features and immunohistochemical reactivity with antibodies to specific types of MUCs was developed [95]. The gastric-type IPMN (MUC 1−; MUC2−, MUC5AC+) usually shows low-grade atypia corresponding to intraductal papillary-mucinous adenoma. The intestinal-type IPMN (MUC1−, MUC2+, MUC5AC+) usually shows moderate- or high-grade atypia corresponding to borderline or in situ carcinoma. The pancreatobiliary and the oncocytic types IPMN (MUC1+, MUC2−, MUC5AC+) usually show severe/high grade atypia corresponding to carcinoma in situ and can progress in 50% to an invasive ductal adenocarcinoma of the pancreas [95].

In a preliminary experience reported in literature, the pattern of phenotypic expression on MUCs in 90 patients with benign and malignant pancreatic lesions, underwent FNA-EUS, was examined [96]. The material was utilized both for cytologic diagnosis and for mucin expression analysis at RNA level. PCR for MUC1, MUC2, MUC3, MUC4, MUC5AC, MUC5B, MUC6 and MUC7 was performed. The aspired material from cysts was amorphous and scanty for cytologic analysis in 52% of cases but RNA extraction was successful n 81% of biopsies. MUC7 expression was highly significant for adenocarcinoma (P=0.007) and borderline for IPMN (P=0.05). Although these are preliminary results, a sufficient quantity of RNA was extracted from EUS-guided FNA [96].

9.7 Rare Cystic Pancreatic Tumors

A variety of other pancreatic tumors with cystic changes is less frequently encountered during routine clinical practice. These rare lesions can be incidentally detected or may present associated with nonspecific symptoms. Some of the most important rare pancreatic tumors with cystic changes are here reported.

Solid-pseudopapillary tumor (SPT) with cystic changes is a rare exocrine tumor of the pancreas with predilection for young (second to fourth decades of life) women (sex ratio 10:1) and indolent biologic behavior. If larger in size, abdominal discomfort and pain can be referred. At imaging examinations, SPT usually presents as a well-defined, round mass with heterogeneous solid and cystic aspect [3, 37, 97, 98]. A thick and fibrous capsule is often observed and the identification of internal hemorrhage is a typical sign [97]. Lamellar calcifications can be clearly recognized [3, 37]. At US the cystic content is impossible to define correctly: CT or better MRI, to avoid radiation dose to these young patients, are required [97, 98]. CT and MRI remain the imaging modalities of choice to demonstrate the hemorrhagic content typical of these lesions, which appear hyperdense on unenhanced CT and varying in signal intensity both on T1- and T2-weighted images at MRI depending on the age of the bleeding [37, 97]. Moreover, areas of hyperintensity are constantly detected on fat-suppressed T1-weighted images [98]. After the administration of contrast medium, the thick capsule and solid portions show progressive enhancement, while the hemorrhagic, necrotic and cystic areas appear avascular. Delayed enhancement of the fibrous capsule on CT and MRI has been described. Although SPT has low malignant potential, it can show local invasion [3].

Endocrine cystic tumors are endocrine tumors with cystic changes. Endocrine tumors with cystic changes are more frequently non-symptomatic tumors, both benign and malignant or of uncertain behavior. At imaging examinations, cystic endocrine tumors usually show 3 cm or larger in size, with calcification and complex features, such as irregular thick wall, septa and nodules [37, 99-103]. A well-encapsulated rounded lesion characterized by a wide central cystic/necrotic area can be demonstrated at US, CT and MRI. After the administration of contrast agent a typically rapid enhancement of the solid components is easily documented around the central unenhanced portion [5, 99-103]. Quantitative perfusion analysis of the enhancement is nowadays possible after CEUS study which shows the high perfusion values of the solid portion (wall, nodules and septa) of the endocrine cystic tumors. In small lesions, the main pancreatic duct is usually regular in caliber or can be involved by larger lesion as a consequence of malignant behavior.

Cystic changes rarely described in adenocarcinoma can be due to the central necrosis and therefore usually observed in poorly differentiated tumors [7, 37]. Macroscopic calcifications are generally absent. After the administration of contrast material, unlike the cystic endocrine tumors, the solid peripheral tissue appears hypovascular compared to the surrounding pancreatic parenchyma. This pattern with more or less tumor enhancement can be present in cases of anaplastic pancreatic tumor [37]. Vascular involvement or regional lymph nodes enlargement, as signs of local invasion, can be very often detected. Moreover, an accurate evaluation of the liver parenchyma after the administration of contrast agent is paramount to exclude hepatic metastases [37].

9.8 Incidental Pancreatic Cyst: Risk Factors and Management

Due to advances in imaging techniques, the detection of pancreatic cystic lesions is significantly increased [3-5]. The lack of symptoms makes these lesions more likely to be anything but pseudocysts. In a series of 212 consecutive patients with pancreatic cysts the rate of pseudocysts was 19.4% in symptomatic and only 3.8% in asymptomatic patients [43]. Malignancy is significantly lower in frequency in asymptomatic pancreatic cystic lesions. While a symptomatic cystic lesion of the pancreas can be a pseudocyst but it is also possible that if it is neoplastic it is already malignant, the asymptomatic lesions are smaller, unlikely to be pseudocysts but less likely to have undergone malignant changes [43]. Hence the frequency of malignancy in small pancreatic cysts is significantly higher in symptomatic patients [41]. Regarding other risk factors, dimensions and inclusions have to be taken into great consideration. Monitoring might be possible for those lesions smaller than 2.5 cm and which spare the main pancreatic duct and demonstrate no solid components [14, 41]. Attention is mainly focused on IPMN. The international consensus guidelines recommended resection for all main-duct IMPNs and mucinous cystic neoplasms and careful observation for asymptomatic branch-duct IPMNs measuring less than 3 cm in the absence of solid components or main-duct dilation [86]. Cystic aspiration is strongly advised by the ACR Incidental Findings Committee before any surgery is undertaken in patients with cystic lesions between 2 and 3 cm. However, most pancreatic cystic tumors should be resected without the need for cystic fluid analysis [104].

The majority of small cysts (<3 cm) are reported to be benign but, regarding cystic intralesional component, also the presence of septa was associated with borderline or in situ malignancy in 20% of cases [105].

However on the basis of imaging alone the correct diagnosis can be very difficult. As a matter of fact, an incorrect preoperative diagnosis is reported in one-third of the incidental pancreatic cystic lesions [106]. Preoperative differential diagnosis is influenced by the frequent overlapping of the imaging features [11, 37]. The most important diagnosis remains the differentiation between neoplastic vs non-neoplastic and mucinous vs nonmucinous cystic pancreatic lesions. MRI with MRCP is reported to be the imaging method of choice [7, 41]. CEUS is however reported to be extremely accurate in the demonstration of the vascularization of inclusions and EUS still provides the highest image resolution of the pancreas. In cases of undetermined lesions, EUS-FNA can supply further diagnostic information on the basis of cytology, fluid viscosity, concentration of tumor glycoproteins, amylase level and molecular analysis [107]. The management of these patients remains complex and correlating imaging findings with clinical data is mandatory [15].

In summary, in the presence of an incidental pancreatic cyst what should be considered are: presence of symptoms, gender and age of the patient, lesion dimensions, intralesional solid vascularized component, main duct dilation and laboratory data.

With regard to follow-up, it is reported in the literature that asymptomatic thin-walled unilocular cysts less than 3 cm in size should be followed by imaging at 6 months, 12 months and then annually for 3 years, while cystic pancreatic lesions with more complex features should be followed more closely [11]. How long the follow-up period should be, needs to take into account the possibility of degeneration of these lesions. This could however also increase over long periods of time (years). In the follow-up of borderline cystic pancreatic lesions CT cannot be proposed owing to the radiation exposure, so to reduce the number of MRI examinations in the subgroup of patients in whom the lesions can be visualized, CEUS can be used because it is less expensive, radiation-free and, as reported [10], an effective imaging method.

References

1. Zhang XM, Mitchell DS, Doohke M et al (2002) Pancreatic cysts: depiction on singleshot fast spin-echo MR images. Radiology 223:547-553.

2. Sahani DV, Kadavigere R, Saokar A et al (2005) Cystic pancreatic lesions: a simple imaging-based classification system for guiding management. Radiographics 25:1471-1484

3. Lewin M, Hoeffel C, Azizi L et al (2008) Imaging of incidental cystic lesions of the pancreas. J Radiol 89:197-207

4. Sahani DV, Kadavigere R, Blake M et al (2006) Intraductal papillary mucinous tumor of the pancreas: Multi–Detector Row CT with 2D Curved Reformations-Correlation with MRCP. Radiology 238:560-569

5. D'Onofrio M, Zamboni G, Faccioli N et al (2007) Ultrasonography of the pancreas. 4. Contrast-enhanced imaging. Abdom Imaging 32:171-181

6. Kim YH, Saini S, Sahani D et al (2005) Imaging diagnosis of cystic pancreatic lesions: pseudocyst versus nonpseudocyst. Radiographics 25:671-685

7. D'Onofrio M, Gallotti A, Pozzi Mucelli R (2010) Imaging techniques in pancreatic tumors. Expert Rev Med Devices 7:257-273

8. D'Onofrio M, Barbi E, Dietrich CF et al (2011) Pancreatic multicenter ultrasound study (PAMUS). Eur J Radiol doi:10.1016/j.ejrad.2011.01.053

9. Rickes S, Wermke W (2004) Differentiation of cystic pancreatic neoplasms and pseudocysts by conventional and echo-enhanced ultrasound. J Gastroenterol Hepatol 19:761-766

10. D'Onofrio M, Megibow AJ, Faccioli N et al (2007) Comparison of contrast-enhanced sonography and MRI in dis-

playing anatomic features of cystic pancreatic masses. Am J Roentgenol 189:1435-1442

11. Sahani DV, Miller JC, del Castillo CF et al (2009) Cystic pancreatic lesions: classification and management. J Am Coll Radiol 6:376-380. Review

12. Pilleul F, Rochette A, Partensky C et al (2005) Preoperative evaluation of intraductal papillary mucinous tumors performed by pancreatic magnetic resonance imaging and correlated with surgical and histopathologic findings. J Magn Reson Imaging 21:237-244

13. Manfredi R, Mehrabi S, Motton M et al (2008) MR imaging and MR cholangiopancreatography of multifocal intraductal papillary mucinous neoplasms of the side branches, MR pattern and its evolution. Radiol Med 113:414-428

14. Megibow AJ, Lombardo FP, Guarise A et al (2001) Cystic pancreatic masses: cross-sectional imaging observations and serial follow-up. Abdom Imaging 26:640-647

15. Morana G, Guarise A (2006) Cystic tumors of the pancreas. Cancer Imaging 6:60-71

16. Goh BK, Tan YM, Thng CH et al (2008) How useful are clinical, biochemical, and cross-sectional imaging features in predicting potentially malignant cystic lesions of the pancreas? Results from a single institution experience with 220 surgically treated patients. J Am Coll Surg 206:17-27

17. Fishman EK, Jeffrey RB Jr (2004) Multidetector CT: Principles, techniques and clinical applications. Lippincott Williams & Wilkins, Philadelphia, p. 85

18. Nino-Murcia M, Jeffrey RB Jr, Beaulieu CF et al (2001) Multidetector CT of the pancreas and bile duct system: value of curved planar reformations. Am J Roentgenol 176:689-693

19. Sahani D, Shah ZK (2006) Soft-organ MDCT imaging: pancreas and spleen. In: Saini S, Rubin GD, Kalra MK (eds) MDCT. A practical approach. Springer-Verlag, Milan

20. Koito K, Namieno T, Nagakawa T et al (1997) Solitary cystic tumor of the pancreas: EUS-pathologic correlation. Gastrointest Endosc 45:268-276

21. Gress F, Gottlieb K, Cummingd O et al (2000) Endoscopic ultrasound characteristics of mucinous cystic neoplasms of the pancreas. Am J Gastroenterol 95:961-965

22. Ahmad NA, Kochman ML, Lewis JD et al (2001) Can EUS alone differentiate between malignant and benign cystic lesions of the pancreas? Am J Gastroenterol 96:3295-3300

23. Ahmad NA, Kochman ML, Bresinger C et al (2003) Interobserver agreement among endosonographers for the diagnosis of neoplastic versus non-neoplastic pancreatic cystic lesions. Gastrointest Endosc 58:59-64

24. Frossard JL, Amouyal P, Amouyal G et al (2003) Performance of endosonography-guided fine needle aspiration and biopsy in the diagnosis of pancreatic cystic lesions. Am J Gastroenterol 98:1516-1524

25. Brugge WR, Lewandrowski K, Lee-Lewandrowski E et al (2004) Diagnosis of pancreatic cystic neoplasm: a report os the cooperative pancreatic cyst study. Gastroenterology 126:1330-1336

26. Al-Haddad M, Wallace MB, Woodward TA et al (2008) The safety of fine-needle aspiration guided by endoscopic ultrasound: a prospective study. Endoscopy 40:204-208

27. Giovannini M, Seitz JF, Monges G et al (1995) Fine-needle aspiration cytology guided by endoscopic ultrasonography; results in 141 patients. Endoscopy 27:171-177

28. Wiersema MJ, Kochman ML, Cramer HM et al (1994) Endosonography-guided real-time fine-needle aspiration biopsy. Gastrointest Endosc 40:700-707

29. Lee LS, Saltzman JR, Bounds BC et al (2005) EUS-guided fine needle aspiration of pancreatic cysts: a retrospective analysis of complications and their predictors. Clin Gastroenterol Hepatol 3:231-236

30. Klapman JB, Logrono R, Dye CE et al (2003) Clinical impact of on-site cytopathology interpretation on endoscopic ultrasound-guided fine needle aspiration. Am J Gastroenterol 98:1289-1294

31. Brandwein SL, Farrell JJ, Centeno BA et al (2001) Detection and tumor staging of malignancy in cystic, intraductal, and solid tumors of the pancreas by EUS. Gastrointest Endosc 53;722-727

32. Sedlack R, Affi A, Vazquez-Sequeiros E et al (2002) Utility of EUS in the evaluation of cystic pancreatic lesions. Gastrointest Endosc 2002;56:543-547.

33. Al-Haddad M, El Hajj I, Eloubeidi M (2010) Endoscopic ultrasound for the evaluation of cystic lesions of the pancreas. JOP 11:299-309

34. Chaya CT, Bhutani MS (2007) Ultrasonography of the pancreas. 6. Endoscopic imaging. Abdom Imaging 32:191-199

35. Mallery JS, Centeno BA, Hahn PF et al (2002) Pancreatic tissue sampling guided by EUS, CT/US, and surgery: a comparison of sensitivity and specificity. Gastrointest Endosc 56:218-224

36. Brugge WR (2004) Pancreatic fine needle aspiration: to do or not to do? JOP 5:282-288

37. Procacci C, Biasiutti C, Carbognin G et al (2001) Pancreatic neoplasms and tumor-like conditions. Eur Radiol 11[Suppl 2]:S167-S192

38. Garcea G, Ong SL, Rajesh A et al (2008) Cystic lesions of the pancreas. A diagnostic and management dilemma. Pancreatology 8:236-251

39. Kloppel G (2000) Pseudocysts and other non-neoplastic cysts of the pancreas. Semin Diagn Pathol 17:7-15

40. Krinsky G (2001) Case 26-2000: intraductal papillary mucinous carcinoma. N Engl J Med 344:141; author reply 141-142

41. Berland LL, Silverman SG, Gore RM et al (2010) Managing incidental findings on abdominal CT: white paper of the ACR incidental findings committee. J Am Coll Radiol 7:754-773

42. Allen PJ, D'Angelica M, Gonen M et al (2006) A selective approach to the resection of cystic lesions of the pancreas: results from 539 consecutive patients. Ann Surg. 244:572-582

43. Fernández-del Castillo C, Targarona J, Thayer SP et al (2003) Incidental pancreatic cysts: clinicopathologic characteristics and comparison with symptomatic patients. Arch Surg 138:427-423; discussion 433-434

44. Adsay NV (2008) Cystic neoplasia of the pancreas: pathology and biology. J Gastrointest Surg 12:401-404. Review

45. Martinez-Noguera A, D'Onofrio M (2007) Ultrasonography of the pancreas. 1. Conventional imaging. Abdom Imaging 32:136-149

46. D'Onofrio M, Gallotti A, Salvia R et al (2010) Acoustic

radiation force impulse (ARFI) ultrasound imaging of pancreatic cystic lesions. Eur J Radiol 39:939-940

47. D'Onofrio M, Gallotti A, Falconi M et al (2010 Acoustic radiation force impulse ultrasound imaging of pancreatic cystic lesions: preliminary results. Pancreas 39:939-940

48. D'Onofrio M, Gallotti A, Mucelli RP (2010) Pancreatic mucinous cystadenoma at ultrasound acoustic radiation force impulse (ARFI) imaging. Pancreas 39:684-685

49. D'Onofrio, Martone E, Malagò R et al (2007) Contrast-enhanced ultrasonography of the pancreas. JOP J Pancreas 8 [Suppl 1]:71-76

50. D'Onofrio M et al (2011) Pancreas. In: Weskott HP (ed) Contrast-enhanced ultrasound. UNI-MED Verlag AG, Bremen

51. D'Onofrio M, Gallotti A, Martone E et al (2009) Solid appearance of pancreatic serous cystadenoma diagnosed as cystic at ultrasound acoustic radiation force impulse imaging. JOP 10:543-546

52. Khurana B, Mortele KJ, Glickman J et al (2003) Macrocystic serous adenoma of the pancreas: radiologic-pathologic correlation. Am J Roentgenol 181:119-123

53. Jacobson BC, Baron TH, Adler DG et al (2005) ASGE guidelines: the role of endoscopy in the diagnosis and the management of cystic lesion and inflammatory fluid collections of the pancreas. Gastrointestinal Endosc 61:363-370

54. Carlson SK, Johnson CD, Brandt KR et al (1998) Pancreatic cystic neoplasms: the role and sensitivity of needle aspiration and biopsy. Abdom Imaging 23:387-393

55. Manfredi R (2010) Benign cystic neoplasms of the pancreas: MR/MRCP imaging appearance and evolution. RSNA VU31-06

56. Buetow PC, Rao P, Thompson LDR (1998) Mucinous cystic neoplasms of the pancreas: radiologic-pathologic correlation. Radiographics 18:433-449

57. Compagno J, Oertel JE (1978) Mucinous cystic neoplasms of the pancreas with overt and latent malignancy (cystadenocarcinoma and cystadenoma). A clinicopathologic study of 41 cases. Am J Clin Pathol 69:573-580

58. Procacci C, Carbognin G, Accordini S et al (2001) CT features of malignant mucinous cystic tumors of the pancreas. Eur Radiol 11:1626-1630

59. D'Onofrio M, Zamboni G, Malagò R et al (2005) Pancreatic pathology. In: Quaia E (ed) Contrast media in ultrasonography. Springer-Verlag, Berlin, pp. 335-347

60. D'Onofrio M, Caffarri S, Zamboni G et al (2004) Contrast-enhanced ultrasonography in the characterization of pancreatic cystadenoma. J Ultrasound Med 23:1125-1129

61. D'Onofrio M, Gallotti A, Principe F et al (2010) Contrast-enhanced ultrasound of the pancreas. World J Radiol 2:97-102

62. EFSUMB Study Group (2008) Guidelines and good clinical practice recommendations for contrast enhanced ultrasound (CEUS) – update 2008. Ultraschall Med 29:28-44

63. Rickes S, Wermke W (2004) Differentiation of cystic pancreatic neoplasms and pseudocysts by conventional and echo-enhanced ultrasound. J Gastroenterol Hepatol 19:761-766

64. Hammond N, Miller FH, Sica GT et al (2002) Imaging of cystic disease of the pancreas. Radiol Clin North Am 40:1243-1262

65. Xu M, Xie XY, Liu GJ et al (2011) The application value of contrast-enhanced ultrasound in the differential diagnosis of pancreatic solid-cystic lesions. Eur J Radiol doi:10.1016/ j.ejrad.2011.03.048

66. Saftoiu A (2011) State of the art imaging techniques in endoscopic ultrasound. World J Gastroenterol 17:691-696

67. Fukukura Y, Fujiyoshi F, Sasaki M et al (2000) Intraductal papillary mucinous tumors of the pancreas. Am J Roentgenol 174:441-447

68. Manfredi R, Graziani R, Motton M et al (2009) Main pancreatic duct intraductal papillary mucinous neoplasms: accuracy of MR imaging in differentiation between benign and malignant tumors compared with histopathologic analysis. Radiology 253:106-115

69. Procacci C, Megibow AJ, Carbognin G et al (1999) Intraductal papillary mucinous tumor of the pancreas: a pictorial essay. Radiographics 19:1447-1463

70. Baiocchi GL, Portolani N, Missale G et al (2010) Intraductal papillary mucinous neoplasm of the pancreas (IPMN): clinico-pathological correlations and surgical indications. World J Surg Oncol 8:25

71. Perez-Johnston R, Lin JD, Fernandez-Del Castillo Carlos C et al (2009) Management of intraductal papillary mucinous neoplasms of the pancreas. Minerva Chir 64:477-487. Review

72. Choi JY, Lee JM, Lee MW et al (2009) Magnetic resonance pancreatography: comparison of two- and three-dimensional sequences for assessment of intraductal papillary mucinous neoplasm of the pancreas. Eur Radiol 19:2163-2170

73. Guarise A, Faccioli N, Ferrari M et al (2008) Evaluation of serial changes of pancreatic branch duct intraductal papillary mucinous neoplasms by follow-up with magnetic resonance imaging. Cancer Imaging 8:220-228

74. Ishida M, Egawa S, Aoki T et al (2007) Characteristic clinicopathological features of the types of intraductal papillary-mucinous neoplasms of the pancreas. Pancreas 35:348-352

75. Schmidt CM, Yip-Schneider MT, Ralstin MC et al (2008) PGE(2) in pancreatic cyst fluid helps differentiate IPMN from MCN and predict IPMN dysplasia. J Gastrointest Surg 12:243-249

76. Pitman MB, Genevay M, Yaeger K et al (2010) High-grade atypical epithelial cells in pancreatic mucinous cysts are a more accurate predictor of malignancy than "positive" cytology. Cancer Cytopathol 118:434-440

77. Takanami K, Yamada T, Tsuda M et al (2010) Intraductal papillary mucininous neoplasm of the bile ducts: multimodality assessment with pathologic correlation. Abdom Imaging 4:447-456

78. Jang JY, Hwang DW, Kim MA et al (2011) Analysis of prognostic factors and a proposed new classification for invasive papillary mucinous neoplasms. Ann Surg Oncol 18:644-650

79. Mimura T, Masuda A, Matsumoto I et al (2010) Predictors of malignant intraductal papillary mucinous neoplasm of the pancreas. J Clin Gastroenterol 44:e224-229

80. Kanno A, Satoh K, Hirota M et al (2010) Prediction of invasive carcinoma in branch type intraductal papillary mucinous neoplasms of the pancreas. J Gastroenterol 45:952-959

81. Ingkakul T, Sadakari Y, Ienaga J et al (2010) Predictors of

the presence of concomitant invasive ductal carcinoma in intraductal papillary mucinous neoplasm of the pancreas. Ann Surg 251:70-75

82. Salvia R, Fernández-del Castillo C, Bassi C et al (2004) Main-duct intraductal papillary mucinous neoplasms of the pancreas: clinical predictors of malignancy and long-term survival following resection. Ann Surg 239:678-685; discussion 685-687

83. Itoh T, Hirooka Y, Itoh A et al (2005) Usefulness of contrastenhanced transabdominal ultrasonography in the diagnosis of intraductal papillary mucinous tumors of the pancreas. Am J Gastroenterol 100:144-152

84. Shapiro RS, Wagreich J, Parsons RB et al (1998) Tissue harmonic imaging sonography: evaluation of image quality compared with conventional sonography. Am J Roentgenol 171:1203-1206

85. Bennett GL, Hann LE (2001) Pancreatic ultrasonography. Surg Clin North Am 81:259-281

86. Tanaka M, Chari S, Adsay V et al (2006) International consensus guidelines for management of intraductal papillary mucinous neoplasms and mucinous cystic neoplasms of the pancreas. Pancreatology 6:17-32

87. Huang ES, Gazelle GS, Hur C (2010) Consensus guidelines in the management of branch duct intraductal papillary mucinous neoplasm: a cost-effectiveness analysis. Dig Dis Sci 55:852-860

88. Buscaglia JM, Shin EJ, Giday SA et al (2009) Awareness of guidelines and trends in the management of suspected pancreatic cystic neoplasms: survey results among general gastroenterologists and EUS specialists. Gastrointest Endosc 69:813-820

89. Jang JY, Kim SW, Lee SE et al (2008) Treatment guidelines for branch duct type intraductal papillary mucinous neoplasms of the pancreas: when can we operate or observe? Ann Surg Oncol 15:199-205

90. Dongbin L, Fei L, Werner Josefin B et al (2010) Intraductal papillary mucinous neoplasms of the pancreas: diagnosis and management. Eur J Gastroenterol Hepatol 22:1029-1038

91. Salvia R, Partelli S, Crippa S et al (2009) Intraductal papillary mucinous neoplasms of the pancreas with multifocal involvement of branch ducts. Am J Surg 198:709-714

92. Sadakari Y, Ienaga J, Kobayashi K et al (2010) Cyst size indicates malignant transformation in branch duct intraductal papillary mucinous neoplasm of the pancreas without mural nodules. Pancreas 39:232-236

93. Gerdes B, Wild A, Wittenberg J et al (2003) Tumor-suppressing pathways in cystic pancreatic tumors. Pancreas 26:42-48

94. Khalid A, McGrath KM, Zahid M et al (2005) The role of pancreatic cystic lesions of the pancreas. Clin Lab Med 3:967-973

95. Furukawa T, Kloppel G, Volkan Adsay N et al (2005) Classifications of type of intraductal papillary mucinous neoplasm of the pancreas: a consensus study. Virchows Arch 447:794-799

96. Carrara S, Cangi MG, Pecciarini L et al (2011) Mucin expression pattern in pancreatic diseases: preliminary experience on material obtained under EUS-guided FNA. Am J Gastroenterol [in print]

97. Cantisani V, Mortele KJ, Levy A et al (2003) MR imaging features of solid pseudopapillary tumor of the pancreas in adult and pediatric patients. Am J Roentgenol 181:395-401

98. Chen SQ, Zou SQ, Dai QB et al (2008) Clinical analysis of solid-pseudopapillary tumor of the pancreas: report of 15 cases. Hepatobiliary Pancreat Dis Int 7:196-200

99. Graziani R, Brandalise A, Bellotti M et al (2010) Imaging of neuroendocrine gastroenteropancreatic tumours. Radiol Med 115:1047-1064. Review

100. Bordeianou L, Vagefi PA, Sahani D et al (2008) Cystic pancreatic endocrine neoplasms: a distinct tumor type? J Am Coll Surg 206:1154-1158

101. Sidden CR, Mortele KJ (2007) Cystic tumors of the pancreas: ultrasound, computed tomography, and magnetic resonance imaging features. Semin Ultrasound CT MR 28:339-356. Review

102. Deshpande V, Lauwers GY (2007) Cystic pancreatic endocrine tumor: a variant commonly confused with cystic adenocarcinoma. Cancer 111:47-53

103. Tamagno G, Maffei P, Pasquali C et al (2005) Clinical and diagnostic aspects of cystic insulinoma. Scand J Gastroenterol 40:1497-1501

104. van der Waaij LA, van Dullemen HM, Porte RJ (2005) Cyst fluid analysis in the differential diagnosis of pancreatic cystic lesions: a pooled analysis. Gastrointest Endosc 62:383-389. Review

105. Sahani D, Saokar A, Hahn PF et al (2006) Pancreatic cysts 3 cm or smaller: how aggressive should treatment be? Radiology 238:912-919

106. Correa-Gallego C, Ferrone CR, Thayer SP et al (2010) Incidental pancreatic cysts: do we really know what we are watching? Pancreatology 10:144-150

107. Petrone MC, Arcidiacono PG (2008) Role of endosocopic ultrasound in the diagnosis of cystic tumours of the pancreas. Dig Liver Dis 40:847-853. Review

Rare Pancreatic Tumors

Roberto Malagò, Ugolino Alfonsi, Camilla Barbiani, Andrea Pezzato and Roberto Pozzi Mucelli

10.1 Introduction

Rare pancreatic tumors are a heterogeneous group of tumors infrequently seen in any given individual clinical practice. These lesions show some clinical and imaging features different from the more common pancreatic adenocarcinoma, islet cell neoplasms or cystic tumors.

In order to make a classification, the main rare tumors were divided into epithelial and non epithelial origin. Many tumors are described in the literature with different names. Pathologic entities will be reported with the accepted World Health Organization (WHO) nomenclature.

10.2 Epithelial Origin Rare Pancreatic Tumors

10.2.1 Solid Pseudopapillary Tumor of the Pancreas

10.2.1.1 Epidemiology and Clinical Features

Different names of this tumor were reported until it was defined by the World Health Organization (WHO) in 1996 as a *solid pseudopapillary tumor* of the pancreas [1-3]. Solid-pseudopapillary tumors (SPTs) have also been known as solid papillary epithelial neoplasms, solid and cystic papillary tumors, and Hamoudi or Frantz [4] due to the variable pattern of presentation at diagnosis. SPTs are epithelial neoplasms with low malignant potential occurring predominantly in young women [5-7]. They usually start as solid tumors and undergo massive degeneration giving rise to a cystic appearance on radiologic imaging [8]. The cystic areas consist of blood, necrotic debris and foamy macrophages [9]. Although the malignant potential of SPT is low, up to 15% of SPT patients develop metastasis. SPTs with clear criteria of malignancy have been described as solid pseudopapillary carcinomas according to the WHO classification [10, 11]. The most common sites of metastasis are the liver, regional lymph nodes, mesentery, omentum, and peritoneum [12].

The female predominance of this lesion is well documented. Buetow et al. [13] reviewed the AFIP experience finding 53 of 56 (94.6%) cases occurring in women. Martin et al. [6] reviewed the experience at Memorial Sloan-Kettering Cancer Center in New York documenting 20 of 24 patients (83.3%) in females. The reason for the female predominance is unclear. The mean age at diagnosis is considerably less than typically seen in patients with pancreatic adenocarcinoma, ranging from 25 years (range 10-74) [13], to 39 years (range 12-79) [6].

Patients typically present with vague abdominal pain occasionally associated with weight loss, anorexia and a palpable abdominal mass [8, 14]. Acute manifestations such as hemoperitoneum caused by the rupture of the tumor capsule are rare.

10.2.1.2 Main Imaging Features

Because of their large size and heterogeneous morphology these lesions are easily recognized on imaging studies (Fig. 10.1). The lesions may appear anywhere within

R. Malagò (✉)
Department of Radiology
G.B. Rossi University Hospital, Verona, Italy
e-mail: roberto.malago@ospedaleuniverona.it

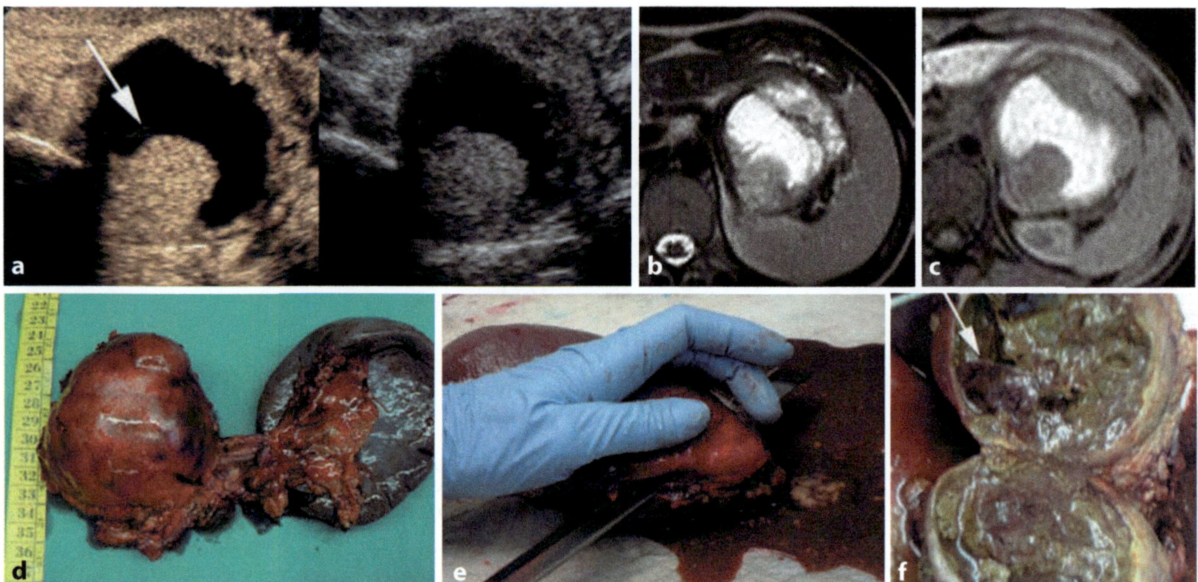

Fig. 10.1 a-f Solid-pseudopapillary pancreatic tumor. **a** Pancreatic tail mass extremely inhomogeneous with irregular vascular thick wall, cystic avascular content and intralesional nodular vegetation (*arrow*) enhancing at CEUS. **b** The mass appears cystic and complex in T2-weighted MRI. **c** The hemorrhagic content of the lesion is better depicted in T1-weighted MRI. **d** Resected specimen. **e** Abundant hemorrhagic content is visible after cutting the lesion. **f** Extremely inhomogeneous content of the lesion that shows thick capsule and intralesional nodular vegetation (*arrow*)

the pancreas although a slight predilection for the pancreatic tail has been reported. When detected, lesions are often quite large at the time of diagnosis, with mean sizes between 7.5 cm, 9 cm [13] to 11 cm [5].

On US examination SPT is usually a well-encapsulated lesion and includes cystic and solid components, but sometimes the mass is solid-looking especially in small lesions. Internal septa or calcifications may be observed [10]. Usually the appearance of SPT is variable [15, 16].

Multidetector CT (MDCT) can show tumor with typical cystic spaces in the center and enhanced solid areas at its surroundings [17]. However, MDCT has inherent limitations in showing certain tissue characteristics, such as hemorrhage and cystic degeneration. Magnetic resonance imaging (MRI) is better than CT in characterizing the cystic or solid components of the tumor (see also Chapter 11). If MRI reveals an encapsulated mass with solid and cystic components as well as hemorrhage without obvious internal septa, SPT of the pancreas should be highly suspected [18]. MR images demonstrate a well-defined lesion with heterogeneous signal intensity on T1- and T2-weighted images (Fig. 10.1), which reflects the complex nature of the mass [10]. The presence of hemorrhage degeneration

is usually easily detected as hyperintense on T1-weighted images (Fig. 10.1).

Contrast-enhanced ultrasonography (CEUS) has been used recently for the study of pancreatic tumors [19, 20]; however, the reported experiences of CEUS in cystic neoplasms of the pancreas are extremely limited [21].

In small lesions CEUS is able to identify a rim enhancement around the lesions related to the presence of a pseudocapsule resulting from compression of the adjacent parenchyma [21]. The presence of a peripheral capsule or pseudocapsule is reported to be suggestive of SPTs [22]. The advantages of CEUS are the possibility of demonstrating the vasculature of the viable portion of the tumor (Fig. 10.1) with high-quality diagnostic images. CEUS enables the dynamic observation of the enhancement and tumor perfusion [20]. In fact, CEUS is the only noninvasive imaging modality that allows a continuous evaluation of the lesion during the contrast-enhanced phases in real-time mode [23, 24]. For this reason, at CEUS, rapid enhancement patterns, especially in a highly vascular parenchyma such as the pancreatic gland, are depicted more clearly [19]. The possibilities of CEUS in the identification of the vasculature of pancreatic tumors are reported in the literature [19, 20, 25-27].

The differential diagnosis of SPT includes microcystic adenoma, mucinous cystic neoplasm, nonfunctioning islet cell tumor with cystic changes, pancreatoblastoma, pancreatic adenocarcinoma, and hemorrhagic pseudocyst [9, 13, 28, 29]. The former 3 tumors occur in older age. Microcystic adenoma is composed of microscopic cystic spaces. A mucinous cystic neoplasm has multilocular cystic spaces. A nonfunctioning islet cell tumor may be indistinguishable from SPT on sonography, but it appears as areas of rapid and intense enhancement at CEUS and MDCT and as low intensity or isointensity on T1-weighted MR images. Pancreatoblastoma is typical for childhood and more aggressive than SPT. Pancreatic adenocarcinoma is seen in older patients and does not grow as large as SPT, and cystic degeneration is extremely rare. A pancreatic pseudocyst is thin-walled and associated with a history of pancreatitis. SPT of the pancreas is obviously not a new tumor, but in the past it has been misclassified as adenocarcinoma, an islet cell tumor, cystadenoma or cystadenocarcinoma [30]. In some instances this may explain long survival after resection for adenocarcinoma.

10.2.2 Acinar Cell Carcinoma

10.2.2.1 Epidemiology and Clinical Features

Acinar cell carcinoma (ACC) is a well described, albeit rare pancreatic neoplasm, and accounts for 1% of pancreatic exocrine neoplasms. In a study of 645 pancreatic tumors, mixed cell type carcinomas are very rare, representing only 0.2% of all cases [31]. The tumor occurs in adults in the 5th-6th decades with white males being predominantly affected and has been also reported in children [32]. ACC shows three different combinations: a tumor with separate acinar and endocrine regions identifiable by light microscopy (collision tumor), a mixture of endocrine and acinar cells (intermingled tumor), as well as a tumor with uniform cell population by light microscopy but with amphicrine features, immunohistochemically [33, 34]. The histogenesis of mixed exocrine-endocrine tumors of the pancreas is still controversial. The co-existence of exocrine and endocrine elements can be attributed to their common embryologic origin [35]. ACC usually presents with nonspecific signs or symptoms such as abdominal pain, weight loss and abdominal mass. Jaundice is rare even in tumors within the pancreatic head and less frequent than in ductal carcinoma [36].

Schmid's triad, a syndrome of subcutaneous fat necrosis, polyarthralgia, and eosinophilia due to increased serum lipase, is typical for ACCs, even if very rare. A widely reported clinical syndrome manifested by any or all of the symptoms including subcutaneous or interosseous fat necrosis, panniculitis, polyarthralgia and eosinophilia has been reported [37-39]. The syndrome occurs in association with elevated serum lipase levels. Despite the widespread knowledge of this association, it has been reported in approximately 16% of cases [32]. CEA and or CA 19-9 levels may remain normal [40]. Elevation of serum alpha-fetoprotein has been reported in tumors characterized by acinar cell differentiation [41]. The prognosis of ACCs is generally poor, with median overall survivals ranging between 5 and 38 months in different institutions but mostly inferior to 36 months [42-44].

10.2.2.2 Main Imaging Features

The typical radiologic findings of ACC of the pancreas are solitary, exophytic, oval or round and well-demarcated masses with or without cystic areas [45, 46]. At US, variably sized hypoechoic regions suggesting necrosis may be seen [39]. Occasionally, intratumoral punctate calcification or hemorrhage have been reported [39, 47]. Usually, MDCT after contrast enhancement will demonstrate the mass becoming hyperdense related to the pancreas during the arterial phase and isodense in the portal venous phase. The brisk enhancement of the tumor results in an imaging appearance which mimics a neuroendocrine neoplasm [48]. On MRI the lesion appears markedly hyperintense on T2-weighted images and hyperintense on enhanced T1-weighted images. However, Tatli et al. reported that ACCs are well-defined hypovascular lesions at both MDCT and MRI with cystic areas in 55% of cases [45] and Chiou et al. described ACCs as hypodense masses at MDCT with well-defined enhancing capsule [49]. The differential diagnosis of a diffuse pancreatic mass also includes diffuse metastasis to the pancreas and pancreatic lymphoma. The presence of a peripheral capsule-like structure, heterogeneous enhancement, including well enhancing areas and hypervascular nodules, and high signal intensity on T2-weighted images, are useful for the differential diagnosis [50, 51]. Peripancreatic venous invasion is common with tumor thrombus found growing into the portal and or splenic veins [52]. The degree of thrombosis can be so prominent that the splenoportal system can appear enlarged.

10.2.3 Pancreatoblastoma

10.2.3.1 Epidemiology and Clinical Features

Pancreatoblastoma is a rare malignant primary tumor of the pancreas, but together with solid and papillary epithelial neoplasms they make up the commonest pancreatic tumors in the pediatric population [53-55]. Pancreatoblastoma usually affects patients between the ages of 1 and 8 years [56, 57], but it has been also reported in neonates [58] and in the elderly [59]. The congenital form is associated with Beckwith-Wiedemann syndrome and has been described as a cystic tumor [60]. It is slightly more common in males, and half of all cases reported in the literature occurred in Asians [58].

Pancreatoblastomas grow slowly, acquire large size at presentation which makes it difficult to identify the organ of origin and differentiate from other abdominal pediatric malignancies [61]. They cause symptoms from mass effect, or endocrine syndromes due to tumor adrenocorticotrophoid secretion and anemia due to duodenal and vascular invasion [62, 63].

Patients most frequently present with an abdominal mass, and consequent vomiting, constipation or early satiety. Pain, weight loss and jaundice occur less frequently [58, 63]. Elevated alpha-fetoprotein (particularly in the presence of liver metastases), alpha-1-antitrypsin, and LDH serum levels may be demonstrated. Elevated levels of adrenal corticotrophic hormone (ACTH) are thought to be responsible for the Cushing-like syndrome or the syndrome of inappropriate ADH secretion.

10.2.3.2 Main Imaging Features

Since pancreatoblastomas are of soft and gelatinous consistency, they rarely cause biliary or duodenal obstruction, but they may encase adjacent vessels, which makes their distinction from neuroblastoma difficult [55, 63, 64].

At US, pancreatoblastomas show mixed or low echogenicity, sometimes containing small fluid areas. At MDCT, they are usually well-defined, hypodense lesions which show mild enhancement and internal enhancing septations. Calcifications within the lesion are either rim-like or clustered. On MRI, pancreatoblastomas usually have non-specifically low to intermediate signal on T1-weighted images and high signal on T2-weighted images, and may show enhancement [54, 55, 63].

Overall pancreatoblastomas are considered malignant due to their capacity to metastasize; however, 75% are resectable and only 14% progress after resection [65].

The differential diagnosis in a child includes a consideration of any large intra- or retroperitoneal mass, such as a neuroblastoma, non-Hodgkin lymphoma, or Wilms tumor.

10.2.4 Rare Endocrine Syndromic Tumors

10.2.4.1 Gastrinoma

Epidemiology and Clinical Features

Gastrinomas are the second most frequently found (approximately 20% of all neuroendocrine tumors) functioning neuroendocrine tumors of the pancreas [66]. They differ from insulinomas by location, size and vasculature [67, 68]. The anatomic area comprising the head of the pancreas, the superior and descending portion of the duodenum and the relevant lymph nodes has been called the "gastrinoma triangle", since it harbors the vast majority of these tumors [69]. They are multiple in 60%, malignant in 60-65% and associated with MEN type I in 20-60%. Approximately 50% of patients with gastrinoma have metastases at the time of diagnosis. The reported incidence of gastrinomas is between 0.5 and 4 per million of the population per year. Zollinger-Ellison syndrome is more common in males than in females, with a ratio of 3:2. The mean age at the onset of symptoms is 38 years, range 7-83 years in some series [70]. Over 90% of patients with gastrinomas have a peptic ulcer disease. Diarrhea is another common symptom caused by the large volume of gastric acid secretion. Abdominal pain from either peptic ulcer disease or gastroesophageal reflux disease remains the most common symptom, occurring in more than 75% of patients [70]. If the patient presents gastric pH below 2.5 and serum gastric concentration above 1000 pg/mL (normal <100 pg/mL), then the diagnosis of Zollinger–Ellison is confirmed and no other diagnostic studies are actually needed; in patients presenting lower values of serum gastric concentration a secretin test should be performed in addition to a determination of basal acid output (BAO) and pentagastrin–stimulated acid output (MAO).

Main Imaging Features

Gastrinomas enhance in the early contrast phase (Fig. 10.2). Because the vascularity of gastrinomas is inferior to that of insulinomas [67, 68], the enhancement of this tumor is slower and more progressive. The same contrast enhancement pattern appears in metastatic liver

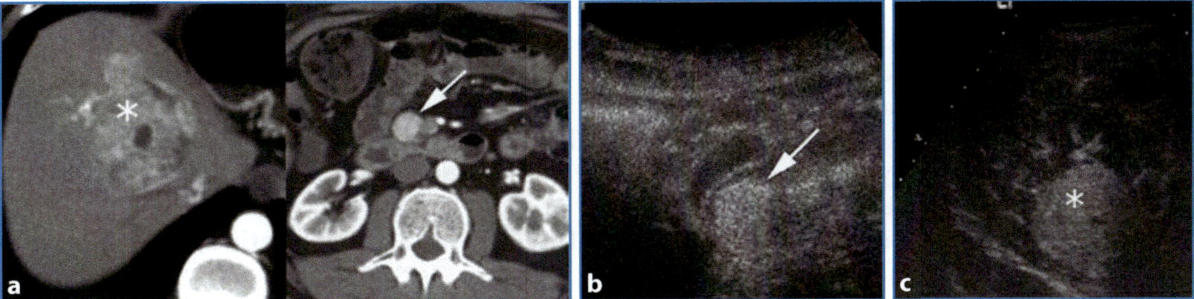

Fig. 10.2 a-c Pancreatic gastrinoma. **a** Voluminous hypervascular liver metastasis (*asterisk*) from small gastrinoma at the pancreatic uncinate process (*arrow*), hyperdense in the pancreatic phase at CT. **b** The pancreatic mass shows intense progressive enhancement in the early contrast phases at CEUS resulting hyperechoic (*arrow*). **c** In the same contrast phases the voluminous liver metastasis (*asterisk*) can also be seen as hypervascular

lesions (Fig. 10.2) present in 60% of cases at the time of diagnosis [66, 71, 72].

Both CT and MRI have the advantage of staging the entire abdomen and pelvis, which is not possible with US. In equivocal or negative cases but high clinical suspicion, somatostatin receptor scintigraphy is very effective in assessing primary tumor in pancreas or ectopic sites and metastatic lesions to the liver. Some reports have shown MRI sensitivities of 20% to 62% [73-75]. In one study, somatostatin receptor scintigraphy showed a sensitivity of 100% for gastrinomas [76] whereas EUS was 90% and CT, MRI and transabdominal US combined only 30%.

Based on the improved results with cross-sectional imaging and scintigraphy, invasive techniques are not currently recommended for this purpose.

10.2.4.2 VIPoma

Epidemiology and Clinical Features

The tumors are usually larger than 3 cm in diameter and, in 60% or more, are malignant [77-79]. Over two thirds of the tumors are located in the body-tail of the pancreas [79]. Occasionally, tumors producing the same symptoms are located in the adrenal gland, the retroperitoneum, the sympathetic chain, the lung and intestinal tract [77, 79]. Females are affected more often than males, and the age of patients ranges from 19 to 79 years (mean 48 years) [70]. These tumors have been associated with the watery diarrhea syndrome, which has also been called Verner–Morrison syndrome. The diarrhea results in severe loss of potassium and bicarbonate, which in turn leads to metabolic acidosis and dehydration [70].

Main Imaging Features

Related to the fact that VIPomas are quite rare, statistical data on the use of imaging are not available. Case reports or series with all types of hyperfunctioning endocrine tumors mixed together have been published. CT, MRI, angiography and somatostatin receptor scintigraphy have been used to localize the primary lesion and to identify metastases [80-82]. On MRI, metastatic lesions to the liver may show intense peripheral enhancement similar to the appearance of primary and metastatic lesions on CT. A combination of CT or MRI with somatostatin receptor scintigraphy currently appears to be the most effective presurgical assessment.

10.2.4.3 Glucagonoma

Epidemiology and Clinical Features

This tumor occurs slightly more often in women and is seen at a mean age of 55 years [83]. In rare instances, the tumor can cause obstructive pancreatitis [84]. The tumor is malignant in about 60% and the five-year survival is 50%. When the tumor becomes symptomatic, its size usually exceeds 5 cm, it is invasive and has metastasized to the regional lymph nodes. Tumors measuring 3 cm or less are often seen as incidental findings. The glucagonoma syndrome will reflect the catabolic action of excessively elevated glucagon levels. The most common presenting feature of the syndrome is necrolytic migratory erythema found in about 70% of all patients. The syndrome also includes mild glucose intolerance, normochromic anemia, weight loss, depression, diarrhea and a tendency to develop deep vein thrombosis [70].

Main Imaging Features

Glucagonomas are intrapancreatic and most occur in the head and neck of the pancreas. CT, MRI, angiography, EUS and F-18 fluorodeoxyglucose positron emission tomography (PET) have been used with success, but all reports included only anecdotal references to this type of tumor largely due to its rarity [85-89]. PET has been used more recently as a reliable tool to localize the primary pancreatic mass and its metastases to the liver [88, 89]. Somatostatin analog (octreotide) imaging serves as an adjuvant to conventional imaging [90].

10.2.4.4 Somatostatinoma

Epidemiology and Clinical Features

Somatostatinoma is usually a solitary lesion and tends to be aggressive with over 70% presenting with metastases, particularly if the primary tumor is larger than 2 cm [91, 92]. This tumor is usually located within the pancreas but it may also arise from the small bowel, the duodenal ampulla or periampullary mucosa. The tumor tends to be large (2 to 10 cm in diameter) and 75% occur in the head of the pancreas [93]. In men, the tumor is more frequently seen in the duodenum and in women more often in the pancreas [94]. When the small bowel is involved, the neoplasm is usually a carcinoid that consists almost completely of somatostatin-containing cells but produces little somatostatin. If the neoplasm is outside of the pancreas, it tends to be smaller (0.5 to 4 cm). This is probably due to the fact that it produces symptoms such as jaundice, bleeding and ulceration and therefore is detected early. The clinical features associated with the somatostatinoma syndrome are: hyperglycemia, cholelithiasis, diarrhea, steatorrhea and hypochlorhydria. The patients may also present with abdominal pain, weight loss and anemia as signs of malignant disease [70]. The tumor occurs in the fourth to sixth decades of life and the prognosis is poor with an average survival time of only 1 to 2 years.

Main Imaging Features

Radiologic features of somatostatinomas resemble those of other neuroendocrine tumors. All studies reported only a few cases or included somatostatinomas in their series of neuroendocrine tumors. Lesions in the pancreas and liver are usually well shown. However, radiologic techniques often fail to demonstrate tumors in the duodenum but may show obstruction of pancreatic or biliary ducts as indirect evidence. The diagnosis in

cases of duodenal localization can be established by endoscopic techniques including biopsy [95].

10.3 Non Epithelial Origin Rare Pancreatic Tumors

10.3.1 Primary Pancreatic Lymphoma

10.3.1.1 Epidemiology and Clinical Features

Pancreatic lymphoma is a rare pancreatic tumor that accounts for only 1% of all pancreatic tumors. The main pathologic type is B-cell non-Hodgkin's lymphoma and the overwhelming majority of cases involve pancreatic infiltration by systemic lymphoma [96]. It can also originate from the pancreas showing primary pancreatic manifestations, being called primary pancreatic lymphoma (PPL). The pancreatic involvement as a part of disseminated disease is more frequent but still relatively unusual [96].

Patients present most commonly with abdominal pain of the severity engendering an imaging examination. Laboratory values are non-specific. Lactate dehydrogenase (LDH) levels may be elevated [97]. Among the pancreatic tumors, there are many similarities in clinical manifestations and imaging characteristics of pancreatic cancer and pancreatic lymphoma and thus they are easy to be misdiagnosed [98-101]. The data show a strong male predominance (male to female ratio 13:3) and an increasing trend with age (median age of 57.5 years) [102].

10.3.1.2 Main Imaging Features

The lesion presents most commonly as a focal mass and less frequently as diffuse pancreatic enlargement [103]. When the lesion presents as a focal mass, it is difficult to distinguish from a primary ductal adenocarcinoma [104, 105]. However, the literature reports show a mean diameter of the pancreatic lymphoma lump usually greater than 70 mm, compared with a mean diameter of the pancreatic cancer usually smaller than 50 mm [100, 106-108]. A possible reason is that the early symptoms of pancreatic lymphoma are not obvious and diagnosis is made relatively late; therefore the lesions are relatively big when they are found.

There are no significant differences in age of onset, gender ratio, weight loss, or nausea and vomiting between the two groups. However the course of disease, back pain, jaundice, CEA and CA19-9 increase, palpable abdominal lump, superficial lymph node enlargement, fever and night sweats significantly different between the two groups of patients. Moreover bile duct dilatation significantly differs between the two diseases, occurring more frequently in pancreatic cancer than in pancreatic lymphoma. Lymph node involvement below the level of the renal veins can be seen in lymphoma, but is unusual in ductal adenocarcinoma. Finally, the intrahepatic metastases occur more easily in patients with pancreatic cancer compared with pancreatic lymphoma [109].

Less frequently, PPL can present as diffuse infiltration and enlargement of the pancreas without clinical signs of acute pancreatitis. These findings may prompt fine needle aspiration biopsy (FNAB) of the pancreatic mass to obtain a diagnosis [50].

10.3.2 Mature Teratoma

10.3.2.1 Epidemiology and Clinical Features
Mature cystic teratomas are lesions comprising a variety of tissues foreign to the organ at the anatomic site in which they arise. They are believed to develop from pluripotential cells and originate in descending order of frequency from ovaries, testes, anterior mediastinum, retroperitoneum, coccygeal and presacral areas, pineal and intracranial regions, neck, and abdominal viscera [3]. Dermoid cysts are true cysts, and as such, the cyst wall is characteristically composed of stratified squamous epithelium and its underlying connective tissue. These are extremely rare tumors arising from intrapancreatic embryonic rests. Less than 20 cases have been described in the literature [110]. The cases that appear to be true dermoid cysts occur in a younger age group (mean age, 23, range, 2 to 53 years), with no gender predominance.

10.3.2.2 Main Imaging Features
The imaging appearance of pancreatic teratoma is similar to those seen elsewhere in the body (such as in the adnexa) and is related to the amount of preponderant tissue within the lesion. Fat with fat/fluid levels are diagnostic, and septations and calcifications have been reported [111, 112].

The radiologic appearance of these lesions depends on the proportions of various tissues of which they are composed.

US initially defines a cystic mass, with distinct margins without septations [112]. The fatty component is expected to appear hyperechoic [113]. MDCT confirms

areas of calcifications and fat and can characterize the fluid as sebum, serous or complex [113]. MRI can also be performed for further characterization: the presence of fat can easily be demonstrated with fat saturated images [113, 114].

10.3.3 Lymphangioma

10.3.3.1 Epidemiology and Clinical Features
Vascular tumors of the pancreas are cystic tumors accounting for 0.1% of all pancreatic tumors [115]. The most frequent of these pancreatic tumors is lymphangioma. Lymphangiomas are congenital abnormalities of the lymphatics that occur predominantly in the pancreatic head and neck [116]. All ages are affected and a female predominance is noted [117]. This tumor has benign behavior, without invasion ability. Abdominal sites account for 1% of all lymphangiomas, with mesentery and retroperitoneum (perirenal) accounting for the vast majority [118]. Lymphangiomas were also reported to be more frequent in the pancreatic tail [119].

The tumors are considered to arise from the pancreas if they are within the parenchyma, adjacent to the gland or attached by a pedicle [119]. However, true peripancreatic lymphangiomas can be considered retroperitoneal. Abdominal pain and distension associated with the enlarged tumor are the most frequent symptoms described.

A complete surgical excision is curative [119-121], with incomplete excision being the only reason for recurrent disease [122].

10.3.3.2 Main Imaging Features
At imaging, the tumor appears as a homogeneous cystic mass. If pedunculated, the mass may appear as a juxtapancreatic cyst. Local mass effects on adjacent organs are present if large in size. On US, they appear as heterogeneous well-defined masses with a mixture of high and low echoic areas.

MRI will confirm the hyperintense cystic content on T2-weighted sequences. Following IV contrast injection, at MDCT and T1-weighted MRI there may be mural enhancement and visualization of fine septa [123-127].

Lymphangiomas are benign, but can be locally invasive. Complete surgical excision is curative. Incomplete excision results in local recurrence [119].

Differential diagnoses include pancreatic pseudocysts, mucinous and serous cystadenomas, other congenital cysts and pancreatic ductal carcinoma with cystic degeneration [124, 128, 129]. The final diagnosis is histological [124], with the endothelial cells showing immunohistochemical reactivity to factor VIII/R antigen, CD 31 (+) positivity and CD 34 (-) negativity [119], as seen in our patient. Aspiration of the cyst content may provide the diagnosis when the fluid is chylous [119].

10.3.4 Pancreatic Lipoma

10.3.4.1 Epidemiology and Clinical Features
These are extraordinarily rare benign tumors. The first case on MDCT was described in 1996 [130]. They are identical to lipomas arising in other locations.

10.3.4.2 Main Imaging Features
The tumors are detected as incidental findings on imaging studies performed for other reasons. MDCT scans show a well-circumscribed mass within the pancreas composed almost entirely of fat, with a few scattered vessels or septa or both [131]. The presence of a capsule is important for the differentiation from pancreatic fatty infiltration [132]; MRI, particularly with gradient recalled echo T1 – weighted sequences, either obtained as opposed or in – phase, may be helpful in the differentiation of these two entities [133]. Regarding US, the typical echofeature of lipoma is considered to be a hyperechoic and homogeneous well-defined mass [134]. Conservative management is indicated.

10.3.5 Schwannoma

10.3.5.1 Epidemiology and Clinical Features
Schwannomas are neurogenic neoplasms derived from Schwann cells of the sheaths of the peripheral nerves [135, 136]. They are basically soft tissue neoplasms, usually found in the head and neck, extremities, mediastinum and retroperitoneum [137, 138], only rarely found in the pancreas. In the literature, only 48 cases of pancreatic schwannoma have been reported from 1948 through 2004. Patient age ranged from 35 to 87 years with a nearly equal gender distribution, and the majority of tumors were located in the head of pancreas [139].

The preoperative diagnosis of a pancreatic schwannoma is difficult, being often confused with cystic neoplasms, such as nonfunctioning endocrine tumors, solid pseudopapillary neoplasms and mucinous cystic lesions [139, 140]. Since malignant transformation of pancreatic schwannoma is uncommon, simple enucleation is usually sufficient [139].

10.3.5.2 Main Imaging Features
MRI can better recognize the cystic component than MDCT. MRI usually shows hypointensity on T1-weighted images and hyperintensity on T2-weighted images [140, 141], and most tumors are gradually enhanced on T1-weighted images after gadolinium administration.

The most characteristic feature on MDCT is the presence of a low density and/or cystic image in various degrees within the tumor. The low density and/or cystic images would reflect the Antoni B component or the degenerative cystic areas of the schwannoma. MDCT shows the difference between the Antoni A and the Antoni B areas based on their vascularity, i.e. well-enhanced areas corresponding to Antoni A, and unenhanced areas corresponding to Antoni B. Therefore, the CT findings of these tumors correlate quite well with the pathologic features [135, 142].

The solid and cystic pattern can also be seen at US, in which hypoechoic and/or cystic findings are described in a high percentage of cases. At CEUS, the enhancement of the solid component is well documented [143].

10.4 Metastases

Primary tumors that most frequently metastasize to the pancreas are from the lung, breast, kidney, or melanoma [144]. Pancreatic metastases can appear as focal, multifocal lesions or diffuse enlargement of the pancreas in a patient with a known primary neoplasm.

Pancreatic metastases are rare; the most common are from renal cell carcinoma. CEUS may demonstrate enhancement of pancreatic metastases from renal carcinoma, being hypervascular, allowing a differential diagnosis with pancreatic ductal adenocarcinoma. However the CEUS features of pancreatic metastases from renal cell carcinoma cannot be differentiated from those of endocrine tumors. The differential diagnosis is therefore based on the clinical history and symptoms, with biopsy often being required.

References

1. Ooi LL, Ho GH, Chew SP et al (1998) Cystic tumours of the pancreas: a diagnostic dilemma. Aust N Z J Surg 68:844-846
2. Papavramidis T, Papavramidis S (2005) Solid pseudopapillary tumors of the pancreas: review of 718 patients reported in English literature. J Am Coll Surg 200:965-972

3. Yu PF, Hu ZH, Wang XB et al (2010) Solid pseudopapillary tumor of the pancreas: a review of 553 cases in Chinese literature. World J Gastroenterol 16:1209-1214

4. Frantz VK (1959) Tumors of the pancreas. Atlas of Tumor Pathology:fasc 27-28, ser 7. Washington DC: Armed Forces Institute of Pathology, pp 32-33

5. Mao C, Guvendi M, Domenico DR et al (1995) Papillary cystic and solid tumors of the pancreas: a pancreatic embryonic tumor? Studies of three cases and cumulative review of the world's literature. Surgery 118:821-828

6. Martin RC, Klimstra DS, Brennan MF, Conlon KC (2002) Solid-pseudopapillary tumor of the pancreas: a surgical enigma? Ann Surg Oncol 9:35-40

7. Yamamoto S, Shiqeyoshi Y, Ishida Y et al (2001) Expression of the Per1 gene in the hamster: brain atlas and circadian characteristics in the suprachiasmatic nucleus. J Comp Neurol 430:518-532

8. Tipton SG, Smyrk TC, Sarr MG, Thompson GB (2006) Malignant potential of solid pseudopapillary neoplasm of the pancreas. Br J Surg 93:733-737

9. Volkan Adsay N (2007) Cystic lesions of the pancreas. Mod Pathol 20[Suppl 1]: S71-S93

10. Coleman KM, Doherty MC, Bigler SA (2003) Solid-pseudopapillary tumor of the pancreas. Radiographics 23:1644-1648

11. Kloppel G, Luttges J (2001) WHO-classification 2000: exocrine pancreatic tumors. Verh Dtsch Ges Pathol 85:219-228

12. Tang LH, Aydin H, Brennan MF, Klimstra DS (2005) Clinically aggressive solid pseudopapillary tumors of the pancreas: a report of two cases with components of undifferentiated carcinoma and a comparative clinicopathologic analysis of 34 conventional cases. Am J Surg Pathol 29:512-519

13. Buetow PC, Buck JL, Pantongrag-Brown L et al (1996) Solid and papillary epithelial neoplasm of the pancreas: imaging-pathologic correlation on 56 cases. Radiology 199:707-711

14. Salvia R, Festa L, Butturini G et al (2004) Pancreatic cystic tumors. Minerva Chir 59:185-207

15. Cantisani V, Mortele KJ, Levy A et al (2003) MR imaging features of solid pseudopapillary tumor of the pancreas in adult and pediatric patients. Am J Roentgenol 181:395-401

16. Lee DH, Yi BH, Lim JW, Kp YT (2001) Sonographic findings of solid and papillary epithelial neoplasm of the pancreas. J Ultrasound Med 20:1229-1232

17. Miao F, Zhan Y, Wang XY et al (2002) CT manifestations and features of solid cystic tumors of the pancreas. Hepatobiliary Pancreat Dis Int 1:465-468

18. Yu CC, Tseng JH, Yeh CN et al (2007) Clinicopathological study of solid and pseudopapillary tumor of pancreas: emphasis on magnetic resonance imaging findings. World J Gastroenterol 13:1811-1815

19. D'Onofrio M, Mansueto G, Vasori S et al (2003) Contrast-enhanced ultrasonographic detection of small pancreatic insulinoma. J Ultrasound Med 22:413-417

20. D'Onofrio M, Mansueto G, Falconi M, Procacci C (2004) Neuroendocrine pancreatic tumor: value of contrast enhanced ultrasonography. Abdom Imaging 29:246-258

21. D'Onofrio M, Malagò R, Vecchiato F et al (2005) Contrast-enhanced ultrasonography of small solid pseudopapillary tumors of the pancreas: enhancement pattern and pathologic correlation of 2 cases. J Ultrasound Med 24:849-854

22. Nishihara K, Nagoshi M, Tsuneyoshi M et al (1993) Papillary cystic tumors of the pancreas. Assessment of their malignant potential. Cancer 71:82-92

23. D'Onofrio M, Rozzanigo U, Caffarri S et al (2004) Contrast-enhanced US of hepatocellular carcinoma. Radiol Med 107:293-303

24. Wu Y, Du LF, Li F (2007) Contrast-enhanced ultrasonographic features of a solid-cystic papillary tumor of the pancreas. J Ultrasound Med 26:853-856

25. D'Onofrio M, Caffarri S, Zamboni G et al (2004) Contrast-enhanced ultrasonography in the characterization of pancreatic mucinous cystadenoma. J Ultrasound Med 23:1125-1129

26. Nagase M, Furuse J, Ishi H, Yoshino M (2003) Evaluation of contrast enhancement patterns in pancreatic tumors by coded harmonic sonographic imaging with a microbubble contrast agent. J Ultrasound Med 22:789-795

27. Kitano M, Kudo M, Maekawa K et al (2004) Dynamic imaging of pancreatic diseases by contrast enhanced coded phase inversion harmonic ultrasonography. Gut 53:854-859

28. Choi BI, Kim KW, Han MC et al (1988) Solid and papillary epithelial neoplasms of the pancreas: CT findings. Radiology 166:413-416

29. Ohtomo K, Furui S, Onoue M et al (1992) Solid and papillary epithelial neoplasm of the pancreas: MR imaging and pathologic correlation. Radiology 184:567-570

30. Sanfey H, Mendelsohn G, Cameron JL (1983) Solid and papillary neoplasm of the pancreas. A potentially curable surgical lesion. Ann Surg 197:272-275

31. Cubilla AL, Fitzgerald PJ (1985) Cancer of the exocrine pancreas: the pathologic aspects. CA Cancer J Clin 35:2-18

32. Klimstra DS, Heffess CS, Oertel JE, Rosai J (1992) Acinar cell carcinoma of the pancreas. A clinicopathologic study of 28 cases. Am J Surg Pathol 16:815-837

33. Kloppel G (2000) Mixed exocrine-endocrine tumors of the pancreas. Semin Diagn Pathol 17:104-108

34. Klimstra DS, Rosai J, Heffess CS (1994) Mixed acinar-endocrine carcinomas of the pancreas. Am J Surg Pathol 18:765-778

35. Ballas KD, Rafailidis SF, Demertzidis C et al (2005) Mixed exocrine-endocrine tumor of the pancreas. JOP 6:449-454

36. Butturini G, Pisano M, Scarpa A et al (2010) Aggressive approach to acinar cell carcinoma of the pancreas: a single-institution experience and a literature review. Langenbecks Arch Surg 396:363-369

37. Kuerer H, Shim H, Perfsemidis D, Unger P (1997) Functioning pancreatic acinar cell carcinoma: immunohistochemical and ultrastructural analyses. Am J Clin Oncol 20:101-107

38. MacMahon HE, Brown PA, Shen EM (1965) Acinar cell carcinoma of the pancreas with subcutaneous fat necrosis. Gastroenterology 49:555-559

39. Radin DR, Colletti PM, Forrester DM, Tang WW (1986) Pancreatic acinar cell carcinoma with subcutaneous and intraosseous fat necrosis. Radiology 158:67-68

40. Chen JD, Wu MS, Tien YW et al (2001) Acinar cell carcinoma with hypervascularity. J Gastroenterol Hepatol 16:107-111

41. Cingolani N, Shaco-Levy R, Farruggio A et al (2000) Alpha-fetoprotein production by pancreatic tumors exhibiting

acinar cell differentiation: study of five cases, one arising in a mediastinal teratoma. Hum Pathol 31:938-944

42. Holen KD, Klimstra DS, Hummer A et al (2002) Clinical characteristics and outcomes from an institutional series of acinar cell carcinoma of the pancreas and related tumors. J Clin Oncol 20:4673-4678

43. Eriguchi N, Aoyagi S, Hara M et al (2000) Large acinar cell carcinoma of the pancreas in a patient with elevated serum AFP level. J Hepatobiliary Pancreat Surg 7:222-225

44. Chen CP, Chao Y, Li CP et al (2001) Concurrent chemoradiation is effective in the treatment of alpha-fetoprotein-producing acinar cell carcinoma of the pancreas: report of a case. Pancreas 22:326-329

45. Tatli S, Mortele KJ, Levy AD et al (2005) CT and MRI features of pure acinar cell carcinoma of the pancreas in adults. Am J Roentgenol 184:511-519

46. Chung WJ, Byun JH, Lee SS, Lee MG (2010) Imaging findings in a case of mixed acinar-endocrine carcinoma of the pancreas. Korean J Radiol 11:378-381

47. Lim JH, Chung KB, Cho OK, Cho KS (1990) Acinar cell carcinoma of the pancreas. Ultrasonography and computed tomography findings. Clin Imaging 14:301-304

48. Mustert BR, Stafford-Johnson DB, Francis IR (1998) Appearance of acinar cell carcinoma of the pancreas on dual-phase CT. Am J Roentgenol 171:1709

49. Chiou YY, Chiang JH, Hwang JI et al (2004) Acinar cell carcinoma of the pancreas: clinical and computed tomography manifestations. J Comput Assist Tomogr 28:180-186

50. Merkle EM, Bender GN, Brambs HJ (2000) Imaging findings in pancreatic lymphoma: differential aspects. Am J Roentgenol 174:671-675

51. Klein, KA, Stephens DH, Welch TJ (1998) CT characteristics of metastatic disease of the pancreas. Radiographics 18:369-378

52. Ueda T, Ku Y, Kanamaru T et al (1996) Resected acinar cell carcinoma of the pancreas with tumor thrombus extending into the main portal vein: report of a case. Surg Today 26:357-360

53. Nijs E, Callahan MJ, Taylor GA (2005) Disorders of the pediatric pancreas: imaging features. Pediatr Radiol 35:358-373; quiz 457

54. Chung EM, Travis MD, Conran RM (2006) Pancreatic tumors in children: radiologic-pathologic correlation. Radiographics 26:1211-1238

55. Montemarano H, Lonergan GJ, Bulas DI, Selby DM (2000) Pancreatoblastoma: imaging findings in 10 patients and review of the literature. Radiology 214:476-482

56. Kloppel G, Maillet B (1989) Classification and staging of pancreatic nonendocrine tumors. Radiol Clin North Am 27:105-119

57. Friedman AC, Edmonds PR (1989) Rare pancreatic malignancies. Radiol Clin North Am 27:177-190

58. Klimstra DS, Wenig BM, Adair CF, Heffess CS (1995) Pancreatoblastoma. A clinicopathologic study and review of the literature. Am J Surg Pathol 19:1371-1389

59. Levey JM, Banner BF (1996) Adult pancreatoblastoma: a case report and review of the literature. Am J Gastroenterol 91:1841-1844

60. Drut R, Jones MC (1988) Congenital pancreatoblastoma in Beckwith-Wiedemann syndrome: an emerging association. Pediatr Pathol 8:331-339

61. Papaioannou G, Sebire NJ, McHugh K (2009) Imaging of the unusual pediatric 'blastomas'. Cancer Imaging 9:1-11

62. Sheng L, Weixia Z, Longhai Y, Jinming Y (2005) Clinical and biologic analysis of pancreatoblastoma. Pancreas 30:87-90

63. Roebuck DJ, Yuen MK, Wong YC et al (2001) Imaging features of pancreatoblastoma. Pediatr Radiol 31:501-506

64. Gupta AK, Mitra DK, Berry M et al (2000) Sonography and CT of pancreatoblastoma in children. Am J Roentgenol 174:1639-1641

65. Barenboim-Stapleton L, Yang X, Tsokos M et al (2005) Pediatric pancreatoblastoma: histopathologic and cytogenetic characterization of tumor and derived cell line. Cancer Genet Cytogenet 157:109-117

66. Rindi G, Capella C, Solcia E (1998) Cell biology, clinico-pathological profile, and classification of gastro-enteropancreatic endocrine tumors. J Mol Med 76:413-420

67. Panzuto F, Nasoni S, Falconi M et al (2005) Prognostic factors and survival in endocrine tumor patients: comparison between gastrointestinal and pancreatic localization. Endocr Relat Cancer 12:1083-1092

68. Rockall AG, Reznek RH (2007) Imaging of neuroendocrine tumours (CT/MR/US). Best Pract Res Clin Endocrinol Metab 21:43-68

69. Stabile BE, Morrow DJ, Passaro E Jr (1984) The gastrinoma triangle: operative implications. Am J Surg 147:25-31

70. Oberg K, Eriksson B (2005) Endocrine tumours of the pancreas. Best Pract Res Clin Gastroenterol 19:753-781

71. Shi W, Johnston CF, Buchanan KD et al (1998) Localization of neuroendocrine tumours with [111In] DTPA-octreotide scintigraphy (Octreoscan): a comparative study with CT and MR imaging. QJM 91:295-301

72. Debray MP, Geoffrey O, Laissy JP et al (2001) Imaging appearances of metastases from neuroendocrine tumours of the pancreas. Br J Radiol 74:1065-1070

73. Pisegna JR, Doppman JL, Norton JA et al (1993) Prospective comparative study of ability of MR imaging and other imaging modalities to localize tumors in patients with Zollinger-Ellison syndrome. Dig Dis Sci 38:1318-1328

74. Frucht H, Doppman JL, Nortman JA et al (1989) Gastrinomas: comparison of MR imaging with CT, angiography, and US. Radiology 171:713-717

75. Tjon A, Tham RTO, Falke TH et al (1989) CT and MR imaging of advanced Zollinger-Ellison syndrome. J Comput Assist Tomogr 13:821-828

76. Zimmer T, Stölzel U, Liehr RM et al (1995) [Somatostatin receptor scintigraphy and endoscopic ultrasound for the diagnosis of insulinoma and gastrinoma]. Dtsch Med Wochenschr 120:87-93

77. Kloppel G, Heitz PU (1988) Pancreatic endocrine tumors. Pathol Res Pract 183:155-168

78. Rothmund M, Stinner B, Arnold R (1991) Endocrine pancreatic carcinoma. Eur J Surg Oncol 17:191-199

79. Jaffe BM (1987) Surgery for gut hormone-producing tumors. Am J Med 82:68-76

80. Sofka CM, Semelka RC, Marcos HB, Woosley JT (1997) MR imaging of metastatic pancreatic VIPoma. Magn Reson Imaging 15:1205-1208

81. Mortele KJ, Oei A, Bauters W et al (2001) Dynamic gadolinium-enhanced MR imaging of pancreatic VIPoma in a patient with Verner-Morrison syndrome. Eur Radiol 11:1952-1955

82. Thomason JW, Martin RS Fincher ME (2000) Somatostatin receptor scintigraphy: the definitive technique for characterizing vasoactive intestinal peptide-secreting tumors. Clin Nucl Med 25:661-664

83. Bloom SR, Polak KM (1987) Glucagonoma syndrome. Am J Med 82:25-36

84. Pech O, Lingenfelser T, Wunsch P (2000) Pancreatic glucagonoma as a rare cause of chronic obstructive pancreatitis. Gastrointest Endosc 52:562-564

85. Solivetti FM, Giunta S, Caterino M et al (2001) [CT findings in a case of glucagonoma with necrolytic migrating erythema]. Radiol Med 102:410-412

86. Phan GQ, Yeo CJ, Hruban RH et al (1998) Surgical experience with pancreatic and peripancreatic neuroendocrine tumors: Review of 125 patients. J Gastrointest Surg 2:473-482

87. Anderson MA, Carpenter S, Thompson NW et al (2000) Endoscopic ultrasound is highly accurate and directs management in patients with neuroendocrine tumors of the pancreas. Am J Gastroenterol 95:2271-2277

88. Fernandez-Represa JA, Fernández Rodríguez D, Perez Contin MJ et al (2000) Pancreatic glucagonoma: detection by positron emission tomography. Eur J Surg 166:175-176

89. Nishiguchi S, Shiomi S, Ishizu H et al (2001) A case of glucagonoma with high uptake on F-18 fluorodeoxyglucose positron emission tomography. Ann Nucl Med 15:259-262

90. Johnson DS, Coel MN, Bornemann M (2000) Current imaging and possible therapeutic management of glucagonoma tumors: a case report. Clin Nucl Med 25:120-122

91. Gower WR Jr, Fabri PJ (1990) Endocrine neoplasms (nongastrin) of the pancreas. Semin Surg Oncol 6:98-109

92. Tanaka S, Yamasaki S, Matsushita H et al (2000) Duodenal somatostatinoma: a case report and review of 31 cases with special reference to the relationship between tumor size and metastasis. Pathol Int 50:146-152

93. Howard TJ, Stabile BE, Zinner MJ et al (1990) Anatomic distribution of pancreatic endocrine tumors. Am J Surg 159:258-264

94. Patel YC, Ganda OP, Benoit R (1983) Pancreatic somatostatinoma: abundance of somatostatin-28(1-12)-like immunoreactivity in tumor and plasma. J Clin Endocrinol Metab 57:1048-1053

95. Guo M, Lemos LB, Bigler S, Baliga M (2001) Duodenal somatostatinoma of the ampulla of vater diagnosed by endoscopic fine needle aspiration biopsy: a case report. Acta Cytol 45:622-626

96. Borrowdale R, Strong RW (1994) Primary lymphoma of the pancreas. Aust N Z J Surg 64:444-446

97. Bouvet M, Staerkel GA, Spitz FR et al (1998) Primary pancreatic lymphoma. Surgery 123:382-390

98. Miura F, Takada T, Amano H et al (2006) Diagnosis of pancreatic cancer. HPB (Oxford) 8:337-342

99. Mulkeen AL, Yoo PS, Cha C (2006) Less common neoplasms of the pancreas. World J Gastroenterol 12:3180-3185

100. Leite NP, Kased N, Hanna RF et al (2007) Cross-sectional imaging of extranodal involvement in abdominopelvic lymphoproliferative malignancies. Radiographics 27:1613-1634

101. Sheth S, Fishman EK (2002) Imaging of uncommon tumors of the pancreas. Radiol Clin North Am 40:1273-1287, vi

102. Lin H, Li SD, Hu XG, Li ZS (2006) Primary pancreatic lymphoma: report of six cases. World J Gastroenterol 12:5064-5067

103. Qiu L, Luo Y, Peng YL (2008) Value of ultrasound examination in differential diagnosis of pancreatic lymphoma and pancreatic cancer. World J Gastroenterol 14:6738-6742

104. Teefey SA, Stephens DH, Sheedy PF 2nd (1986) CT appearance of primary pancreatic lymphoma. Gastrointest Radiol 11:41-43

105. Van Beers B, Lafonde L, Soyer P et al (1993) Dynamic CT in pancreatic lymphoma. J Comput Assist Tomogr 17:94-97

106. Sata N, Kurogochi A, Endo K et al (2007) Follicular lymphoma of the pancreas: a case report and proposed new strategies for diagnosis and surgery of benign or low-grade malignant lesions of the head of the pancreas. JOP 8:44-49

107. Shah S, Mortele KJ (2007) Uncommon solid pancreatic neoplasms: ultrasound, computed tomography, and magnetic resonance imaging features. Semin Ultrasound CT MR 28:357-370

108. Ji Y, Kuang TT, Tan YS et al (2005) Pancreatic primary lymphoma: a case report and review of the literature. Hepatobiliary Pancreat Dis Int 4:622-626

109. Peeters E, Op de Beeck B, Osteaux M (2001) Primary pancreatic and renal non-Hodgkin's lymphoma: CT and MR findings. JBR-BTR 84:108-110

110. Fernandez-Cebrian JM, Carda P, Morales V, Galindo J (1998) Dermoid cyst of the pancreas: a rare cystic neoplasm. Hepatogastroenterology 45:1874-1876

111. Ferrozzi F, Zuccoli G, Bova D, Calculli L (2000) Mesenchymal tumors of the pancreas: CT findings. J Comput Assist Tomogr 24:622-627

112. Jacobs JE, Dinsmore BJ (1993) Mature cystic teratoma of the pancreas: sonographic and CT findings. Am J Roentgenol 160:523-524

113. Strasser G, Kutilek M, Mazai P, Schima W (2002) Mature teratoma of the pancreas: CT and MR findings. Eur Radiol 12[Suppl 3]:S56-S58

114. Koomalsingh KJ, Fazylov R, Chorost MI, Horovitz J (2006) Cystic teratoma of the pancreas: presentation, evaluation and management. JOP 7:643-646

115. Le Borgne J, de Calan L, Partensky C (1999) Cystadenomas and cystadenocarcinomas of the pancreas: a multiinstitutional retrospective study of 398 cases. French Surgical Association. Ann Surg 230:152-161

116. Khandelwal M, Lichtenstein GR, Morris JB et al (1995) Abdominal lymphangioma masquerading as a pancreatic cystic neoplasm. J Clin Gastroenterol 20:142-144

117. Toyoki Y, Hakamada K, Narumi S et al (2008) A case of invasive hemolymphangioma of the pancreas. World J Gastroenterol 14:2932-2934

118. Abe H, Kubota K, Noie T et al (1997) Cystic lymphangioma of the pancreas: a case report with special reference to embryological development. Am J Gastroenterol 92:1566-1567

119. Paal E, Thompson LD, Heffess CS (1998) A clinicopathologic and immunohistochemical study of ten pancreatic lymphangiomas and a review of the literature. Cancer 82:2150-2158

120. Igarashi A, Maruo Y, Ito T et al (2001) Huge cystic lymphangioma of the pancreas: report of a case. Surg Today 31:743-746

121. Letoquart JP, Marcorelles P, Lancien G et al (1989) [A new case of cystic lymphangioma of the pancreas]. J Chir (Paris) 126:650-658

122. Daltrey IR, Johnson CD (1996) Cystic lymphangioma of the pancreas. Postgrad Med J 72:564-566
123. Bishop MD, Steer M (2001) Pancreatic cystic lymphangioma in an adult. Pancreas 22:101-102
124. Gray G, Fried K, Iraci J (1998) Cystic lymphangioma of the pancreas: CT and pathologic findings. Abdom Imaging 23:78-80
125. Koenig TR, Lover EM, Whitman GJ et al (2001) Cystic lymphangioma of the pancreas. Am J Roentgenol 177:1090
126. Pandolfo I, Scribano E, Gaeta M et al (1985) Cystic lymphangioma of the pancreas: CT demonstration. J Comput Assist Tomogr 9:209-210
127. Viola G, Frontera D, Bellantone R et al (1997) Lymphangiomas of the pancreas: a case report. Pancreas 14:207-210
128. Schneider G, Seidel R, Altmeyer K et al (2001) Lymphangioma of the pancreas and the duodenal wall: MR imaging findings. Eur Radiol 11:2232-2235
129. Casadei R, Minni F, Selva S et al (2003) Cystic lymphangioma of the pancreas: anatomoclinical, diagnostic and therapeutic considerations regarding three personal observations and review of the literature. Hepatogastroenterology 50:1681-1686
130. Di Maggio EM, Solcia M, Dore R et al (1996) Intrapancreatic lipoma: first case diagnosed with CT. Am J Roentgenol 167:56-57
131. Katz DS, Nardi PM, Hines J et al (1998) Lipomas of the pancreas. Am J Roentgenol 170:1485-1487
132. Jacobs JE, Coleman BG, Arger PH, Langer JE (1994) Pancreatic sparing of focal fatty infiltration. Radiology 190:437-439
133. Secil M, Iqci E, Goktay AY, Dicle O (2001) Lipoma of the pancreas: MRI findings. Comput Med Imaging Graph 25:507-509
134. Suzuki R, Irisawa A, Hikichi T et al (20099 Pancreatic lipoma diagnosed using EUS-FNA. A case report. JOP 10:200-203
135. Ferrozzi F, Bova D, Garlaschi G (1995) Pancreatic schwannoma: report of three cases. Clin Radiol 50:492-495
136. Paranjape C, Johnson SR, Khwaja K et al (2004) Clinical characteristics, treatment, and outcome of pancreatic Schwannomas. J Gastrointest Surg 8:706-712
137. Kim SH, Choi BI, Han MC, Kim YI (1992) Retroperitoneal neurilemoma: CT and MR findings. Am J Roentgenol 159:1023-1026
138. Feldman L, Philpotts LE, Reinhold C et al (1997) Pancreatic schwannoma: report of two cases and review of the literature. Pancreas 15:99-105
139. Soumaoro LT, Teramoto K, Kawamura T et al (2005) Benign schwannoma of the pancreas. J Gastrointest Surg 9:288-290
140. Okuma T, Hirota M, Nitta H et al (2008) Pancreatic schwannoma: report of a case. Surg Today 38:266-270
141. Morita S, Okuda J, Sumiyoshi K et al (1999) Pancreatic Schwannoma: report of a case. Surg Today 29:1093-1097
142. Yu RS, Sun JZ (2006) Pancreatic schwannoma: CT findings. Abdom Imaging 31:103-105
143. Suzuki S, Kaji S, Koike N et al (2010) Pancreatic schwannoma: a case report and literature review with special reference to imaging features. JOP 11:31-35
144. Merkle EM, Braz T, Kolkythas O et al (1998) Metastases to the pancreas. Br J Radiol 71:1208-1214

Imaging Correlation

Marie-Pierre Vullierme and Enrico Martone

11.1 Introduction

Ultrasonography (US), multidetector computed tomography (MDCT) and magnetic resonance imaging (MRI) often represent complementary imaging modalities, covering different roles in diagnosing focal or diffuse disease. US is an increasingly powerful imaging technique especially after intravenous injection of contrast agent for lesion characterization or with endoscopic approach for lesion detection. MDCT is still the modality of choice in studying solid tumors, and is mandatory for achieving adequate preoperative staging. On the other hand, MRI is the criterion standard for accurately evaluating both the ductal system and cystic lesions. Therefore, US and contrast-enhanced US (CEUS) could be seen to be at the center in choosing between MDCT and MRI, if a lesion is detected especially given that US is very often the first-line examination. This chapter provides a diagnostic algorithm based on US findings, and also discusses both the advantages and disadvantages of the US study compared to the other imaging modalities.

11.2 Pancreas Visualization and Lesion Detection

11.2.1 Location

US evaluation is usually accurate in studying the head, the isthmus and the proximal portion of the body of the

M.P. Vullierme (✉)
Department of Radiology, Beaujon Hospital, Clichy, Paris, France
e-mail: mpvullierme@gmail.com

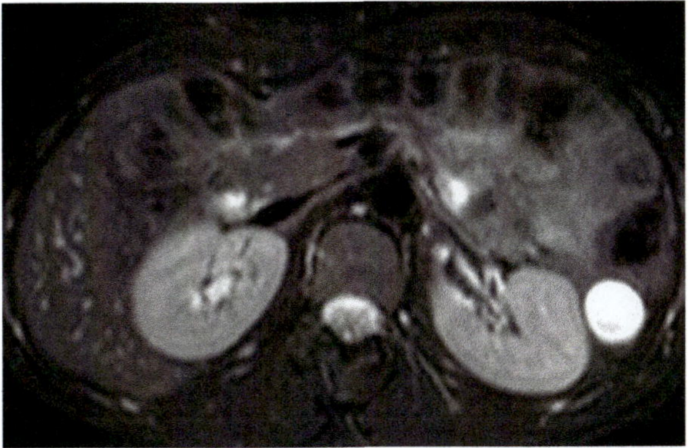

Fig. 11.1 MEN 1 patient with cystic endocrine pancreatic tumor. MRI, axial T2-weighted image. Round hyperintense 2 cm tumor of the tail. This lesion was missed by endoscopic US

pancreas. The distal pancreatic body and the tail of the gland are often obscured by the stomach, and/or the left colonic flexure. As reported in previous chapters, the left portion of the gland can be evaluated through the splenic window. Moreover, many technical tools have been proposed to improve the transabdominal US visualization of the pancreas, such as filling the stomach with degassed water. However, MDCT or MRI remain the most accurate techniques for studying the whole gland (Fig. 11.1).

11.2.2 Obesity

Obesity can be responsible for a difficult US examination of the pancreas, as well as of other abdominal organs. As previously described, the application of several attempts could allow the visualization of the pancreas even in overweight patients or in patients with high body mass index (BMI). However, patient BMI cannot predict the result of

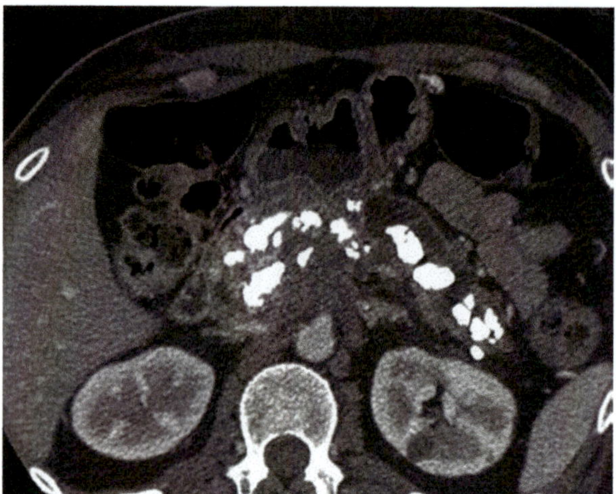

Fig. 11.2 Pancreatic calcification and unresectable adenocarcinoma. MDCT with intravenous contrast. Axial slice. Macroscopic calcifications >1 cm occupying the MPD, which is enlarged

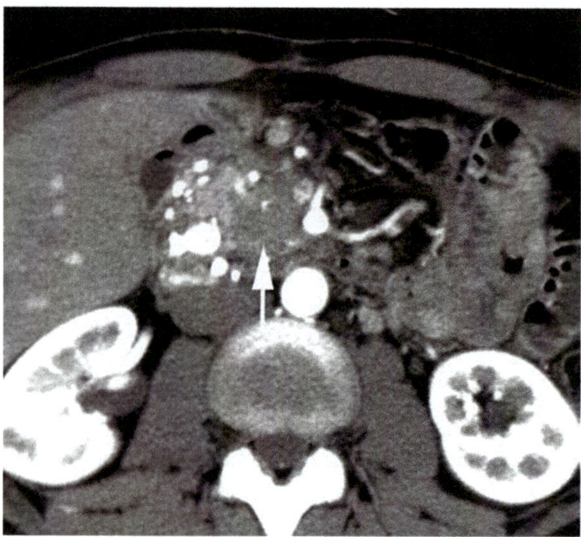

Fig. 11.3 Pancreatic adenocarcinoma in chronic pancreatitis. MDCT with intravenous contrast. Axial slice. Small hypodense lesion (*arrow*) can be seen displacing multiple pancreatic calcifications in chronic pancreatitis

the US exploration of the pancreas. MDCT and MRI can overcome this limitation, generating high quality images substantially unconstrained by the BMI of patients.

11.2.3 Fatty Infiltration

Fatty infiltration of the pancreas limits contrast between the gland and the surrounding fat. In fact, a reduction

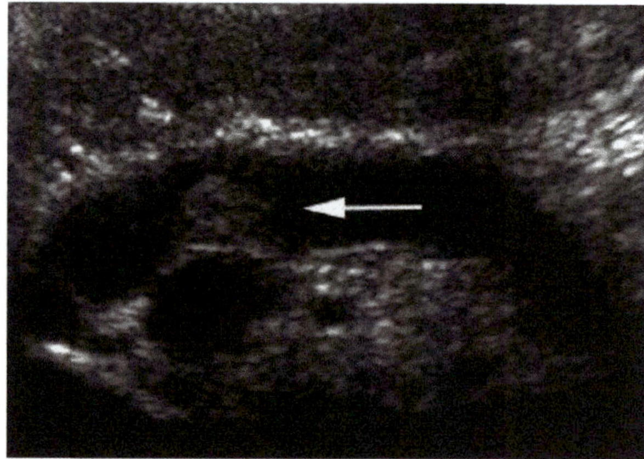

Fig. 11.4 Non calcified intraductal plug. Axial US scan showing atrophy of the pancreatic parenchyma with dilated main pancreatic duct containing small echoic plug (*arrow*)

in the US conspicuity of the pancreatic gland in respect to the retroperitoneal fat is observed (see Chapter 6) according to the degree of fatty infiltration (hyperechoic). Also in this case, MDCT and MRI can overcome the limitation and so these examinations should be suggested in cases of doubt.

11.2.4 Calcifications and Plugs

Intraductal and parenchymal calcifications can impair the US pancreatic study due to the strong acoustic shadow generated behind them. MDCT is the most specific imaging method to assess calcifications (Fig. 11.2) and to allow an accurate evaluation of the surrounding parenchyma (Fig. 11.3). In contrast, even if at MRI they show signal void on T2-weighted sequences, some can be missed. However, non calcified protein plugs are better depicted at MRCP and US (Fig. 11.4) than at MDCT, especially if located in the main pancreatic duct (MPD).

11.2.5 Lesions Conspicuity

The administration of contrast agent usually follows the identification of a focal lesion at conventional US. In fact, most pancreatic lesions are detected without the administration of contrast agent. This is due to the high conspicuity of focal pancreatic masses compared to the adjacent parenchyma. Ductal adenocarcinoma almost always shows high difference in acoustic impedance with respect to the adjacent pancreatic gland (see Chapter 8). As reported in the literature, pancreatic adenocarcinomas isodense at MDCT where they may

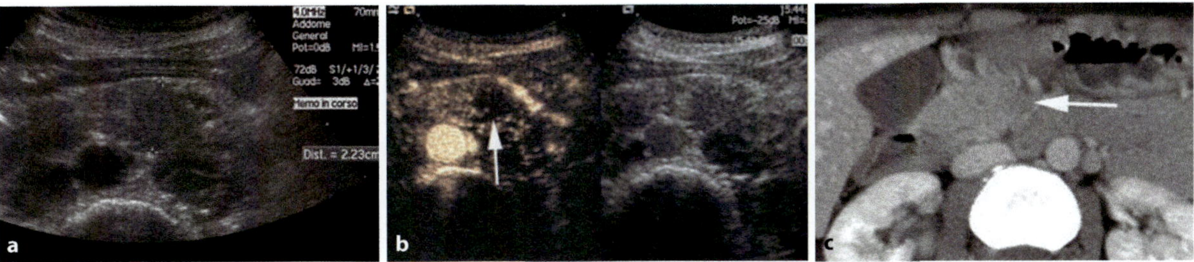

Fig. 11.5 a-c Pancreatic adenocarcinoma. Axial US scan (**a**) showing pancreatic hypoechoic mass in the uncinate process (*caliper*) (**b**) appearing markedly hypovascular (*arrow*) at CEUS (**c**). The same conspicuity is not present at MDCT where the lesion appears slightly hypodense (*arrow*)

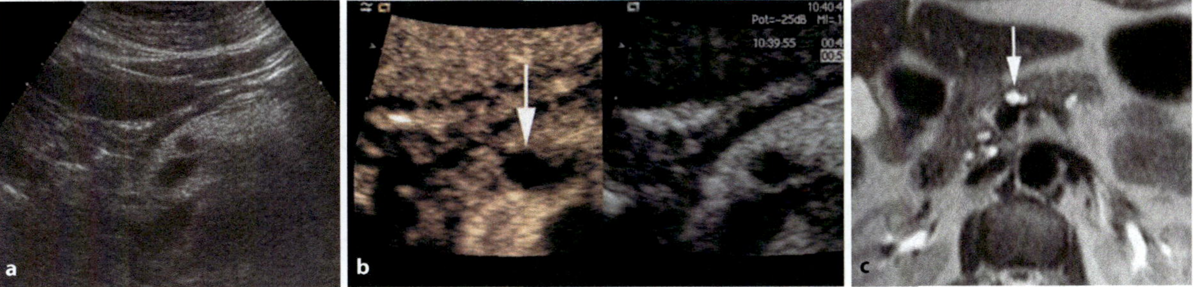

Fig. 11.6 a-c IPMN. Axial US scan (**a**) showing very small pancreatic hypoechoic pseudosolid lesions of the pancreatic neck which appear completely avascular (*arrow*) at CEUS (**b**) with final diagnosis of cystic lesion (**c**). Directly After CEUS an MRI examination with T2 sequence was performed with confirmation of the cystic nature of the lesion (*arrow*) and final diagnosis of IPMN of the branch duct

show typical secondary signs [1] can be easily detected [2, 3] at US (Fig. 11.5). Cystic lesions are usually clearly anechoic compared to the surrounding soft tissue. In these cases, MRI still remains the imaging modality of choice, characterized by the highest capability in detecting fluid components and giving fundamental information regarding the relationship of the cystic lesion with the ductal system (see Chapter 9). However, the accuracy of US in distinguishing between solid and cystic lesions can be improved by the administration of contrast agent.

11.3   CEUS vs CT and MRI

State-of-the-art US provides high spatial resolution images [4], thus enabling the visualization of the smallest details. Furthermore, the introduction of new technologies like tissue harmonic imaging (THI) extensively reduces artifacts, thus providing enhanced overall image quality [5] and improved lesion conspicuity [6]. This is the reason why a small pancreatic lesion which appears ill-defined at CT and MRI can be easily depicted

at US [7, 8]. As stated above, the lesion detection is the result of the difference in acoustic impedance [2] which is always present between pancreatic parenchyma and ductal adenocarcinoma (Fig. 11.5). Unlike other imaging modalities, Doppler study provides the evaluation of flow velocity of the main peripancreatic vascular structures. Other technologies only allow the evaluation of their patency. However, flow velocity is an important information since an infiltration of the vascular wall could generate an alteration in blood speed [9].

CEUS of the pancreas has lead to great developments in the diagnostic capabilities of conventional US, which is usually applied in the initial evaluation of pancreatic diseases [4]. After US detection of a focal pancreatic lesion, the immediate injection of microbubbles is a relatively new, safe and feasible technique to immediately better characterize and stage the disease during the same examination [2, 8]. CEUS is able to provide a more accurate differentiation between solid and cystic lesions (Figs. 11.6, 11.7), during the first evaluation, thus influencing the choice of further examinations [2]. Moreover, a faster diagnosis, i.e. immediate diagnosis of ductal adenocarcinoma (see Chapter 8), can be obtained [2, 8].

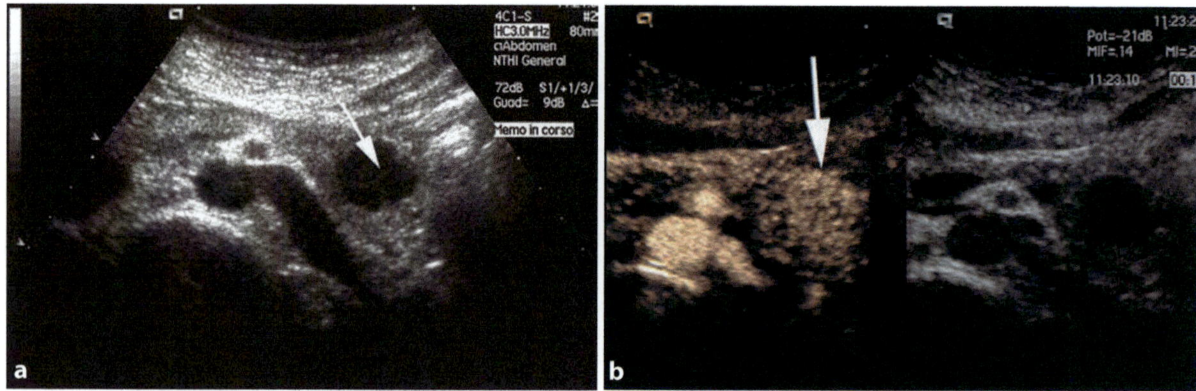

Fig. 11.7 a,b Endocrine tumor. Axial US scan (**a**) showing markedly hypoechoic pancreatic mass with pseudocystic appearance containing small septa (*arrow*). At CEUS (**b**) the lesion appears solid and hypervascular (*arrow*)

Harmonic microbubble-specific software applications which filter all the background tissue signals allow maximum contrast resolution, making the vascular enhancement only due to the presence of microbubbles [8]. Differing from the other contrast agents (used with other modalities such as MDCT or MRI), microbubbles have a purely intravascular (*blood pool*) distribution, without any interstitial phase [10]. The macrovasculature and microvasculature can be accurately imaged [11]. The small mean diameter of the microbubbles, able to reach the microcirculation, allows the visualization of the pancreatic tumor microvasculature even if *silent* at Doppler study [10]. Moreover, a strict correlation between the degree of enhancement at CEUS and the mean vascular density at pathology has been reported in the literature [11, 12]. An undifferentiated ductal adenocarcinoma usually appears as markedly hypovascular at CEUS [12]. This is due to the abundant fibrosis and desmoplasia typical for this kind of lesion, which are typically hypovascular during all the dynamic phases at CEUS. Therefore applications of CEUS for prognostic stratification based on enhancement patterns have been reported in the literature [12]. In contrast, at MDCT and MRI the fibrous content provide delayed enhancement after the administration of contrast agents.

The dynamic evaluation of the enhancement at CEUS differs from the dynamic study at MDCT and MRI being the only imaging technique able to allow a continuous evaluation of the enhancement in real-time [8]. Furthermore, the high temporal resolution is one of the most important features of CEUS. Therefore, immediately after the injection of contrast medium [8], the enhancement of a pancreatic lesion can be monitored [13], and unlike contrast-enhanced MDCT and MRI, the rapid enhancement of hypervascular lesions such as endocrine tumors can be better detected [10]. However, MRI and especially MDCT are more panoramic imaging techniques, mandatory in the staging of abdominal diseases. Lastly, after completion of the pancreatic study, the liver should be assessed in the late phase [14], exploiting the same contrast injection, to identify potential liver metastases [8].

The high contrast resolution together with the real-time study play an important role in the evaluation of the enhancement even in hypovascular and cystic lesions. In fact, especially with regard to cystic lesions (see Chapter 9), the visualization of the enhancement of thin internal inclusions (like septa and nodules) is often difficult at CE-MDCT and MRI, but mandatory in making a differential diagnosis between pseudocysts and cystic tumors [8, 15]. Single microbubble can be easily detected passing through thin septa or mural nodules. As just reported above, this is also due to the utilization of specific software which filters all the background tissue signals [8, 15].

Pancreatic CEUS may be considered a new imaging modality with complementary results to contrast-enhanced CT and MRI [2].

11.4 Tissue Characterization: Is the Lesion Solid or Cystic?

11.4.1 Solid Tissue Contrast Resolution

The normal pancreatic parenchyma often shows similar or slightly greater echogenicity than the liver. A solid lesion is very often hypoechoic. Especially pancreatic adenocarcinoma is usually hypoechoic, thus immediately detectable at US usually with a good conspicuity. However, its correct characterization is not so accurate and immediate. Sometimes cystic pancreatic lesions can appear as solid at basal US (see Chapter 1), especially if small in size (Fig. 11.6), but also solid pancreatic lesions can appear as cystic masses (Fig. 11.7). The use of THI can improve the differentiation between solid and cystic masses, enhancing the overall image quality as previously described. However, real advantages have been added with the introduction of microbubbles, which improve tissue characterization, thus contributing to choose the next most appropriate imaging modality (i.e. MRI and/or EUS for cystic lesions; MDCT for solid lesions) as recently reported in the literature [2].

As mentioned above, in chronic pancreatitis the presence of calcifications can impair the detection of focal masses and MDCT and MRI remain the imaging modalities of choice (Fig. 11.3).

11.4.2 Fluid Content

US remains an accurate imaging technique for assesing a fluid lesion, which appears anechoic with posterior reinforcement. Sometimes, however, fluids can be modified by hemorrhage, infection or dehydration and lose their typical US appearance becoming complex heterogeneous lesions characterized by internal echoes (Fig. 11.8). Mucin too is a complex, corpuscular and viscous fluid, which produces inhomogeneous echoes at US study (see Chapter 9). Hence mucinous tumors appear as lesions with cystic content and fine internal echoes due to the presence of mucin or hemorrhagic fluid-fluid levels. The heterogeneous echoes may impair the detection of intralesional septa and/or parietal nodules, which is fundamental for the differential diagnosis between cystic tumors and pseudocysts. CEUS may significantly improve the US identification of septa and parietal nodules (see Chapter 9) mainly by detecting their potential vasculature. Pseudocysts on the other hand can show heterogeneous content, with debris and internal echoes, which never appear vascular at CEUS. With regard to the intraductal mucinous papillary neoplasm (IPMN) study, the communication with the main pancreatic duct is usually not visible at US/CEUS. MDCT can easily define the hemorrhagic content, which appears hyperdense compared to the simple fluid, but is not as accurate as its depiction of internal inclusions. This is the reason why MRI still remains the imaging modality of choice in studying pancreatic cystic lesions. The hemorrhagic fluid typically presents varying signal intensity on T1-weighted and T2-weighted se-

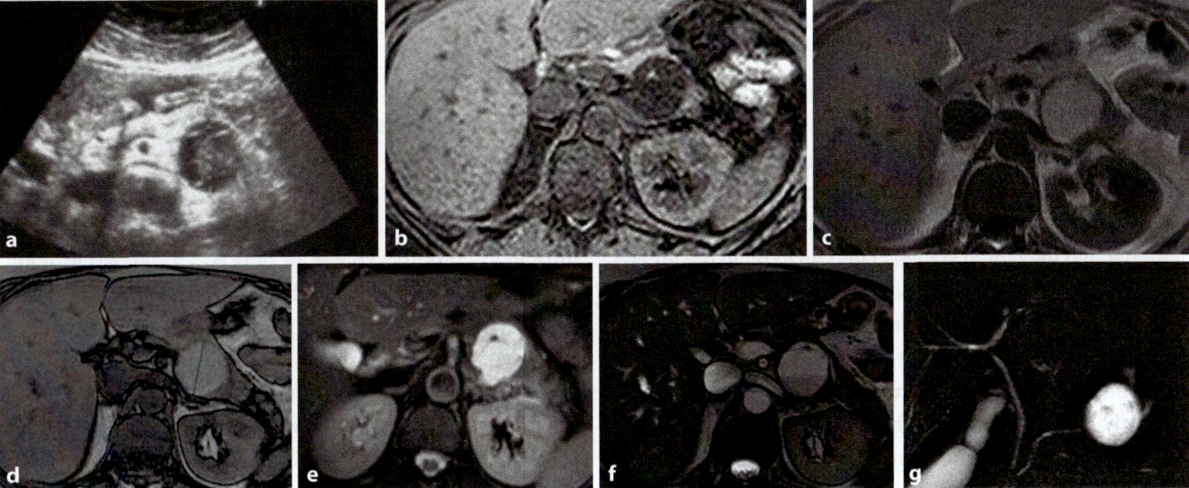

Fig. 11.8 a–g Pseudocyst with hemorrhagic content. **a** Transabdominal US. The round cyst of the body of the pancreas as heterogeneous echoic content mimicking tissue content. **b** The patient had an MRI with T1-weighted sequences a few months before, which showed a normal hypointense (*black*) content. **c** MRI control with T1-weighted in phase sequences the same day as US shows a hyperintense signal within the cyst. **d** MRI T1-weighted out of phase sequences shows the persistent hyperintensity, indicating hemorrhagic content (fat content would have had a drop in signal with this T1-weighted out of phase sequence). **e** MRI with axial T2-weighted sequence showing fibrinous septa within the hemorrhagic cyst. **f** MRI with axial T2-weighted sequence showing a fluid/fluid level also typical of hemorrhagic content. **g** Thick slice 2D MRCP showing the cyst and a normal MPD

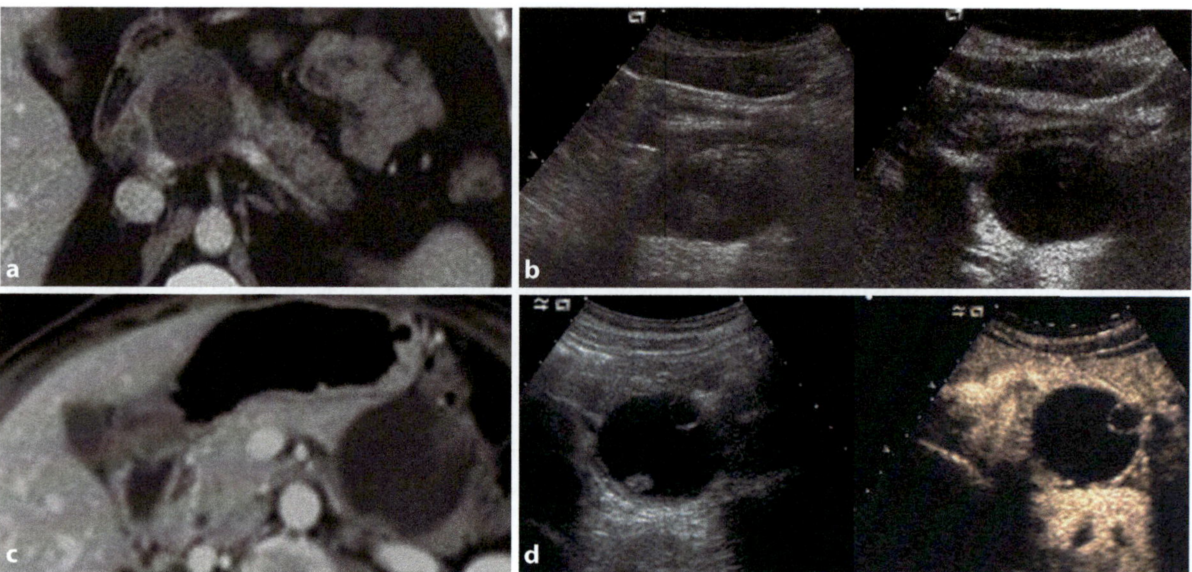

Fig. 11.9 a-d Pseudocystic vs non-pseudocystic lesions. **a** Pseudocyst at CT with intralesional dense debris mimic vegetations. The debris is echoic at conventional US (**b**, *left*) but completely avascular and therefore no longer visualized at CEUS (**b**, *right*). **c** Mucinous cystadenoma at CT with small intralesional dense vegetations. The vegetations are echoic at conventional US (**d**, *left*) and visible as hyperechoic with moving microbubbles during dynamic phase at CEUS and thus vascular, confirming the neoplastic diagnosis (**d**, *right*)

quences according to the time of hemorrhage (Fig. 11.8). Moreover, MRI with MRCP is the criterion standard for evaluating the communication with the main pancreatic duct, as happens in cases of IMPN.

11.4.3 Contrast Agents

Microbubbles and contrast agents used in MDCT and MRI mainly differ from their distribution. US contrast agents have a blood pool supply so remain in the vascular lumen without any interstitial diffusion. On the other hand, contrast materials used both in MDCT and MRI show vascular and interstitial spread. This can explain the greater accuracy of CEUS with respect to MDCT or MRI in distinguishing between recurrence and fibrotic changes, as happens after radiotherapy. At CEUS, even if hypovascular, recurrence shows some degree of enhancement differing from the absence of microbubbles in fibrosis. At CE-MDCT or MRI a delayed and progressive enhancement is usually observed. Therefore the arterial phase is similar in all imaging modalities, while the delayed phases differ from one another. In particular, the fibrous tissue will not show any contrast uptake at CEUS, and thus appears unenhanced [2], whereas it shows progressive enhancement at CE-MDCT and MRI. The evaluation of potential liver metastases is not so different since they present as hypoe-

choic, hypodense or hypointense in all delayed phases. At CE-MDCT and MRI they can be evaluated during all the dynamic phases, whereas at CEUS the arterial phase is focused on the pancreatic lesion and only the late phase is used to study the liver. However good accuracy of the late phase of CEUS in the study of liver metastatic lesions is reported [14, 16]

11.4.4 Septa and Nodules

As just mentioned, the cystic content of a lesion may be heterogeneous [2] due to the presence of mucin or intralesional hemorrhage, or debris. Unlike MDCT and MRI, harmonic microbubble-specific software filters all the background tissue signals and only vascularized tissues (where microbubbles are present) are visible at CEUS, making the examination extremely accurate in distinguishing enhanced and non-enhanced inclusions (Fig. 11.9). Therefore, CEUS covers an important role in distinguishing between cystic tumors and pseudocysts, in which all inclusions are always completely avascular [15]. This differential diagnosis can be more difficult at CE-MDCT and MRI owing to the absence of real-time evaluation and, mainly, the absence of software able to filter all the background signals. In fact, the dynamic phases are superimposed on the unenhanced images.

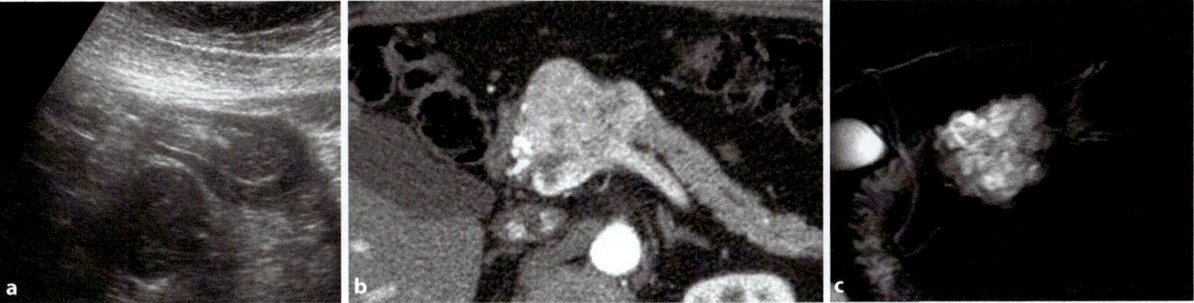

Fig. 11.10 a-c Pseudosolid serous cystadenoma. **a** Transabdominal US. Well circumscribed soft tissue lesion appearing hypoechoic compared with pancreas parenchyma, without upstream MPD enlargement. **b** Enhanced MDCT in the arterial phase. The contrast uptake of the lesion is homogeneous, marked, simulating a neuroendocrine tumor. Upstream the pancreas parenchyma is normal. **c** 2D MRCP showing a lobulated marked hyperintense lesion, indicating cystic liquid content

In IPMN, CEUS shows greater accuracy in detecting the presence and potential enhancement of nodules, septa and focal parietal or septal thickening than other imaging methods. However, a communication with the ductal system, as mentioned above, usually cannot be documented and MRI with MRCP still remains the criterion standard. Lastly, the differential diagnosis between plugs, clots and true mural nodules in simple fluid or complex lesions with cystic pattern can be avoided after the injection of contrast agent.

11.4.5　Pseudosolid Lesion

Extremely microcystic serous cystadenoma (SCA) may mimic a solid lesion (see Chapter 9), both at conventional US and CEUS, appearing as an echogenic hyperenhanced lesion owing to the extremely compact multiple thin septa [2]. In contrast, also in this rare case MRI can solve the problem, as the lesion is cystic in nature, albeit extremely microcystic, and typically appears hyperintense on T2-weighted images (Fig. 11.10). Moreover, the confirmation of lack of communication with the main pancreatic duct allows a non invasive differential diagnosis between SCA and IPMN.

11.5　Lesion Characterization

11.5.1　Solid Tumors

11.5.1.1 Adenocarcinoma

At conventional US, pancreatic ductal adenocarcinoma usually presents as a solid mass, with infiltrative margins, markedly hypoechoic (see Chapter 8) to the adja-

cent pancreatic parenchyma due to the very low US acoustic impedance of the tumor [2]. Furthermore, US conspicuity, coming from the difference in impedance between the lesion and the pancreatic adjacent parenchyma, is sometimes greater than CT as previously reported [2]. At CEUS, ductal adenocarcinoma is typically hypoenhanced in all phases (see Chapter 8) and this is related to the typical presence of high desmoplastic reaction and low mean vascular density [17-20]. This pattern is reported in up to 93% of cases [18-22]. As reported in the multicenter study called PAMUS (Pancreatic Multicenter Ultrasound Study) 90% of the adenocarcinoma were hypovascular at CEUS [23]. Moreover, US can easily and precisely guide fine needle aspiration or biopsy of pancreatic adenocarcinoma [24].

MDCT remains the criterion standard for solid tumor staging [25]. Ductal adenocarcinoma is often isodense to the adjacent parenchyma on unenhanced scan and hypodense during dynamic study [26]. The maximum difference in conspicuity is reached during the pancreatic phase [27]. In the portal/venous phase the conspicuity of the lesion is reduced (see chapter 8) The main pancreatic duct is usually markedly dilated and double duct sign can be observed in tumors located on the head of the gland.

MRI shows superior tumor conspicuity than MDCT [28], even if it is usually not required for solid masses. As some studies show, it seems that diffusion-weighted imaging (DWI) is able to differentiate between normal pancreatic parenchyma and solid tumors in 92 % of cases [29], helping also in detecting distant metastases.

Furthermore, occult carcinoma could be depicted both at CEUS and CE-MDCT with reference to indirect signs, such as MPD dilation, the double duct sign, an abrupt

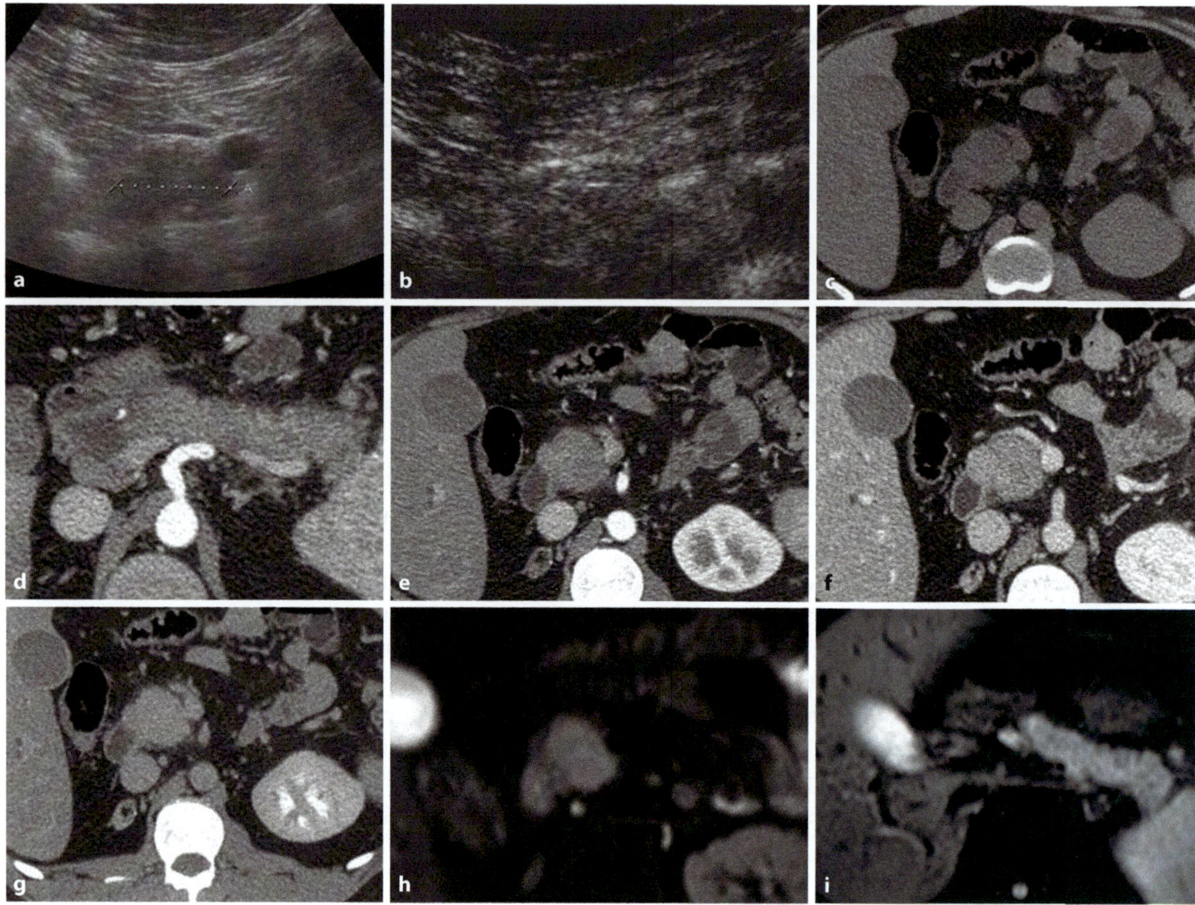

Fig. 11.11 a-r Autoimmune pancreatitis. Pseudotumor of the head of the pancreas. Stenosis of the MPD and MBD that must be diagnosed as dubious adenocarcinoma. CEUS and DW-MRI were the only pattern suggesting autoimmune pancreatitis. **a** Transabdominal US. Solid hypoechoic mass of the head of the pancreas (*calipers*). **b** CEUS showing contrast uptake similar than the rest of the pancreas. **c** Unenhanced MDCT: the lesion is isodense. **d** Enhanced MDCT in the arterial phase. Upstream pancreas is delobulated, with a thin edematous ring surrounding the entire pancreas. **e** Enhanced MDCT in the arterial phase. The lesion of the head is not visible, with a small portion of the normal parenchyma at the right side of the lesion appearing hyperdense. Thin edematous rim surrounding the parenchyma. **f** Enhanced MDCT in the venous phase. The lesion of the head is not visible with a small portion of the normal parenchyma at the right side of the lesion appearing hyperdense. **g** Enhanced MDCT in the late phase. Enhancement of the lesion of the head, with a small portion of the normal parenchyma at the right side of the lesion appearing hypodense. **h** Diffusion-weighted MRI at b=600: restriction of diffusion associated with the lesion of the head. **i** Diffusion-weighted MRI at b=600: restriction of diffusion associated with the lesion of the body and tail, indicating a diffuse inflammatory disease related with AIP and not adenocarcinoma   (*cont.*→)

cutoff of the MPD, focal different echogenicity/density in the gland [2, 30].

11.5.1.2 Endocrine Tumor

Endocrine tumors are typically hypervascular lesions (see Chapter 8). CEUS is an accurate imaging method in demonstrating pancreatic tumor vasculature. The high capability of CEUS in demonstrating pancreatic tumor vasculature [11] is a result of the high resolution power of state-of-the-art US imaging, combined with the size and the distribution (blood pool) of the microbubbles. CEUS may improve the identification and characterization of endocrine tumors [10, 31] allowing accurate locoregional and hepatic staging as reported by Malagò et al. [31]. In some pancreatic neuroendocrine tumors hypodense at dynamic CT, a clear enhancement is visible at CEUS thanks to the real-time evaluation [10]. Endocrine tumors typically present as homogeneous isodense well-demarcated masses in the pre-contrast phase. Very small intralesional calcifications may be detected especially in

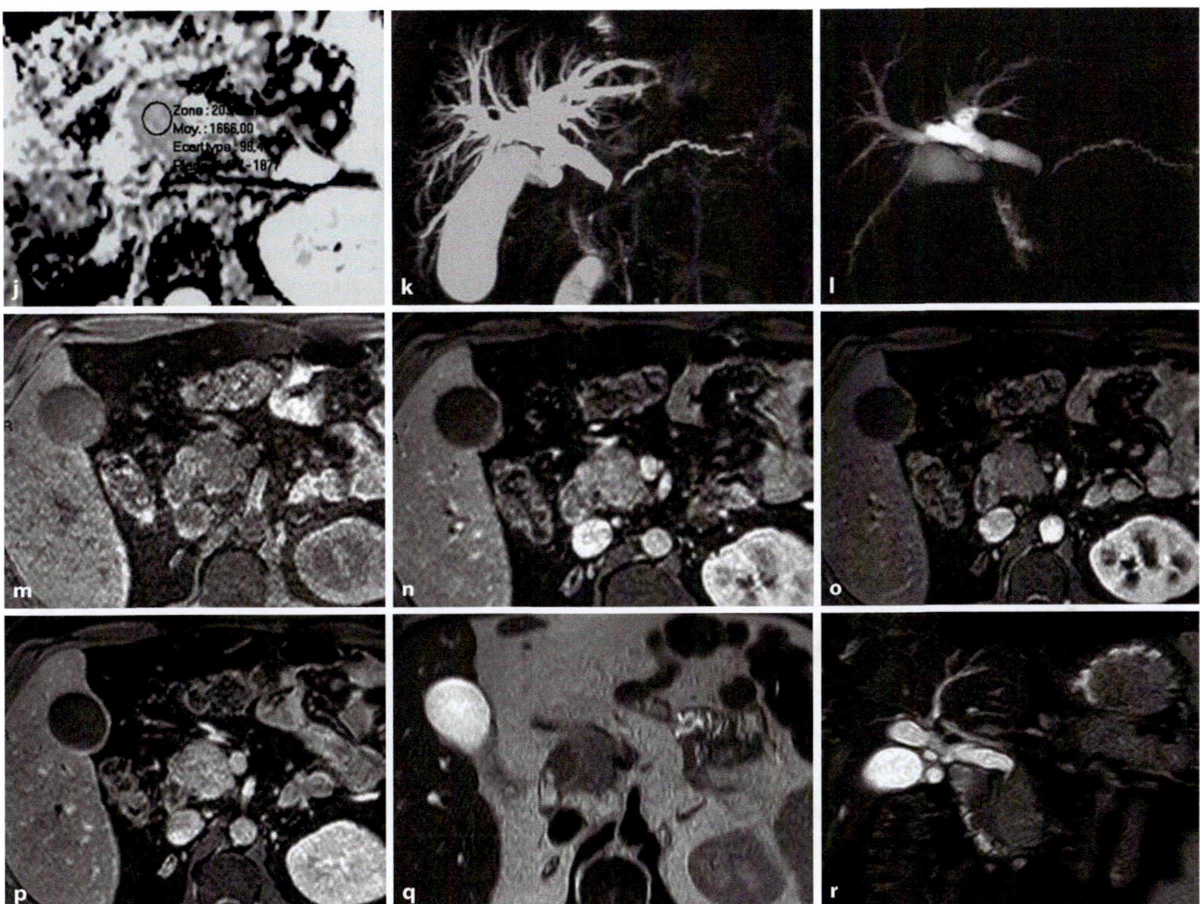

(*continued*) **j** Diffusion-weighted MRI with ADC measure inside the lesion: 1.666, similar to normal parenchyma. **k,l** 3D and 2D MRCP showing the biliary and pancreatic stenosis. **m** Unenhanced MRI: the lesion is hypointense with a small portion of the normal parenchyma at the right side of the lesion, having a normal hyperintense signal. **n** Enhanced MRI in the arterial phase. The lesion of the head is not visible. **o** Enhanced MRI in the venous phase. The lesion of the head is hypointense with a small portion of the normal parenchyma at the right side of the lesion appearing hyperintense. **p** Enhanced MDCT in the late phase. Enhancement of the lesion of the head, with a small portion of the normal parenchyma at the right side of the lesion appearing hypointense. **q,r** Axial and coronal T2-weighted MRI showing the lesion with moderate hyperintensity

the largest nonfunctioning masses [26]. These rarely cause infiltration of the main pancreatic duct. During the earlier dynamic phases, they typically appear homogeneously hyperdense [32], being hyperdense or isodense in the delayed phases. A recent paper shows the application of perfusion CT in studying endocrine tumors and demonstrates the positive correlation between the results and prognostic factors [33]. Rarely are they characterized by cystic degeneration, showing a central avascular portion, surrounded by a thick enhanced wall. Endocrine tumors may also present as hypovascular masses lacking the typical arterial enhancement, making their correct characterization more difficult [10].

11.5.2 Solid Inflammatory Pseudotumors

11.5.2.1 Autoimmune Pancreatitis

Autoimmune pancreatitis (AIP) (Fig. 11.11) can be focal or diffuse throughout the entire gland. The typical pancreatic imaging findings include the usually diffuse enlargement of the pancreatic parenchyma with the typical *sausage* appearance, and the MPD is narrowed, due to a lymphoplasmacytic infiltrate and pancreatic fibrosis. At US, mass-forming pancreatitis is often similar to ductal adenocarcinoma [2, 4, 8], usually presenting as a hypoechoic mass with lumpiness of the gland contour. The presence of small calcifications within the lesion may suggest its inflammatory nature [4], even though poorly specific. On the other hand, the glandular parenchymal enhancement at CEUS is strongly suggestive of an inflammatory mass. A nodular shape is also significantly more frequent in pancreatic cancer, and a longitudinal shape suggests AIP. Moreover, it has been observed that the more the inflammatory process is chronic and long-standing, the less intense is the intralesional parenchymal enhancement, probably in relation to the entity of the associated fibrosis. One of the CT signs that may be helpful in differentiating focal AIP from ductal adenocarcinoma is its contrast enhancement pattern during the late venous phase (Fig. 11.11). However, during the pancreatic phase, the focal forms of AIP may appear hypoattenuating like pancreatic adenocarcinoma. A peripheral rim of hypodensity due to the oedematous fat is also highly suggestive of AIP (Fig. 11.11). The MPD is usually not visible within the lesion, most likely reflecting the periductal inflammatory cell infiltration centered around the pancreatic ducts. In focal forms, there is a normal-size upstream MPD, differing from ductal adenocarcinoma. A marked narrowing of MPD without any upstream enlargement is typical (Fig. 11.11) (if enlarged, MPD must not be >5 mm). For a correct differential diagnosis with adenocarcinoma, MRI with MR cholangiopancreatography (MRCP) can be considered the most accurate non invasive imaging method allowing a dynamic evaluation of the MPD before and after secretin stimulation, which demonstrates the presence of the *duct penetrating sign*. The dynamic aspect after the administration of contrast agent is similar to that described for CE-MDCT. DWI seems helpful in differentiating between AIP and ductal

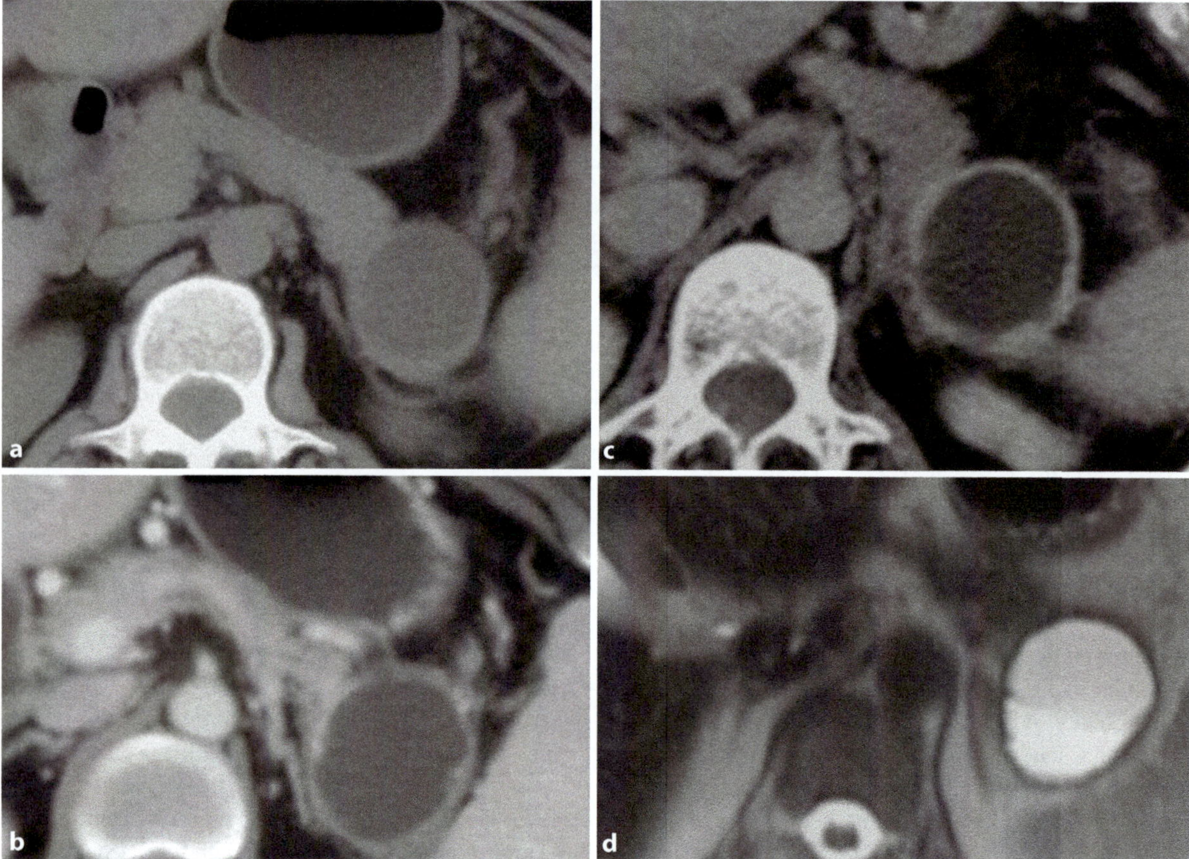

Fig. 11.12 a-d Mucinous cystadenoma. Three phase MDCT. **a** Unenhanced phase showing a unilocular round cyst at the junction of body and tail of the pancreas, with a thick wall. **b** Portal phase showing no enhancement of the cyst. **c** Late phase of injection showing marked enhancement of the cystic wall, indicating its fibrous nature. **d** T2-weighted MRI. Axial slice. Water content of the cyst appearing hyperintense in T2. A thin septa is seen in the middle of the cyst

adenocarcinoma: they are both detected as high-signal intensity areas, but diffuse and/or multiple in AIP patients (Fig. 11.11). ADC values are significantly lower in AIP ($1.012+/-0.112 \times 10^{-3}$ mm²/s) than in pancreatic cancer ($1.249+/-0.113 \times 10^{-3}$ mm²/s) and normal pancreas ($1.491+/-0.162 \times 10^{3}$ mm²/s) ($p<0.001$). An optimal ADC cutoff value of 1.075×10^{-3} mm²/s must be evaluated to distinguish AIP from pancreatic cancer (Fig. 11.11). After steroid therapy, high-intensity areas on DWI disappear or are markedly decreased, and the ADC values of the reduced pancreatic lesions increase almost to the values of normal pancreas [34], as well the US and CEUS and MDCT features disappear with a *restitutio ad integrum*.

11.5.2.2 Focal Pancreatitis

Focal pancreatitis typically involves the pancreatic head. Differential diagnosis with ductal adenocarcinoma can be a challenge. At US calcification may be present suggesting the diagnosis. However, the displacement of previously monitored calcification should raise suspicion of ductal adenocarcinoma in chronic pancreatitis. For the diagnosis, contrast-enhanced examinations and biopsy are often mandatory. At CEUS, an isovascular pattern of parenchymal enhancement has been described and reported with a good accuracy in the literature, but more reliable for the focal form of AIP. Focal mass-forming pancreatitis associated with chronic pancreatitis is much often studied with MDCT or MRI. As reported above, at MRCP the presence of pancreatic ducts inside

the focal mass (*duct penetrating sign*) is a sign of benign lesion [35].

11.5.3 Cystic Tumors

11.5.3.1 Mucinous Cystadenoma/ Cystadenocarcinoma

CEUS improves the US differential diagnosis [23] between pseudocysts and cystic tumors of the pancreas (e.g. mucinous cystadenoma, cystadenocarcinoma) by accurately revealing the vasculature of intralesional vegetations (see Chapter 9) and favorably compares with MRI in displaying the anatomic features of the pancreatic cystic masses [15]. Mucinous cystadenoma is usually unilocular (Fig. 11.12), mainly (up to 90%) located at the junction of pancreatic body and tail of the pancreas, developing outside the posterior margin of the parenchyma.

Mucinous cystadenoma (MCA) is a potentially malignant lesion that may degenerate into cystadenocarcinoma. It appears as a round (unique) macrocystic lesion with (thick wall > 2 mm and enhancement of the wall with contrast) internal septa and when malignant with thick septa and parietal nodules enhanced at CEUS [8]. On unenhanced MDCT it may present hypodense or slightly hyperdense content, depending on the mucin concentration. Peripheral calcifications can be observed in 10-25% of cases. MRI with MRCP should be performed to confirm the lack of communication with the MPD. The signal intensity on T1-weighted images can be different according to the mucin content, usually

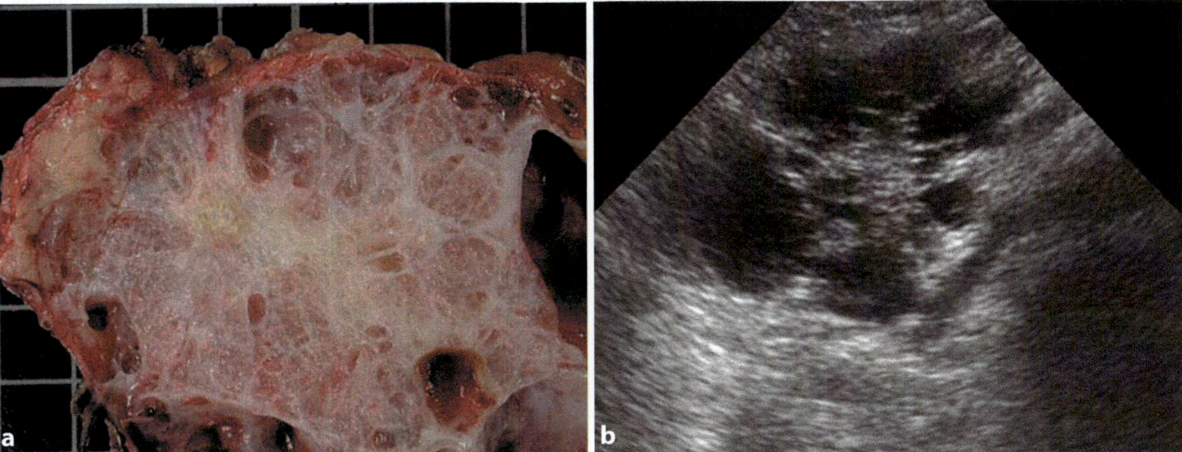

Fig. 11.13 a,b Typical microcystic serous cystadenoma. **a** Resected specimen showing the tiny cysts and central scar. **b** Corresponding US appearance characterized by multiple intralesional thin septa in another case

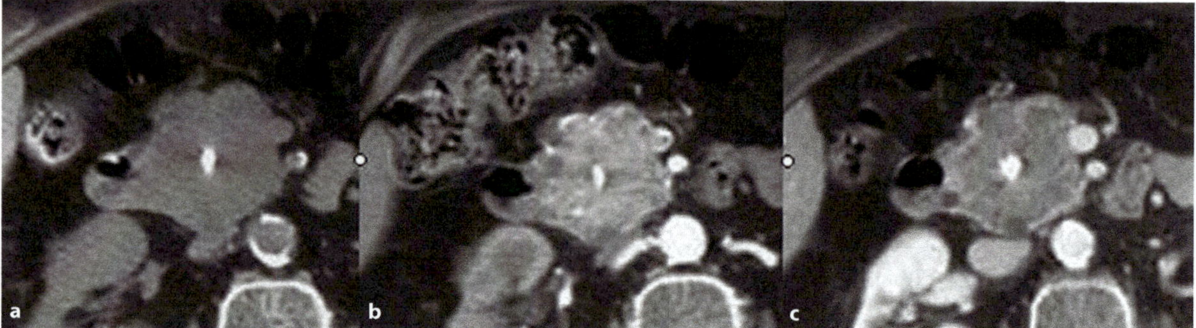

Fig. 11.14 a-c Typical microcystic serous cystadenoma. **a** Unenhanced MDCT showing calcification in the central scar. **b** Enhanced MDCT in the arterial phase showing the microcystic component with cysts measuring 1 cm at the periphery. **c** Enhanced MDCT in the venous phase: the cysts are very well seen, due to the enhancement of the cysts wall

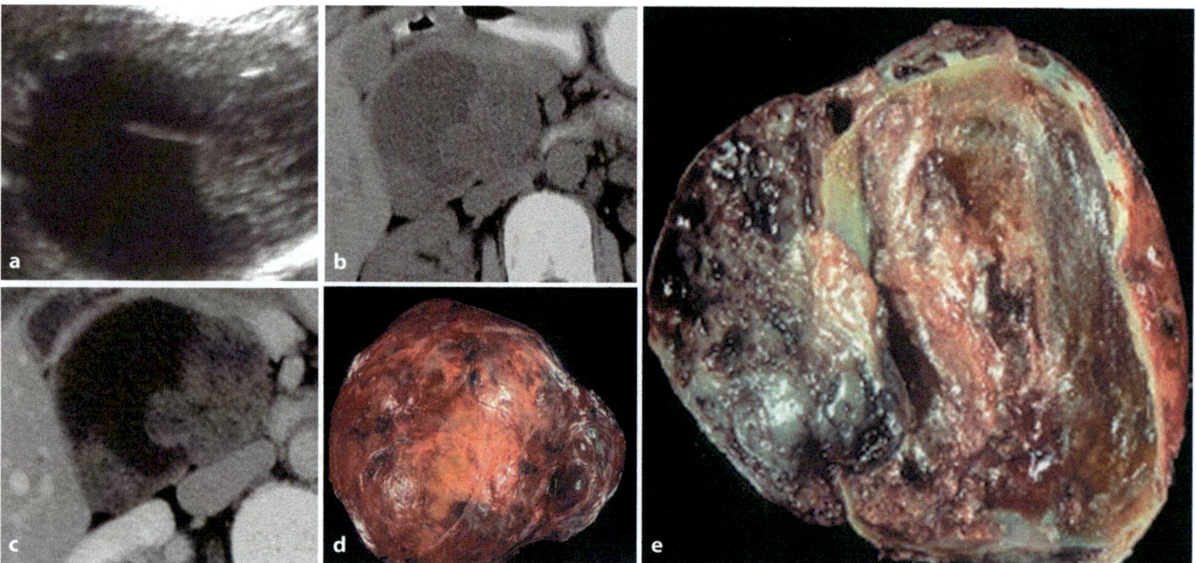

Fig. 11.15 a-e Pseudopapillary and solid tumor. **a** Transabdominal US showing a cystic part at the right, and a solid part at the right portion of the lesion. **b** Unenhanced MDCT showing the two parts of the lesion. **c** Enhanced MDCT showing the two parts of the lesion with moderate enhancement of the tissue portion. **d** Resected specimen showing the well circumscribed lesion with its capsule. **e** Opened specimen (right placed at left side) showing the tissue portion with hemorrhagic component, the cystic part and the thick capsule

showing different degrees of hyperintensity on T2-weighted sequences.

11.5.3.2 Serous Cystadenoma

Serous cystadenoma typically presents as a solitary multilocular microcystic lesion (Fig. 11.13), without communication with the MPD, with thin septa orientated towards the center (see also Chapter 9). In 15% of cases, a central scar, sometimes calcified (Fig. 11.14), is present [2]. As reported above, the extremely microcystic type may mimic a solid hypervascular lesion [2]. The less common macrocystic type (see Chapter 12) presents features often indistinguishable from those of the other macrocystic tumors of the pancreas.

On CE-MDCT the hypervascularity of internal septa is clear, but MRI is the criterion standard as it is able to depict the *honeycomb* multilocular architecture on T2-weighted sequences (see Chapter 9) and the lack of communication with the MPD [2].

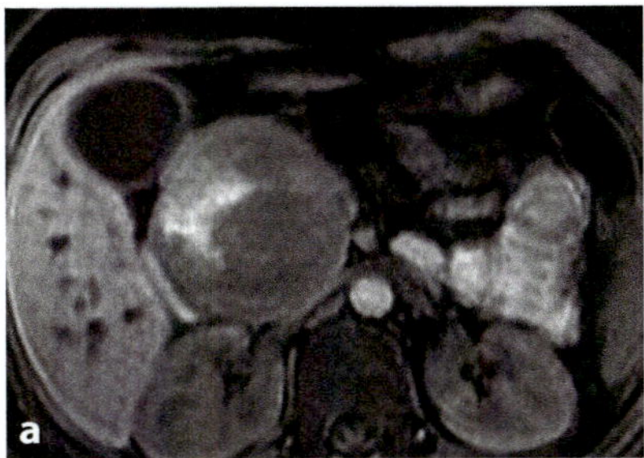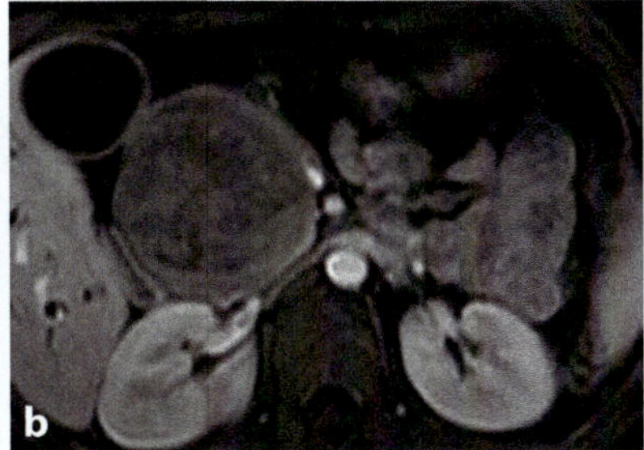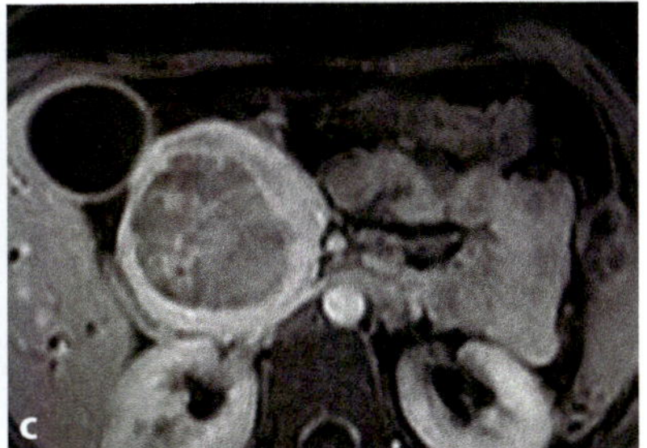

Fig. 11.16 a-c Pseudopapillary and solid tumor. MRI. T1-weighted axial slices. **a** Without intravenous contrast. The lesion of the head of the pancreas is round, with a heterogeneous signal. Hyperintensity is due to partial hemorrhagic content. **b** Arterial phase of injection. The contrast uptake is moderate, showing a hypointense thick rim. **c** Late phase of injection. The contrast uptake of the capsule is marked related to its fibrous nature

11.5.3.3 Pseudopapillary and Solid Tumor

Solid pseudopapillary tumor typically presents as a solitary well-defined round solid-cystic mass, without communication with the MPD. The heterogeneous aspect due to hemorrhagic or necrotic components and cystic degeneration appears as inhomogeneous echo-texture at US (Fig. 11.15), slightly hyperdense at MDCT [2] and with different signal intensity at MRI both on T1-weighted and T2-weighted images depending on the age of the bleeding. Peripheral or central calcifications may be present and well depicted both on US and MDCT. Solid components can also be enhanced at CEUS, CE-MDCT and MRI (Fig. 11.16). Heterogeneous enhancement of the thickened peripheral fibrous capsule is a quite specific feature of this lesion (Fig. 11.16).

11.5.3.4 Multiple Cysts

Intraductal papillary mucinous neoplasms (IPMN) are the most frequent multicystic diseases (see also Chapter 9). They are divided into main-duct and branch-duct types. CEUS is helpful in differentiating perfused (nodules) and non-perfused (clots) inclusions [8]. As reported in the PAMUS multicenter study (Pancreatic Multicenter Ultrasound Study), cystic tumor can be correctly diagnosed at CEUS with an accuracy of 97.1% [23]. MRI and endoscopic US (EUS) are the imaging methods of choice for the study of these tumors to better demonstrate their communication with the pancreatic ducts [2]. In fact, MRI with MRCP is much more sensitive in depiction of branch duct IPMN, remaining the best imaging method for evaluating and staging the disease, which is based on the number of branch duct cysts and involvement of the MPD [36]. 3D MRCP showed higher image quality than 2D MRCP but did not increase the diagnostic accuracy for predicting ductal communication of the lesion [37]. At any rate, the addition of MRCP to axial CT images may improve diagnostic performance and decrease interobserver variability of MDCT for the determination of MPD communication with macrocystic pancreatic neoplasms and differentiation between IPMN and non-IPMN [38]. In a nutshell, MRI enables more confident assessment of the morphology of small cysts than MDCT [39], but the accuracy of the two imaging techniques for cyst characterization is comparable, with a specificity of 71-84% for the differentiation between mucinous and nonmucinous lesions. However, a higher sensitivity is associated with MRI with MRCP to rule out the multiple character of the pancreatic cystic disease [40]. Imaging features suggestive of malignant degeneration and well detected throughout all imaging modalities are: mural nodule, irregular thick septa and mural calcification, together with a MPD larger than 1 cm.

11.5.4 Pseudocyst

US is the first imaging technique used to study the content of a cyst. The debris is always not visible during CEUS study because the background tissue is filtered by the software. Thus pseudocyst appears avascular at CEUS. CEUS is reported to be highly accurate in the characterization of pseudocysts with 100% specificity [41]. MRI still remains the imaging modality of choice for cystic lesions. T2-weighted sequences show great accuracy for this diagnosis (Fig. 11.17), while MDCT has poor sensitivity and specificity.

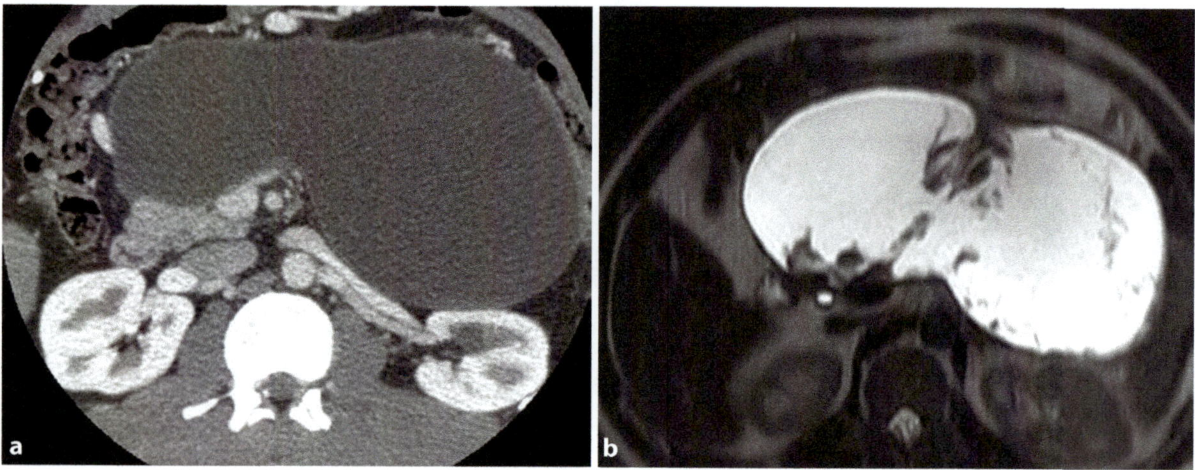

Fig. 11.17 a,b Pseudocyst. Percutaneous drainage planning. **a** MDCT showing a homogeneous cyst. **b** Axial T2-weighted MRI sequences. Some plugs are present inside the cyst (not visible at MDCT), but most of the content is of liquid nature, indicating a possible efficacy of drainage

11.6 Specific Applications

11.6.1 Ultrasound

- A focal pancreatic lesion is well detectable at US and can therefore be immediately characterized by means of CEUS. As the exploration always optimal at EUS, the detection of focal lesions with this modality is superior, although it does require the mini-invasive approach.
- Elastography is a relatively new US-based technique able to improve the differential diagnosis of pancreatic masses by displaying the proper stiffness of the examined pancreatic lesions. In essence, according to the marked fibrosis very often present in pancreatic adenocarcinoma, this tumor appears stiffer at elastographic evaluation than the surrounding parenchyma.
- US-guidance is the procedure of choice if available, because it is sensitive, safe and accurate for tissue sampling in solid un-resectable tumors [2, 24]. MDCT-guidance is always more complex and time consuming. Some important US technical features, such as the continuous monitoring of the ongoing procedure, the oblique approach, the high spatial resolution and the low-cost make this imaging method particularly suitable for targeting percutaneous pancreatic interventional procedures.
- CEUS can accurately demonstrate the vasculature of pancreatic tumors. Correlations between CEUS enhancement patterns and mean vascular density have been reported. Prognostic stratifications based on the CEUS appearance of pancreatic tumors can therefore be expected in the future. Correlation between vascular patterns of pancreatic tumors at CEUS and prognosis is reported for adenocarcinoma [12, 42] and for endocrine tumors [31] of the pancreas. CEUS can demonstrate changes in pancreatic tumor vascularization during therapy [43, 44].

11.6.2 MDCT

- Unenhanced MDCT is the best tool for depicting pancreatic calcification.
- Acute pancreatitis is explored with MDCT at 48 hours after the beginning of the disease. It is the best tool for depicting: pancreas necrosis (enhancement defect of pancreatic parenchyma) and extra-pancreatic collection. The modified prognosis score (CTSI-CT severity index) used is derived from the Balthazar score. US is not accurate for this study. Furthermore, pleural effusion or venous thrombosis could be present and not depicted with US.
- In contrast, the study of pseudocystic content, making possible transcutaneous drainage if purely fluid, is accurate with US, or MRI, but not at MDCT. Hemorrhage into a pseudocyst appears hyperdense on unenhanced MDCT slices. Arterial acquisition with reconstruction could show blood effusion and/or

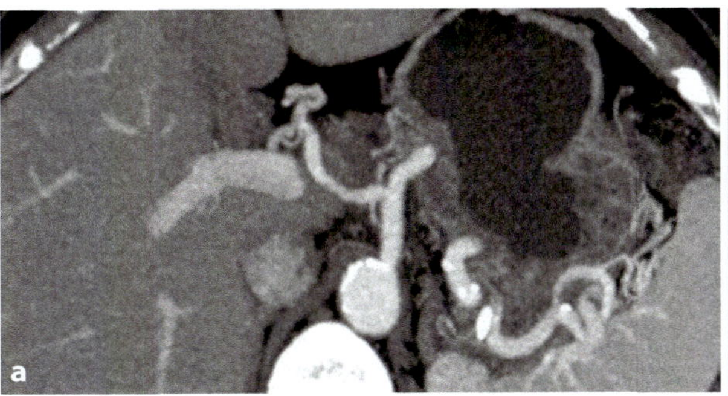
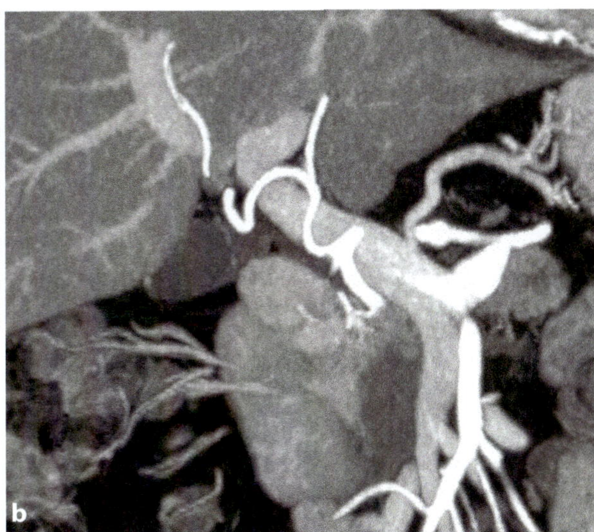

Fig. 11.18 a,b MDCT. **a** Staging of pancreatic ductal adenocarcinoma with irregular wall of the hepatic artery related to vascular involvement. **b** Coronal reformatting maximal intensity projection (MIP) of the vascular enhancement in the portal phase showing hepatic arteries in front of the main portal vein and superior mesenteric artery in front of the superior mesenteric vein with a normal pattern

aneurysm and MDCT (arterial phase with bolus track) is the technique of choice.

- Malignant lesions require a precise assessment of their locoregional extension [25, 28] and MDCT is the most frequently recommended tool (Fig. 11.18). Coronal plane seems better than axial plane in showing stenosis or irregular vascular walls.
- Enhancement of neuroendocrine pancreatic tumors, part of the prognostic factor of WHO grade, is well studied with all techniques.

11.6.3 MRI

- Studies of the pancreatic duct as well as the biliary duct are part of pancreatic imaging. The imaging study of pancreatic disease is probably not complete without MRI and particularly MRCP. With particular reference to branch-duct IPMN (see Chapter 9), MRCP is mandatory for performing an accurate staging of the disease, showing the number of enlarged branched ducts with high sensitivity [45]. The communication of a cyst with the MPD is well shown, especially using 3D MRCP [37, 38]. This communication with the ductal system cannot be established by US.
- MRCP is able to assess the presence of chronic pancreatitis, with a good specificity and sensitivity. This technique can probably differentiate an enlargement of the MPD related with IPMN (marked >1 cm, regular, parallel MPD wall) from chronic pancreatitis (less dilated, irregular MPD with string-of-beads

appearance). If chronic pancreatitis is present, MRCP is also useful for the diagnosis of a single round cyst showing that it is a pseudocyst related to an acute pancreatitis associated with chronic pancreatitis. A focal chronic pancreatitis could be upstream to a stenosis related with a focal lesion such as adenocarcinoma. Patterns associated with autoimmune pancreatitis are of great impact for the diagnosis of such disease (see below). Furthermore, enhancement of the MPD wall related with malignant IPMN has been reported [46].

- DWI may help in the differential diagnosis of cancer and autoimmune pancreatitis pseudotumor (Fig. 11.11) and of pancreatic cysts. On visual evaluation, all cystic lesions are hyperintense on DWI with b factors of 0 and 500 s/mm^2. On DWI with a b factor of 1,000 s/mm^2, all abscesses and hydatid and neoplastic cysts are hyperintense, whereas most of the simple and pseudocysts are isointense. With a b factor of 1,000 s/mm^2, the cyst-to-pancreas signal intensity ratios of the abscesses and hydatid and neoplastic cysts are significantly higher than those of the simple cysts and pseudocysts. Setting the cutoff value of signal intensity ratio at 1.9, the cyst-to-pancreas signal intensity ratio had a sensitivity of 70% and a specificity of 90% for differentiating neoplastic cysts from simple cysts and pseudocysts. The ADC and the ADC ratios of neoplastic cysts were significantly lower than those of simple cysts and pseudocysts [47].
- MRCP is the imaging modality of choice for the study of the pancreatic ductal system, thus being

mandatory in the evaluation of the narrowed MPD in AIP patients. It also plays an important role in patients with acute or chronic pancreatitis to rule out the presence of stones in the MPD.

References

1. Prokesch RW, Chow LC, Beaulieu CF et al (2002) Isoattenuating pancreatic adenocarcinoma at multi-detector row CT: secondary signs. Radiology 224:764-768
2. D'Onofrio M, Gallotti A, Pozzi Mucelli R (2010) Imaging techniques in pancreatic tumors. Expert Rev Med Devices 7:257-273
3. Oshikawa O, Tanaka S, Ioka T et al (2002) Dynamic sonography of pancreatic tumors: comparison with dynamic CT. Am J Roentgenol 178:1133–1137
4. Martínez-Noguera A, D'Onofrio M (2007) Ultrasonography of the pancreas. 1. Conventional imaging. Abdom Imaging 32:136-149
5. Shapiro RS, Wagreich J, Parsons RB et al (1998) Tissue harmonic imaging sonography: evaluation of image quality compared with conventional sonography. Am J Roentgenol 171:1203-1206
6. Hohl C, Schmidt T, Honnef D et al (2007) Ultrasonography of the pancreas. 2. Harmonic imaging. Abdom Imaging 32:150-160. Review
7. Minniti S, Bruno C, Biasiutti C et al (2003) Sonography versus helical CT in identification and staging of pancreatic ductal adenocarcinoma. J Clin Ultrasound 31:175-182
8. D'Onofrio M, Zamboni G, Faccioli N et al (2007) Ultrasonography of the pancreas. 4. Contrast-enhanced imaging. Abdom Imaging 32:171-181
9. Bertolotto M, D'Onofrio M, Martone E et al (2007) Ultrasonography of the pancreas. 3. Doppler imaging. Abdom Imaging 32:161-170
10. D'Onofrio M, Mansueto GC, Falconi M et al (2004) Neuroendocrine pancreatic tumor: value of contrast enhanced ultrasonography. Abdom Imaging 29:246-258
11. D'Onofrio M, Malagò R, Zamboni G et al Contrast-enhanced ultrasonography better identifies pancreatic tumor vascularization than helical CT. Pancreatology 5:398-402
12. D'Onofrio M, Zamboni G, Malagò R et al (2009) Resectable pancreatic adenocarcinoma, is the enhancement pattern at contrast-enhanced ultrasonography a pre-operative prognostic factor? Ultrasound Med Biol 35:1929–1937
13. Takeda K, Goto H, Hirooka Y et al (2003) Contrast-enhanced transabdominal ultrasonography in the diagnosis of pancreatic mass lesions. Acta Radiol 44:103–106
14. D'Onofrio M, Martone E, Faccioli N et al (2006) Focal liver lesions, sinusoidal phase of CEUS. Abdom Imaging 31:529-536
15. D'Onofrio M, Megibow AJ, Faccioli N et al (2007) Comparison of contrast-enhanced sonography and MRI in displaying anatomic features of cystic pancreatic masses. Am J Roentgenol 189:1435-1442
16. Claudon M, Cosgrove D, Albrecht T et al (2008) Guidelines and good clinical practice recommendations for contrast enhanced ultrasound (CEUS) – update. Ultraschall Med 29:28-44
17. Numata K, Ozawa Y, Kobayashi N et al (2005) Contrast-enhanced sonography of pancreatic carcinoma, correlation with pathological findings. J Gastroenterol 40:631-640
18. Sofuni A, Iijima H, Moriyasu F et al (2005) Differential diagnosis of pancreatic tumors using ultrasound contrast imaging. J Gastroenterol 40:518-525
19. Nagase M, Furuse J, Ishii H et al (2003) Evaluation of contrast enhancement patterns in pancreatic tumors by coded harmonic sonographic imaging with a microbubble contrast agent. J Ultrasound Med 22:789–795
20. D'Onofrio M, Zamboni G, Tognolini A et al (2006) Mass-forming pancreatitis: value of contrast-enhanced ultrasonography. World J Gastroenterol 12:4181-4184
21. Kitano M, Kudo M, Maekawa K et al (2004) Dynamic imaging of pancreatic diseases by contrast enhanced coded phase inversion harmonic ultrasonography. Gut 53:854-859
22. Hocke M, Schmidt C, Zimmer B et al (2008) Contrast enhanced endosonography for improving differential diagnosis between chronic pancreatitis and pancreatic cancer. Dtsch Med Wochenschr 133:1888-1892
23. D'Onofrio M, Barbi E, Dietrich CF et al (2011) Pancreatic multicenter ultrasound study (PAMUS). Eur J Radiol doi:10.1016/j.ejrad.2011.01.053
24. Zamboni GA, D'Onofrio M, Idili A et al (2009) Ultrasound-guided percutaneous fine-needle aspiration of 545 focal pancreatic lesions. Am J Roentgenol 193:1691-1695
25. Schima W, Ba-Ssalamah A, Kölblinger C et al (2007) Pancreatic adenocarcinoma. Eur Radiol 17:638–649
26. Procacci C, Biasiutti C, Carbognin G et al (2001) Pancreatic neoplasms and tumor-like conditions. Eur Radiol 11[Suppl 2]:S167–S192
27. Sahani DV, Shah ZK, Catalano OA et al (2008) Radiology of pancreatic adenocarcinoma, current status of imaging. J Gastroenterol Hepatol 23:23–33
28. Park HS, Lee JM, Choi HK et al (2009) Preoperative evaluation of pancreatic cancer: comparison of gadolinium-enhanced dynamic MRI with MR cholangiopancreatography versus MDCT. J Magn Reson Imaging 30:586-595
29. Kartalis N, Lindholm TL, Aspelin P et al (2009) Diffusion-weighted magnetic resonance imaging of pancreas tumours. Eur Radiol 19:1981-1990
30. Miller FH, Rini NJ, Keppke AL (2006) MRI of adenocarcinoma of the pancreas. Am J Roentgenol 187:365-374
31. Malagò R, D'Onofrio M, Zamboni GA et al (2009) Contrast-enhanced sonography of nonfunctioning pancreatic neuroendocrine tumors. Am J Roentgenol 192:424–430
32. Procacci C, Carbognin G, Accordini S et al (2001) Non-functioning endocrine tumors of the pancreas: possibilities of spiral CT characterization. Eur Radiol 11:1175-1183
33. D'Assignies G, Couvelard A, Bahrami S et al (2009) Pancreatic endocrine tumors: tumor blood flow assessed with perfusion CT reflects angiogenesis and correlates with prognostic factors. Radiology 250:407-416
34. Kamisawa T, Takuma K, Anjiki H et al (2010) Differentiation of autoimmune pancreatitis from pancreatic cancer by diffusion-weighted MRI. Am J Gastroenterol 105:1870-1875
35. Ichikawa T, Sou H, Araki T et al (2001) Duct-penetrating sign at MRCP: usefulness for differentiating inflammatory pancreatic mass from pancreatic carcinomas. Radiology 221:107-116
36. Song SJ, Lee JM, Kim YJ et al (2007) Differentiation of intra-

ductal papillary mucinous neoplasms from other pancreatic cystic masses: comparison of multirow-detector CT and MR imaging using ROC analysis. Magn Reson Imaging 26:86-93

37. Yoon LS, Catalano OA, Fritz S et al (2009) Another dimension in magnetic resonance cholangiopancreatography: comparison of 2- and 3-dimensional magnetic resonance cholangiopancreatography for the evaluation of intraductal papillary mucinous neoplasm of the pancreas. J Comput Assist Tomogr 33:363-368

38. Choi JY, Lee JM, Lee MW et al (2009) Magnetic resonance pancreatography: comparison of two- and three-dimensional sequences for assessment of intraductal papillary mucinous neoplasm of the pancreas Eur Radiol 19:2163-2170

39. Sainani NI, Saokar A, Deshpande V et al (2009) Comparative performance of MDCT and MRI with MR cholangiopancreatography in characterizing small pancreatic cysts. Am J Roentgenol 193:722-731

40. Waters JA, Schmidt CM, Pinchot JW et al (2008) CT vs MRCP: optimal classification of IPMN type and extent. J Gastrointest Surg 12:101-109

41. Rickes S, Wermke W (2004) Differentiation of cystic pancreatic neoplasms and pseudocysts by conventional and echoenhanced ultrasound. J Gastroenterol Hepatol 19:761-766

42. Masaki T, Ohkawa S, Amano A et al (2005) Noninvasive assessment of tumor vascularity by contrast-enhanced ultrasonography and the prognosis of patients with nonresectable pancreatic carcinoma. Cancer 103:1026-1035

43. Tawada K, Yamaguchi T, Kobayashi A et al (2009) Changes in tumor vascularity depicted by contrast-enhanced ultrasonography as a predictor of chemotherapeutic effect in patients with unresectable pancreatic cancer. Pancreas 38:30-35

44. Kobayashi A, Yamaguchi T, Ishihara T et al (2005) Evaluation of vascular signal in pancreatic ductal carcinoma using contrast enhanced ultrasonography: effect of systemic chemotherapy. Gut 54:1047

45. Schmidt CM, White PB, Waters JA et al (2007) Intraductal papillary mucinous neoplasms: predictors of malignant and invasive pathology. Ann Surg 246:644-651

46. Manfredi R, Graziani R, Motton M et al (2009) Main pancreatic duct intraductal papillary mucinous neoplasms: accuracy of MR imaging in differentiation between benign and malignant tumors compared with histopathologic analysis. Radiology 253:106-115

47. Inan N, Arslan A, Akansel G et al (2008) Diffusion-weighted imaging in the differential diagnosis of cystic lesions of the pancreas. Am J Roentgenol 191:1115-1121

Paola Capelli and Alice Parisi

12.1 Introduction

In recent years the evolution of imaging technology has made possible a more detailed identification of the structural features of pancreatic cancers, facilitating the differential diagnosis between different tumor histologies and pancreatic diseases in relation to other *tumor-forming* lesions. At the same time pathologists have provided a most accurate definition of the different tumor histologies with the development of the most recent WHO classification (2010) [1].

The aim of this chapter is to report the pathologic, macroscopic and microscopic characteristics of pancreatic tumors and lesions that mimic tumors, focusing particularly on those aspects that affect imaging findings.

A simple diagnostic algorithm that integrates gross and radiographic features with histologic and immunohistochemical findings to reach a proper diagnosis has been proposed and adopted by the recent WHO classification [1, 2].

We have subdivided pancreatic lesions into solid and cystic according to clinical presentation as it is imaged by radiologists, which firstly gives a morphologic description of the clinical problem which draws attention to the pancreas (Table 12.1).

P. Capelli (✉)
Department of Pathology
G.B. Rossi University Hospital
Verona, Italy
e-mail: paola.capelli@ospedaleuniverona.it

12.2 Solid Lesions - Solid Tumors

12.2.1 Ductal Adenocarcinoma

Ductal adenocarcinoma and its variant are the most frequent neoplasms of the pancreas (approximately 85-90% of all pancreatic neoplasms). The incidence varies from 1 to 10 in 100,000 people in developed countries. As many as 80% of cases are between 60 to 80 years of age.

Given the very poor survival, mortality rates closely parallel incidence rates [1], with a 5-year survival of 10-20 months for patients who underwent surgical resection and 3-5 months for inoperable patients.

The vast majority of cases are inoperable at diagnosis, mostly due to their usually advanced stage when they give symptoms such as pain, loss of weight, diabetes and ascites.

It is still very unusual to have an early diagnosis. About 10-20% of cases undergo surgery to reach a radical resection of the tumor, but they will still have a high rate of local relapse or distant metastasis too [2]. For these tumors, surgical resection currently remains the only potentially curative approach, and the prognosis is primarily dependent on the anatomic extent of disease and performance status of the patient.

Gross Findings
The majority (60-70%) of ductal adenocarcinomas are located in the head of the pancreas; the prevalence of head location is due to earlier detection and easier resection as they produce symptoms earlier (jaundice or pancreatitis). Thus the average tumor size of the head (2-3 cm) is considerably smaller than tumors of the body and tail (5-7 cm).

Table 12.1 Solid and cystic classification of pancreatic lesions

Solid lesions	Cystic lesions
Solid tumors	Cystic tumors
• Ductal adenocarcinoma and variants	• Serous neoplasms
• Neuroendocrine neoplasm	- Serous cystadenoma
• Acinar cell carcinoma	- Macrocytic serous cystadenoma
• Pancreatoblastoma	- Solid serous adenoma
• Solid-pseudopapillary tumor	- Von Hippel-Lindau (VHL)-associated
• Metastasis	• Cystic tumor with mucinous epithelium
	- Mucinous cystic neoplasms (MCNs)
Non neoplastic solid lesions	- Intraductal papillary mucinous neoplasms (IPMNs)
• Autoimmune pancreatitis	• Squamous-lined cysts
• Paraduodenal pancreatitis	- Lymphoepithelial cysts (LECs)
• Infectious pseudotumors	- Epidermoid cysts within intrapancreatic accessory spleen
• Ampullary adenomyoma	- Dermoid cysts
• Heterotopia (splenic)	- Squamoid cyst of pancreatic ducts
• Lipomatous hypertrophy	• Acinar tumor
• True hamartomas	- Acinar cell cystadenocarcinomas
• Pseudolymphoma	- Acinar cell cystadenomas
• Deposits of foreign substance	• Endothelial cystic tumor
• Granulomatous inflammations	- Lymphangiomas
• Congenital lesions	
	Cystic variant of solid tumors
	• Solid-pseudopapillary tumor (SPT)
	• Cystic change in ordinary ductal adenocarcinoma
	• Cystic pancreatic neuroendocrine tumors
	• Cystic mesenchymal neoplasms
	• Secondary tumor with cyst
	Non-neoplastic cystic lesions
	• Enterogenous (congenital; duplication)
	• Endometriotic cyst
	• Congenital or developmental cysts
	• Pseudocyst - no lining
	• Paraduodenal wall cyst (cystic dystrophy)
	• Inflammatory related pseudocysts

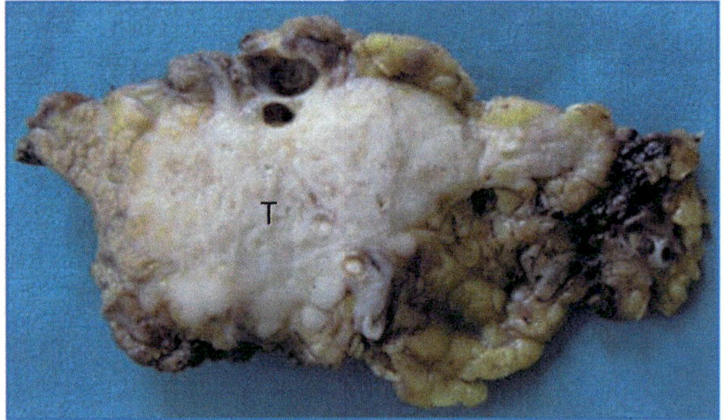

Fig. 12.1 Ductal adenocarcinoma of the body-tail of the pancreas. A large ill-defined tumor (*T*)

On the cut surface, the tumor usually appears as a solid mass with infiltrative ill-defined margins, whitish color and hard consistency (Fig. 12.1). The tumor rarely appears with degenerative cystic changes (necrosis and hemorrhage). Carcinoma of the head of the pancreas, with the exception of those arising in the uncinate process, almost always infiltrate the common bile duct and the duct of Wirsung, leading to a variable degree of stenosis, and ultimately resulting in complete stenosis and upstream dilatation (radiologic finding of the *double-duct*) (Fig. 12.2), causing jaundice and upstream obstructive chronic pancreatitis (Fig. 12.3) with fibrosis and atrophy of the pancreatic parenchyma.

The involvement of the duodenum and/or of the ampulla of Vater causes retraction of the wall and eventually mucosal ulceration. Retroperitoneal tissue infiltration with neural, lymphatic and vascular invasion is considered a relatively early event.

The pathologic evaluation of the retroperitoneal resection margin (so-called posterior lamina) provides the most important information about local recurrence

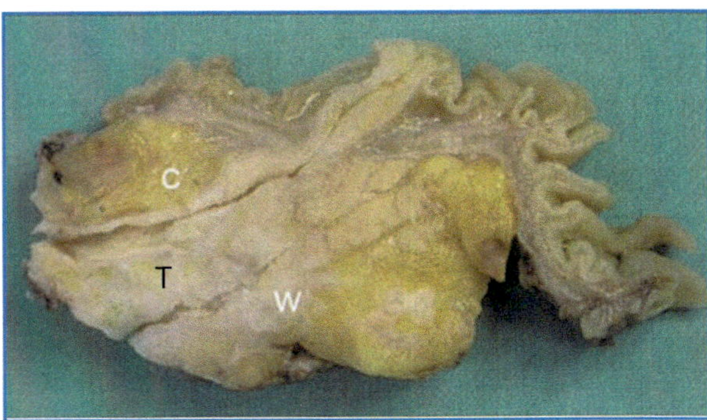

Fig. 12.2 Ductal adenocarcinoma (*T*) of the head of the pancreas causing stenosis of the main duct (*W*) and of the intrapancreatic portion of the common bile duct (*C*) with upstream dilatation (double-duct radiologic sign)

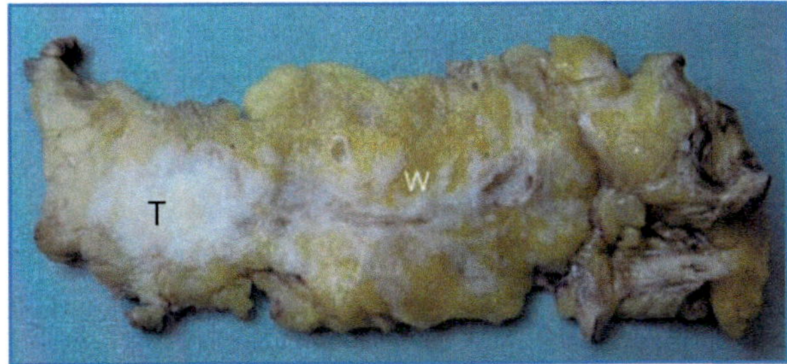

Fig. 12.3 Ductal adenocarcinoma (*T*) of the body of the pancreas with chronic obstructive pancreatitis with duct of Wirsung dilatation (*W*)

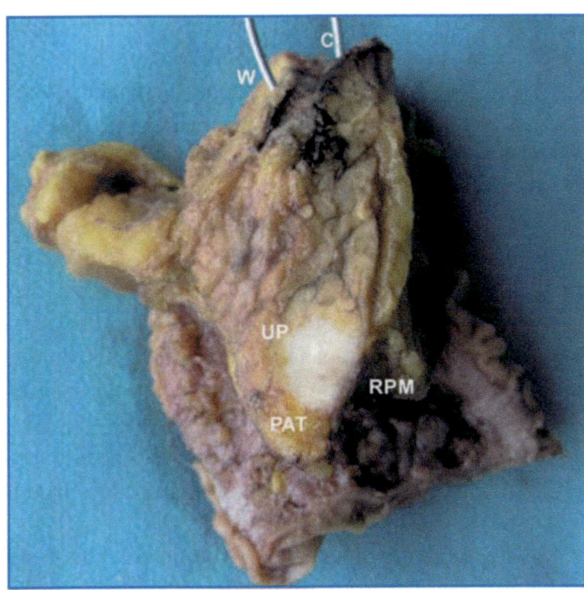

Fig. 12.4 Infiltration of the peripancreatic adipose tissue (*PAT*) and of the retroperitoneal pancreatic margin (*RPM*) of a small adenocarcinoma of the uncinate process (*UP*); probes inside the main duct (*W*) and in the intrapancreatic common bile duct (*C*)

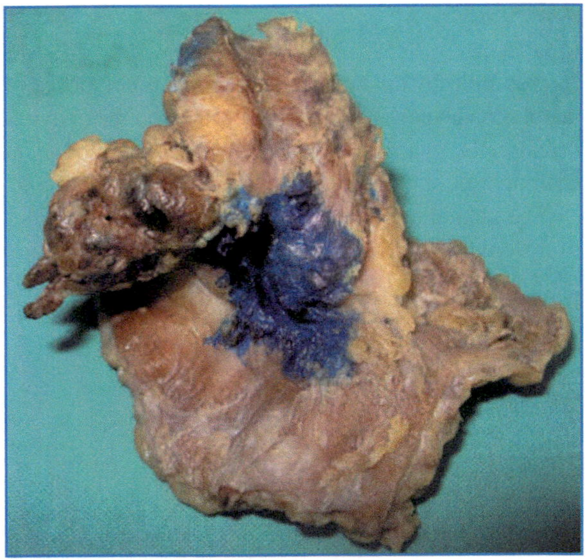

Fig. 12.5 Infiltration of the peripancreatic adipose tissue by a relatively small ductal adenocarcinoma, located in the inferior part of mesenteric vessel's bed (*colored blue*)

and patient survival. This margin is defined as the peripancreatic adipose tissue behind the head of the pancreas that is located dorsal and lateral to the superior mesenteric artery (Figs. 12.4, 12.5). Because local recurrences of pancreatic adenocarcinoma arise in the pancreatic bed corresponding to the retroperitoneal margin and to the retroperitoneal posterior surface of the pancreas, inking the mesenteric vessel's bed and submitting sections through the tumor at its closest approach to this surface as well as the retroperitoneal margin is recommended.

The so-called *posterior lamina* is a very important surgical resection margin and an important lymph node station too.

When the tumor involves the celiac axis or the superior mesenteric artery, it is considered unresectable, so that involvement is rarely encountered in surgical pathology specimens. A focal and partial adhesion of the mesenteric vein to the posterior pancreatic surface, if partial and not circumferential, can lead to a surgical resection of a fragment of vessel wall. Only the histologic examination can prove if that kind of adhesion is caused by a real neoplastic infiltration or by a fibro-inflammatory tumor-associated response.

In advanced cases the tumor infiltrates the stomach, gallbladder and peritoneum, leading to carcinomatosis and ascites. Carcinoma of the head of the pancreas frequently metastasizes in peripancreatic lymph nodes, as almost all ductal adenocarcinoma of the pancreas resected with a good number of lymph nodes are N1.

Carcinoma of the body and tail of the pancreas have the same macroscopic appearance as those arising in the head, with the exception of their usually larger size (due to more space for tumors to grow before they become symptomatic). The extrapancreatic invasion of the tumor involves the mesocolon, transverse colon with encasement of the celiac trunk and splenic vessels, the peritoneum, the stomach, the spleen and left adrenal gland.

Hematologic spread via the portal vein explains the frequent metastasis in the liver.

Most importantly ductal adenocarcinoma of the head of the pancreas has to be differentiated from ampullary carcinoma, characterized by better prognosis. Unfortunately the two lesions have similar microscopic features and the unequivocal establishment of ampullary origin is possible only in small lesions applying strict topographic criteria.

Microscopy

Microscopically ductal adenocarcinoma is composed of neoplastic tubules or glands lined with cuboidal or cylindrical cells, characteristically embedded in abundant desmoplastic stroma, with low vascularity (Fig. 12.6a,b).

The glandular component can have different grades of differentiation from duct-like structure and medium size neoplastic gland in well differentiated cases to a mixture of densely packed, small irregular glands, solid sheets and nests as well as individual cells in poorly differentiated ones.

The stromal component gives the lesion its scirrous and firm appearance and it is responsible for the low vascular density that leads to radiologic detection. Nevertheless such phenomena may become less evident due to the development of a marked peritumoral fibrotic reaction (obstructive chronic pancreatitis). Perineural and vascular invasion is seen in most cases. Even in resectable cases the lesion is rarely confined to the pancreas and the prognosis is related to pathologic parameters (pTN). The tumor is usually T3 for extrapancreatic extension and N1 for lymph nodes metastases.

Variants of Ductal Adenocarcinoma

Rare variants of ductal adenocarcinoma and mixed form exist, like adenosquamous (Fig. 12.7a), signet ring and medullary carcinoma, some of them with well defined distinct clinical and prognostic significance. Most variants have the same macroscopic and radiologic aspect of ductal adenocarcinoma and cannot be distinguished at imaging.

Nevertheless there are some rare exceptions with special gross characteristics, different from those of ductal adenocarcinoma that may pose a differential diagnosis with a less aggressive form than ductal adenocarcinoma.

Hepatoid Carcinoma

This rare variant has the same imaging characteristics as

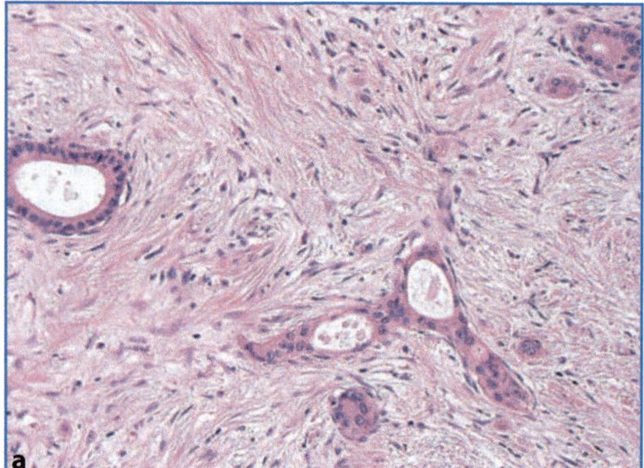
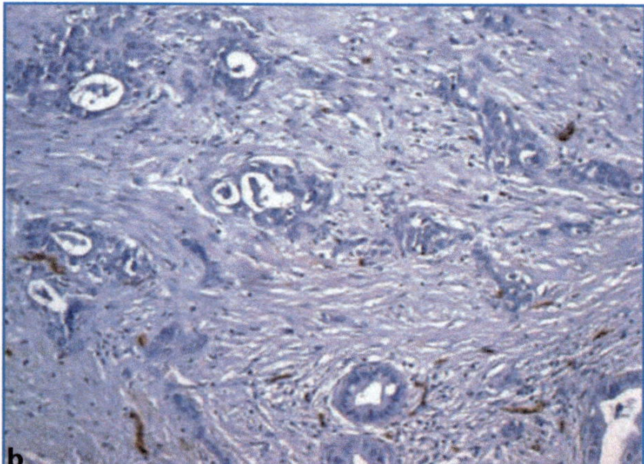

Fig. 12.6 a,b Neoplastic ductal glands with intense desmoplastic reaction (**a**). CD34 (endothelial marker) immunohistochemical reaction showing low intratumoral vascularity (**b**)

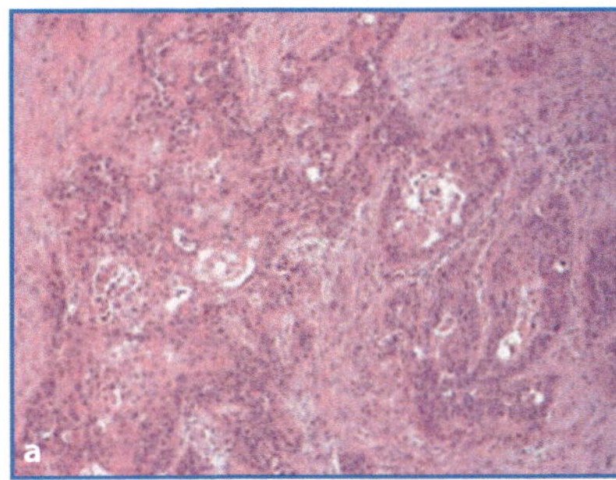
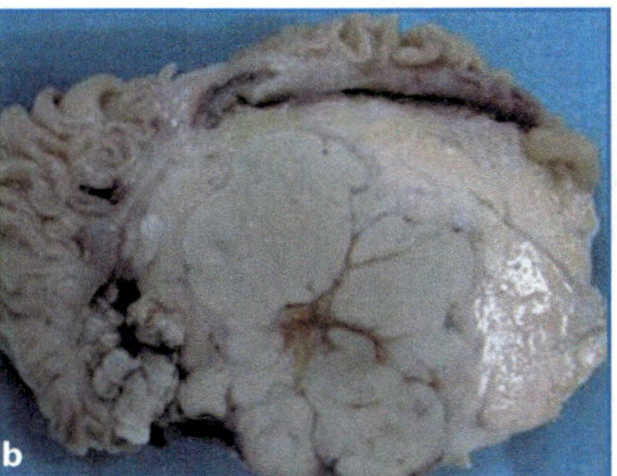
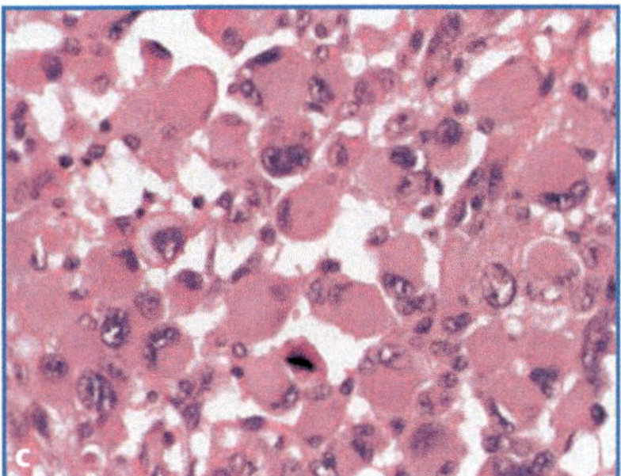

Fig. 12.7 a-c Adenosquamous carcinoma variant (**a**). Hepatoid carcinoma of the head of the pancreas (**b**). Anaplastic variant with bizarre and pleomorphic cells (**c**)

hepatocellular carcinoma, so much closer to an endocrine tumor than to ductal adenocarcinoma (Fig. 12.7b).

Mucinous Noncystic Carcinoma

The incidence of this carcinoma is 1-3% of all ductal adenocarcinomas. The lesion is composed of well differentiated glands floating in abundant (>50%) extracellular mucin and is macroscopically characterized by a gelatinous mass, better demarcated than the ductal carcinoma. Owing to the rich mucinous content, its imaging appearance is different to that of ductal adenocarcinoma.

Undifferentiated (Anaplastic) Carcinoma

Its incidence is 5-7% of all pancreatic tumors. The preferential location is in the tail of the pancreas. Macroscopically it is characterized by a voluminous mass with a variegated aspect on cut section because of the presence of degenerative changes (necrosis and hemorrhage).

At imaging the most significant differential findings are the marked enhancement of the tumor, with the exception of the area of necrosis. This carcinoma is composed of pleomorphic large cells, giant cells or spindle cells (Fig. 12.7c). Its prognosis is poorer than that of conventional ductal adenocarcinoma, with distant metastases frequently present at the time of diagnosis.

12.2.2 Neuroendocrine Neoplasms

Endocrine tumors are rare, accounting for approximately 2% of all pancreatic neoplasms. They commonly affect adults between the ages of 40 and 60 years with no sex predilection. They are epithelial tumors with endocrine differentiation.

Pancreatic endocrine tumors (PETs) are usually sporadic but may be part of hereditary syndromes mostly including multiple endocrine neoplasm type 1 (MEN-1)

and more rarely, von Hippel-Lindau (VHL) syndrome, neurofibromatosis type 1 (NF1), and tuberous sclerosis complex (TSC). Sporadic PETs are solitary, whereas the hereditary forms may be multifocal.

PETs can be located anywhere within the pancreas. Clinical classification is made upon symptoms related to hormones which may be secreted by the tumor. We can have functional (syndromic) tumors (F-PETs) and nonfunctional (nonsyndromic) tumors (NF-PETs). Insulinomas account for the vast majority of F-PETs, and are small non-aggressive tumors.

Patients presenting with metastatic or mass-related symptoms are those with NF-PETs and report abdominal pain, nausea, weight loss or, exceptionally, jaundice. Half of clinically observed PETs and more than 50% of surgically resected cases are NF-PETs.

PETs are classified according to the WHO (2010) criteria and assigned to a TNM-based stage according to ENETS recommendations/AJCC/UICC TNM classification.

The new WHO classification is based on the proliferative index defined by the number of mitoses and the ki-67 percentage of the tumor cells:

- neuroendocrine tumor G1 (less than 2 mitoses x 10 HPF and/or ki67 ≤2%)
- neuroendocrine tumor G2 (2-20 mitoses x 10 HPF and/or ki-67 between 3-20%)
- neuroendocrine carcinoma G3 (>20 mitoses x 10 HPF and/or ki-67 >20%).

The AJCC/UICC and ENETS TNM, with some differences, are based on tumor size and extrapancreatic extension of the tumor.

Imaging procedures address the diagnosis by recognizing the characteristic hypervascular pattern of these lesions, which is present in about 70% of cases. Large size and smooth regular margins with lack of dilation of the biliary and main pancreatic ducts contribute to the differentiation of PET from adenocarcinoma. Most PETs express receptors for somatostatin and can be easily identified by somatostatin receptor scintigraphy. Most F-PETs, with the exception of insulinomas, are diagnosed when they are already advanced staged diseases, and liver metastases are common. NF-PETs have a wide range of aggressiveness. At diagnosis they are also frequently advanced, as more than 50% of patients have liver metastases at diagnosis and almost 40% are not candidates for radical surgery because of either locally advanced disease or unresectable metastases. Patients with well-differentiated NF-PETs have a 5-year survival rate of approximately 65% and a 10-year survival rate of 45%. Moreover, the current and more sensitive imaging techniques increasingly detect small and asymptomatic tumors, the so-called pancreatic endocrine *incidentalomas*.

Unlike the fast proliferating and deadly pancreatic ductal adenocarcinoma, the typical PET grows slowly and impairs patient quality of life only very late in the course of the disease, even when metastatic. It is thus important to distinguish PET from ductal adenocarcinoma, because its prognosis is largely more favorable [3, 4].

Gross Findings

PETs usually present as solitary, solid, homogeneous masses, with medium size from 1 to 5 cm in diameter, rounded and sharp borders (Fig. 12.8 a,b) and rarely surrounded by a fibrotic pseudocapsule. Their expansive pattern of growth differs from the infiltrative pattern of the ductal adenocarcinoma.

When located in the pancreatic head, they usually compress and deviate, but do not infiltrate, the main pancreatic and biliary ducts. As long as PETs grow outside the pancreas, they usually displace rather than invade the adjacent structures including large vessels. Their color and consistency depend on the amount of stroma and vascularity; the usual PET is very rich in small vessels and poor in fibrotic stroma. The color varies from brown to reddish and the consistency is slightly firmer than that of the surrounding parenchyma. Brownish hemorrhagic or necrotic yellowish foci can be observed in large masses.

PET may have an unusual macroscopic appearance that can be difficult to diagnose preoperatively. When the appearance is cystic, they are often interpreted as being a cystic tumor, but they usually retain a normal highly vascular appearance at the periphery.

PET with fibrotic appearance can have firm consistency, whitish color, and ill-defined borders, thus they can mimic a ductal adenocarcinoma. These cases are usually identified as small infiltrative lesions that lead to duct of Wirsung obstruction with consequent pancreatitis episodes.

Microscopy

PET typically has an organoid pattern of growth, characterized by solid nests and macrotrabecular or microtrabecular/gyriform patterns with cords, festoons, and ribbons. Glandular, acinar, and cribriform features can also be observed. Although one pattern is generally prevalent, more than one can be seen in different regions of the same tumor.

A rich vasculature characterizes most PETs and is responsible for their hyperdense radiologic appearance.

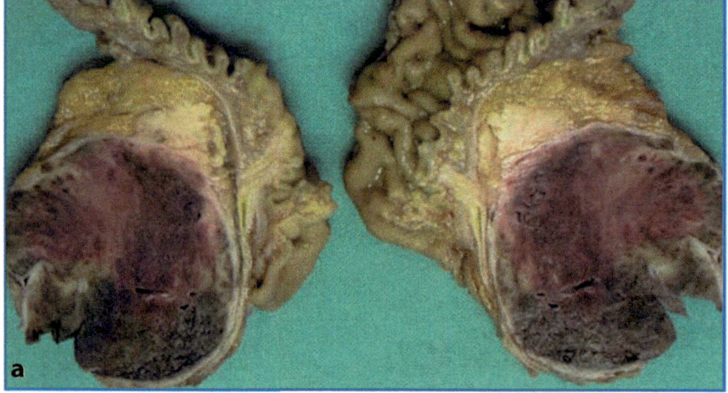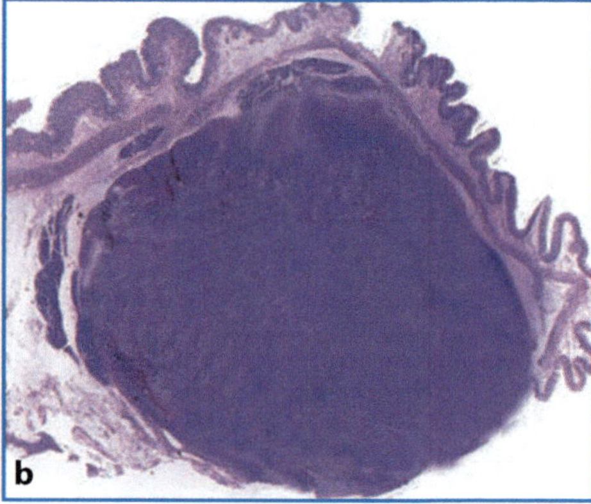

Fig. 12.8 a,b Gross image of a pancreatic endocrine tumor appearing as a large, soft and fleshy mass with well-defined borders in the head of the pancreas (**a**). Macrosection of an endocrine tumor (**b**)

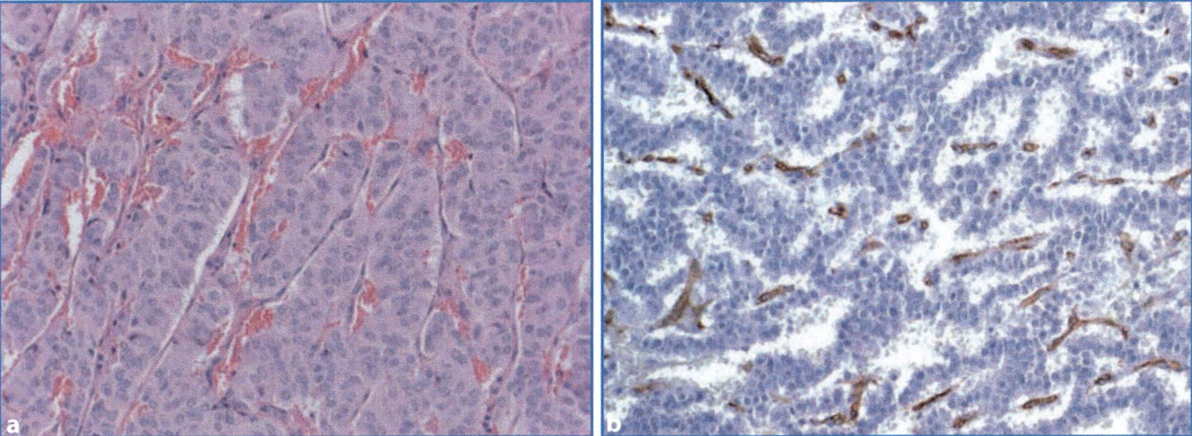

Fig. 12.9 a,b Well-differentiated endocrine tumor. Small-medium size cells arranged in trabeculae or nests with low stroma (**a**). CD34 immunohistochemical reaction showing rich intratumoral vasculature (**b**)

Typically, numerous small vessels encircle the neoplastic nests (Fig. 12.9). These vessels are embedded in a variable amount of stroma, which rarely forms sclerohyaline bands and only occasionally shows calcified foci. Necrosis can be present either as large and confluent areas ("infarct-like"), especially in large tumors, or as punctate foci recognized at microscopic observation in the centre of neoplastic nests.

Regardless of the growth pattern, the neoplastic cells have similar cytologic features: small to medium sized cells with eosinophilic to amphophilic and finely granular cytoplasm, with centrally located, round or oval, nuclei, uniform in size that show finely stippled chromatin referred to as *salt-and-pepper*. In some tumors, the neoplastic cells show a plasmacytoid appearance due to peripherally located nuclei.

12.2.3 Acinar Cell Carcinoma

Acinar cell carcinoma accounts for 1-2% of the tumors of the exocrine pancreas, with lymph nodes and liver metastases in 50% of the cases at the time of diagnosis [5, 6].

Macroscopically the head seems to be more commonly involved, but unlike ductal adenocarcinoma jaundice is very rare. Usually the lesion presents as a well circumscribed, soft mass with an average size of 10 cm. The cut surface demonstrates the presence of bands of dense connective tissue that circumscribe nodules of tumor cells, which can have necrotic foci.

Histologically, the carcinoma is a highly cellular neoplasm composed of cells, with the characteristic of acinar cells (round nuclei and abundant eosinophilic, granular PAS-positive cytoplasm), arranged at least focally in small acinar units. Desmoplastic stroma characteristic of ductal adenocarcinoma is generally absent. Immunohistochemical analysis confirms acinar differentiation with variable positivity for pancreatic enzymes.

The prognosis is midway between that of the ductal adenocarcinoma and that of endocrine tumors.

12.2.4 Pancreatoblastoma

Pancreatoblastoma is a rare tumor, which is prevalent in males and the most common pancreatic tumor in children.

Macroscopically they are solitary large and well circumscribed tumors, without preferential location in the pancreas. In late stage the tumor extensively infiltrates the peripancreatic soft tissue and the adjacent organs and the margins are no longer clearly demarcated.

Histologically the neoplasm consists of lobules of relatively uniform cells, separated by dense fibrous tissue and blended with the characteristic squamoid corpuscles. The pattern of growth can be solid, trabecular or acinar. The tumor may show foci of necrosis as well as, in rare cases, the presence of a conspicuous mesenchymal component with chondroid and osseus differentiation.

The prognosis of the tumor is variable. In one third of patients metastases have been described, usually in the liver [7].

12.2.5 Solid-Pseudopapillary Tumor (see below in cystic tumor)

12.2.6 Metastases

Pancreatic metastases are rare and the most common are those from renal carcinoma. Pancreatic metastases from renal carcinoma are hypervascular, allowing a particular imaging characterization and differential diagnosis with pancreatic ductal adenocarcinoma, but sometimes leading to a wrong diagnosis of neuroendocrine neoplasm (Fig. 12.10) [8]. The patient's clinical history may be necessary to help establish the correct diagnosis.

Other metastases can be found in the pancreas, but they are even rarer. Pancreatic metastases from lung cancer, colon cancer and breast cancer have been reported. Although extremely rare, lymphoma can localize in the pancreas either as primary or as systemic involvement. Mesenchymal tumors such as leiomyosarcoma can also metastasize to the pancreas (Fig. 12.11).

12.3 Solid Lesions - Non Neoplastic

Up to 5% of pancreatectomies performed with the preoperative diagnosis of carcinoma will prove to be non-neoplastic at pathologic examination, although this figure is decreasing with improved diagnostic modalities [9].

Among chronic inflammatory lesions of the pancreas, the two main subtypes that are particularly prone to form pseudotumors are autoimmune (lymphoplasmacytic sclerosing) pancreatitis and paraduodenal pancreatitis.

12.3.1 Autoimmune Pancreatitis [10]

Pseudotumor formation is a characteristic features of autoimmune pancreatitis (AIP). A substantial percentage of cases with full-blown AIP are diagnosed clinically and by imaging as pancreatic cancer. The characteristic pathologic features of AIP include dense lymphoplasmacytic infiltrate around the pancreatic duct, a distinctive cellular fibroinflammatory stroma with storiform ap-

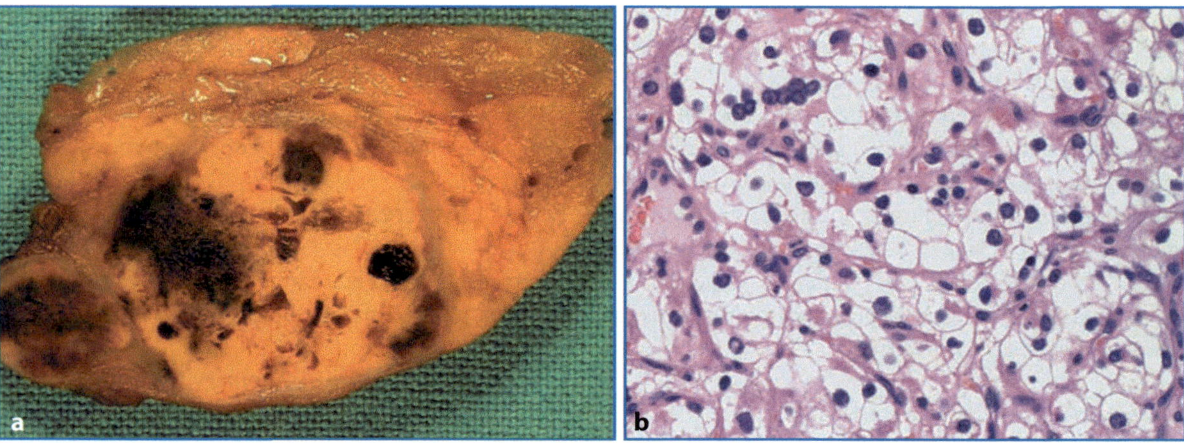

Fig. 12.10 a,b Gross image of clear cell renal cell carcinoma metastasis in the pancreas (**a**). Microscopic image of a metastasis of RCC (**b**)

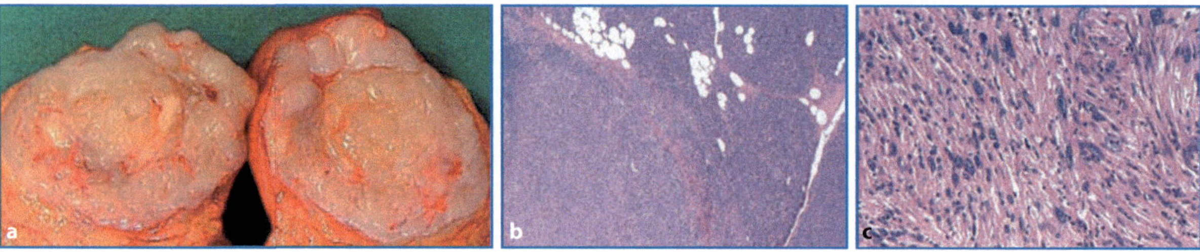

Fig. 12.11 a-c Pancreatic metastasis of a leiomyosarcoma **a** Gross image. Microscopic image at low (**b**) and high (**c**) magnification

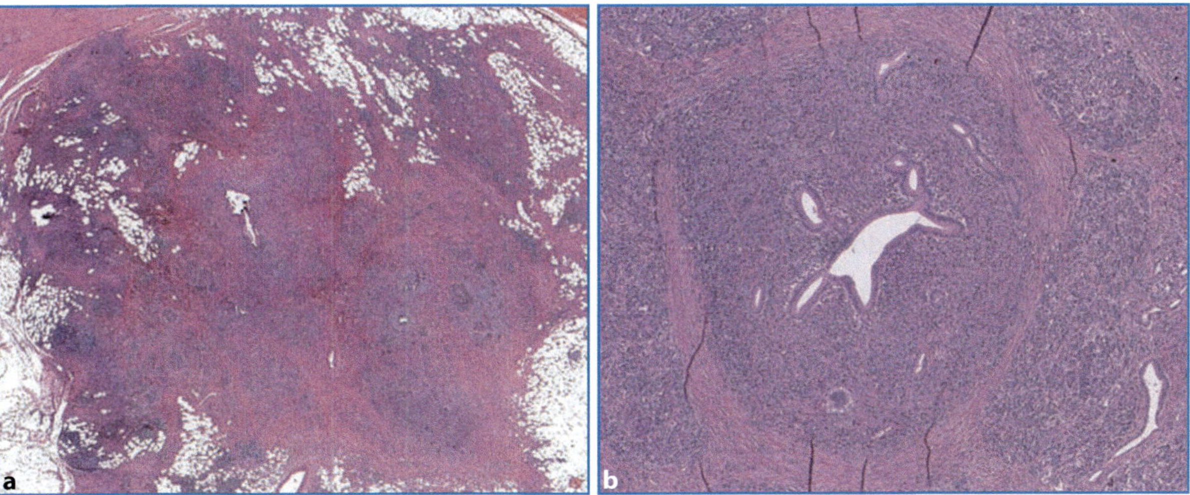

Fig. 12.12 a,b Macrosection of autoimmune pancreatitis (**a**). Microscopic detail of periductal inflammatory infiltration (**b**)

pearance and obliterative venulitis (Fig. 12.12 a,b). In-traepithelial neutrophils (granulocytic epithelial lesions – GEL) may be found in some cases.

The typical AIP is characterized by the presence of a localized mass lesion in the head of the pancreas with stenosis of the bile duct; usually there is no upstream di-latation of the main pancreatic duct. In some cases there may be diffuse, firm enlargement of the pancreas (*sausage* appearance) without discrete mass. If AIP is suspected, serum IgG4 levels may be very helpful in the diagnosis, and avoid an unnecessary pancreatectomy. Autoimmune diseases (or idiopathic inflammatory dis-eases) of practically any type are noted at the time of di-agnosis in about 25% of cases, and some others prove to have autoimmune disorders in the subsequent follow-up. In addition, these patients may have similar *pseudo-tumors* in other organs, in particular, the biliary tract.

12.3.2 Paraduodenal Pancreatitis (see also Paraduodenal Wall Cyst/Cystic Dystrophy/Groove Pancreatitis below)

This is a distinct form of chronic pancreatitis that in-volves the duodenal wall particularly the area corre-sponding to minor papilla (area in which the duct of Santorini connects to the duodenal lumen). There are two distinct gross variants of paraduodenal pancreatitis, the cystic variant is largely more common than the solid one, which is even more rare.

Predominantly solid examples of paraduodenal pan-creatitis (Fig. 12.13) are more prone to be misdiagnosed as carcinoma than the predominantly cystic ones. In these cases the macroscopic features include thickening and scarring of the duodenal wall and fibrosis of the groove region (area located between the common bile duct, pancreas and duodenum). Enlarged lymph nodes may be present in the region of the head of the pancreas. Careful radiologic and endoscopic US (EUS) studies may help to distinguish paraduodenal pancreatitis from ductal adenocarcinoma and avoid unnecessary surgery.

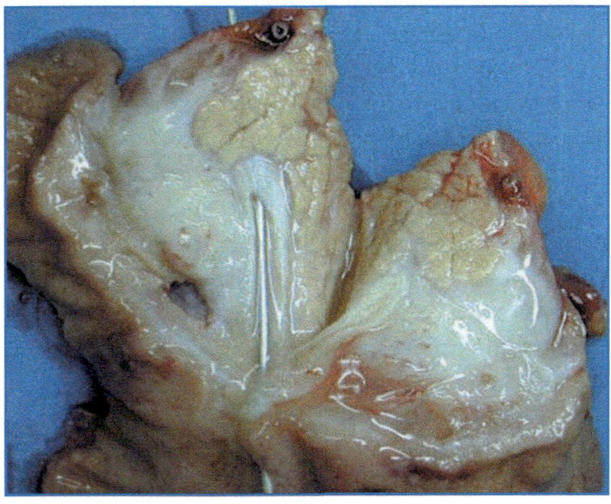

Fig. 12.13 Gross appearance of the solid variant of paraduodenal pancreatitis. A probe is inside the intrapancreatic portion of the common bile duct; groove area with whitish fibrotic tissue

In addition, paraduodenal pancreatitis is seen almost exclusively in males with a mean age of 50, and history of alcohol abuse is characteristic. On the other hand, the presenting symptoms often include abdominal pain and weight loss, which renders the differential diagnosis with adenocarcinoma difficult.

12.3.3 Infectious Pseudotumors

Mycobacterial infections with granulomatous inflammation are particularly prone to form mass lesions and to be misdiagnosed as carcinoma. Other infections such as fungal, parasitic and syphilitic may also occasionally mimic adenocarcinoma in this organ. Malakoplakia may also form a pseudotumor in this organ, like sarcoidosis.

12.3.4 Ampullary Adenomyoma

In some patients with signs and symptoms attributed to pancreatic cancer, the only identifiable *pathologic* finding is a thickened ampulla of Vater, a condition that is referred to as Vaterian adenomyoma (adenomyomatosis, myoepithelial hamartoma, or adenomyomatous hyperplasia). Histologic examination in such cases reveals an accentuated and sometimes slightly disorganized version of normal histologic components of the ampulla of Vater, showing lobules of ducts (of peribiliary type) lying within thickened muscle bundles. Thus, the microscopic findings of this condition are fairly subtle, and by no means specific. The correct diagnosis can only be achieved by careful gross evaluation of the ampulla, and correlation with the clinical and radiologic findings.

EUS shows an intra-ampullary heterogeneous lesion. Since adenomyoma is a benign and slow-growing lesion, it is possible to manage it conservatively; however, it is often difficult to distinguish it from cancer preoperatively with the current diagnostic methods. In addition, since the diagnosis of the entity requires evaluation of the amount of smooth muscle and glands in the deep regions of the ampulla, the diagnosis is extremely difficult to confirm on the basis of an endoscopic biopsy.

12.3.5 Heterotopia (Splenic)

Accessory spleens are noted in about 10% to 15% of necropsies and reported in 16% of abdominal CTs. 1-2% of these are located within the tail of the pancreas, and almost invariably, they are misdiagnosed as pancreatic tumor. Although a few of these harbor epidermoid cysts and fall in the differential diagnosis of cystic lesions, most are composed entirely of splenic tissue and mimic solid tumors. Because they are relatively homogenous, round, and well-demarcated, they tend to be mistaken for endocrine tumors rather than ductal adenocarcinomas. The age group in which intrapancreatic accessory spleen comes to clinical attention is 50 to 70 years, largely because this is the age group that more commonly undergoes radiologic studies, and these lesions, which are typically asymptomatic, are detected incidentally during workup for other conditions. They are usually smaller than 2 cm. The histologic diagnosis is straightforward, revealing ordinary splenic tissue.

12.3.6 Lipomatous Pseudohypertrophy

Lipomatous pseudohypertrophy (pseudolipomatous hypertrophy or lipomatosis) is characterized by the replacement of pancreatic tissue by mature, benign fat. This condition is very uncommon. Although those occurring in children or in association with syndromes are easily diagnosed, others sometimes present as a pseudotumor, particularly if they are associated with enlargement of the pancreas, which can be massive, or have a heterogeneous appearance. Rare examples show mass-effect and cause obstructive jaundice. Microscopically, this entity is characterized by atrophic pancreatic tissue replaced by fat. No fibrotic changes or morphologic alteration in acinar or islet cells are noted (i.e. usually there is no evidence of pancreatitis). Some of the so-called lipomas of the pancreas probably represent lipomatous pseudohypertrophy.

12.3.7 True Hamartomas

A hamartomatous appearance is common in pancreatic injury because chronic pancreatitis is typically associated with acinar atrophy, ductal irregularities and aggregation of islets: the haphazard distribution of the normal pancreatic elements leads to a picture reminiscent of hamartoma. There are, however, rare lesions that would qualify as true hamartomas in the pancreas. Some of these occur in neonates and young children, but they have been recently reported in adults. There appears to be two distinct types of these hamartomas in adults. One is a sharply delimited solid and cystic lesion similar to the multicystic hamartoma of children and is composed of haphazardly distributed cystic ductal elements lined by

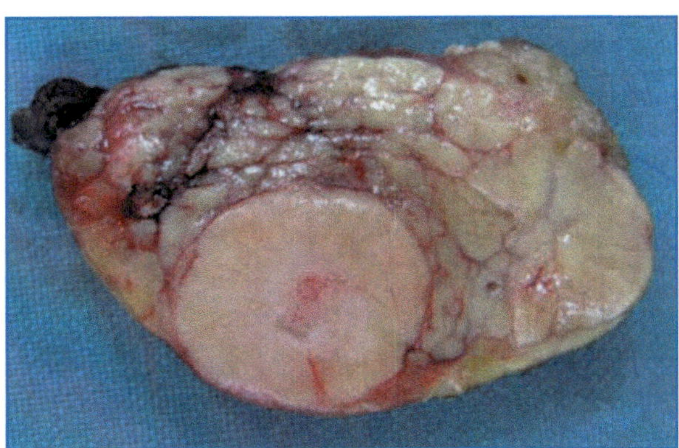

Fig. 12.14 Pancreatic solid hamartoma, seen as a small, firm well-defined whitish mass

cuboidal to flattened epithelium, surrounded by well-differentiated acini embedded in fibroinflammatory stroma. Scattered ill-formed clusters of endocrine cells composed predominantly of PP-cell type and unaccompanied by any insulin positive cells are also present and support the hamartomatous nature of the process. The second type of hamartoma is a solid lesion in which well differentiated ducts and acini are embedded in a fibrous or spindle cell stroma (Fig. 12.14).

12.3.8 Pseudolymphoma

Unlike in the salivary glands, there are no lymph nodes in the pancreas itself, although many lymph nodes are embedded in the surfaces of the pancreas. Localized nodules of reactive lymphoid tissue (with germinal centers) have been reported to form 2- to 3-cm soft, yellow nodules in this organ. Autoimmune pancreatitis, lymphoepithelial cysts, and true lymphomas (including MALT type) ought to be considered high in the differential diagnosis of such cases.

12.3.9 Deposits of Foreign Substance

Rarely, foreign material may accumulate in the pancreas and form a pseudotumor.

12.3.10 Congenital Anomalies

Congenital anomalies of the pancreas are very uncommon and some may present as pseudotumors. For example, annular pancreas sometimes mimics adenocarcinoma.

12.3.11 Granulomatous Inflammations

Granulomatous inflammations (such as sarcoidosis or tuberculosis, Wegener's vasculitis), and congenital lesions may form tumoral lesions.

12.4 Cystic Lesions - Cystic Tumors [11, 12]

Cystic tumors of the pancreas are rare and account for 20% of pancreatic tumors. Their epithelial lining distinguishes them from pseudocysts which are much more frequent as the consequence of inflammatory and necrotic process.

Cystic tumors are usually resectable (80-90% of cases) and usually have a much better prognosis than ductal adenocarcinoma, with a high level of curable disease after resection.

In pancreatic disease cystic tumors are the most frequent indication for surgery. As pathologists we are interested in cystic tumors due to their heterogeneity: in cystic tumors we can find different morphology, different pathogenesis and different clinical behavior. We should also always keep in mind that solid tumors can have necrotic or hemorrhagic events that lead to cystic formation.

According to the kind of epithelium of the cyst the WHO classifies different lesions with different clinical and pathologic characteristics. It is very important to reach a correct preoperative radiologic diagnosis to avoid unnecessary surgery and then to make a proper pathologic diagnosis to find the right prognosis.

12.4.1 Serous Neoplasms

Serous cystic neoplasms are epithelial neoplasms with cystic features, characterized by uniform, cuboidal glycogen-rich, clear cells without atypia. They are relatively uncommon (1-2% of all pancreatic neoplasms) benign neoplasms in most cases. Malignant cases are extremely rare. In these cases the diagnosis of malignancy was established only after metastases to the liver were detected. There is a slight prevalence in females aged 50-60 years old.

The lesions are usually sporadic, although there is an association with von Hippel-Lindau syndrome, and they usually appear with multifocal lesions within the pancreas.

In 20-50% cases they are diagnosed incidentally at routine physical examination, as they are mostly clinically silent.

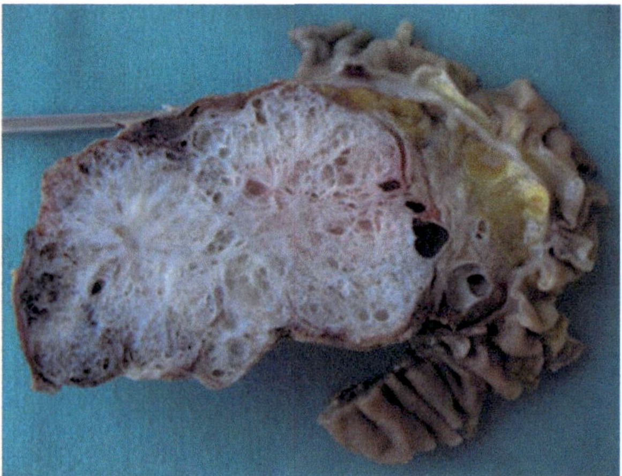

Fig. 12.15 Gross image of a microcystic serous cystadenoma. Note the central scar and sponge-like appearance

Different variants have been described:
- Microcystic serous cystic neoplasm (serous cystadenoma)
- Macrocystic serous cystic neoplasm (macrocystic serous cystadenoma)
- Solid serous adenoma
- Von Hippel-Lindau (VHL)- associated serous cystic neoplasms

12.4.1.1 Serous Cystadenoma

Microcystic serous cystic neoplasms are the most common type (70% of serous neoplasms) [13]. They usually (50-70%) occur in the body-tail of the pancreas.

The gross appearance is characteristic: well-defined lesion, slightly bosselated, with honeycomb appearance on cut surface due to the presence of numerous, tightly packed small cysts. They are often arranged around a central scar, which is often calcified, from which fibrous septa radiate to the periphery creating a sponge-like appearance (Fig. 12.15). This finding is almost diagnostic and allows easy radiologic identification. The radiologic detection is crucial as they are completely benign lesions. Owing to the huge dimensions microcystic cystadenoma usually grow producing a mass effect on adjacent organs without infiltration. Thus even if they occupy the head of the pancreas they do not cause jaundice.

12.4.1.2 Macrocystic Serous Cystadenoma

This form is rarer than the microcystic type. The lesions occur more frequently in males and are mainly found

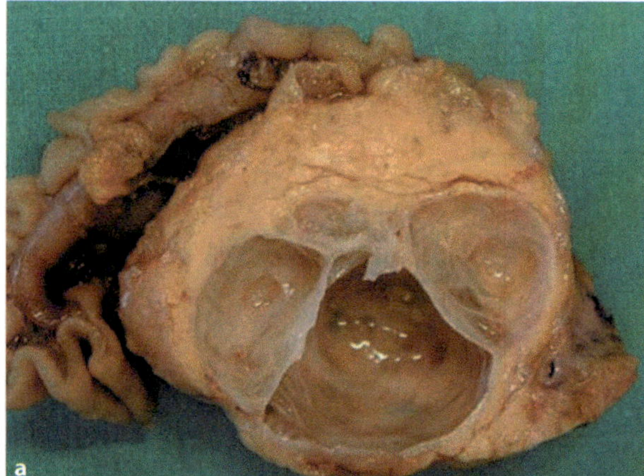

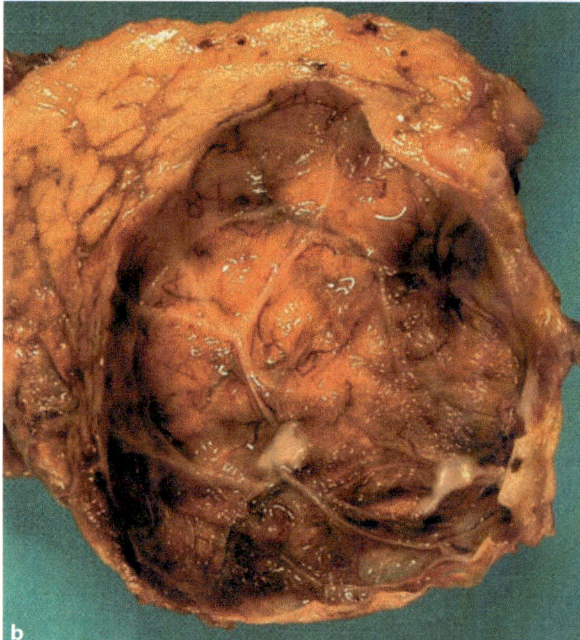

Fig. 12.16 a,b Oligocystic variant of serous cystadenoma (a) Unilocular variant of serous cystadenoma (b)

in the head of the pancreas. Macroscopically they are composed of few but numerable cysts (Fig. 12.16a) usually more than 2 cm in diameter, which can reach 15-20 cm. They may be unilocular (Fig. 12.16b) as well.

The macroscopically visible cysts sometimes are separated by broad septa without a central stellate scar. Generally these lesions are poorly demarcated, with small cysts extending into the adjoining pancreatic tissue. Due to the absence of a central scar, the frequent large size and the not well-defined tumor border, radiologic detection is difficult, and it is difficult to distinguish them from other neoplasms such as mucinous neoplasms or pseudocysts.

When the cysts are large and unilocular, they usually have a thick capsule, the fluid is not as usual typically watery but it may be hemorrhagic. In 40% of cases the epithelial lining may become denuded, making the histologic diagnosis difficult. The lesion must be extensively sampled and examined carefully to identify the characteristic glycogen-rich, clear cells.

12.4.1.3 Solid Serous Adenoma

These are very rare lesions. The solid gross appearance is due to the presence of clear cells arranged in small acini within stromal framework. These tumors are usually well circumscribed and small (2-4 cm). The differential diagnosis includes neuroendocrine tumors.

12.4.1.4 Von Hippel-Lindau (VHL)-Associated Serous Cystic Neoplasms

As many as 90% of patients with Von Hippel-Lindau syndrome develop serous neoplasms. They are frequently multiple and may involve the entire pancreatic gland.

12.4.2 Cystic Tumors with Mucinous Epithelium

These tumors are currently subdivided into two groups with distinct clinical-pathologic characteristics namely mucinous cystic neoplasm (MCN) and intraductal mucinous papillary neoplasm (IPMN).

It is well known that IPMNs and MCNs encompass a spectrum of lesions from mild atypia to invasive carcinoma. The WHO classification classifies the noninvasive tumors on the basis of the highest degree of cytoarchitectural atypia (low-grade/intermediate-grade or high-grade dysplasia). The presence of invasive carcinoma leads to the designation IPMN/MCN with an associated invasive carcinoma.

12.4.2.1 Mucinous Cystic Neoplasms (MCNs)

- MCN with low or intermediate grade dysplasia
- MCN with high-grade dysplasia
- MCN with an associated invasive carcinoma

MCNs are epithelial neoplasms with cystic features that characteristically do not communicate with the ductal system of the pancreas. They make up about 8% of surgically resected cystic lesions of the pancreas [12].

MCNs have distinctive clinical-pathologic features:

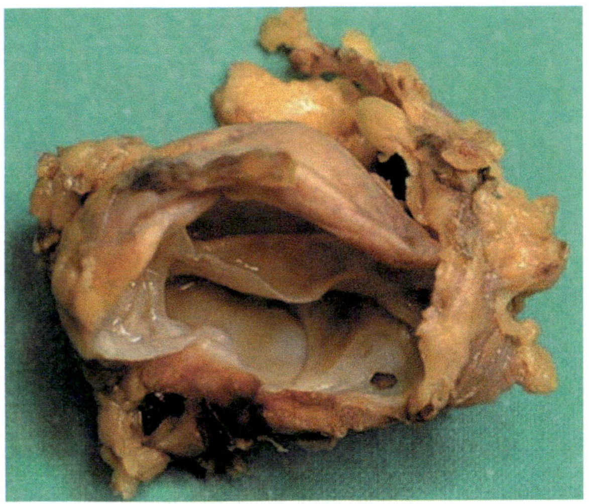

Fig. 12.17 Mucinous cystic tumor with rare thin septa

this neoplasm occurs almost exclusively in women (median age: 40-50 years); it is located in the body-tail of the pancreas; it is characterized by columnar mucin-producing cells with various degrees of atypia, associated with ovarian-like subepithelial stroma. A MCN should be suspected whenever a cystic lesion is seen by imaging in the pancreatic body-tail of a young or middle aged woman, especially in the absence of a history of pancreatitis.

The pathogenetic theory is that of heterotopic ovarian tissue dislocated in the pancreas during embryogenesis, on which a mucinous cystic tumor subsequently arises. Clinical presentation depends on the size of the tumors: small tumors are usually found incidentally; in larger ones symptoms depend on the abdominal mass.

Gross Findings

Usually these neoplasms are composed of sharply demarcated cystic masses ranging in size from one to several centimeters with thick fibrotic walls, with occasional calcifications. Unless there is fistula formation, the lesions do not communicate with the pancreatic ductal system.

On the cut surface, the tumors are unilocular or multilocular; sometimes there are rare thin septa (Fig. 12.17). The cyst often contains mucin, but hemorrhagic content and a more watery fluid may also be noted.

The internal surface may be smooth and glistening, sometimes with trabeculae, especially in low grade lesions, or it may have papillary projections (Fig. 12.18). Unilocular cases can be extensively denudated, thus

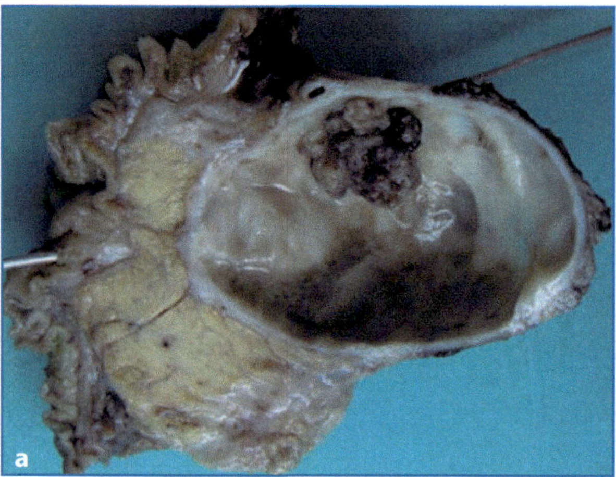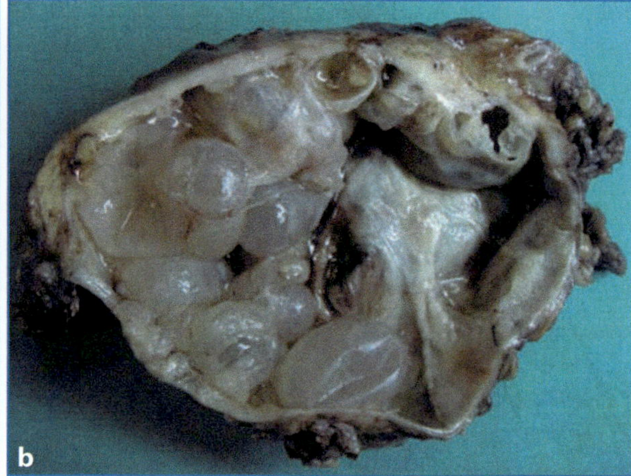

Fig. 12.18 a,b Mucinous cystic tumor with unilocular cyst and focal papillary vegetations (**a**). Multilocular mucinous lesion (**b**)

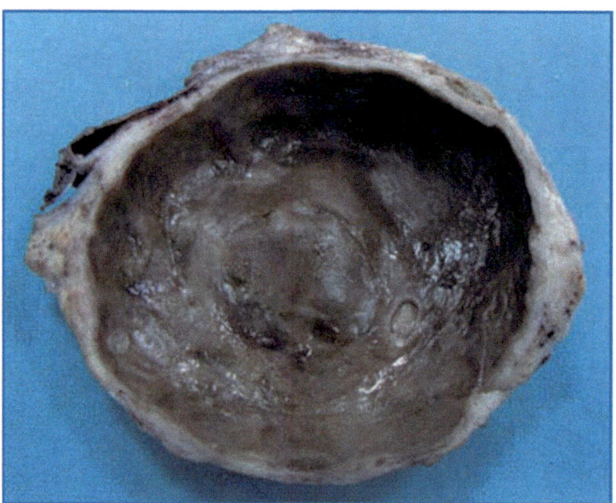

Fig. 12.19 Unilocular denudated case of mucinous cystic tumor

stroma (referred to as ovarian-like) [14]. This stroma is an entity-defining feature of these neoplasms, to the extent that it has almost become a requirement for the diagnosis. The mucin-producing epithelium may exhibit pseudopyloric, gastric foveolar, small or large intestinal differentiation; squamous differentiation may be present. Inflammation may impart a more complex architecture to an otherwise simple mucinous cystic neoplasm and raise the suspicion of malignancy at imaging.

The WHO classification recognizes a noninvasive MCN with low-intermediate and high grade dysplasia and mucinous cystic neoplasm with an associated invasive carcinoma (present in up to one third of MCNs). Patients with invasive carcinoma are 5-10 years older, on average, than those with a noninvasive tumor, suggesting a progression from curable noninvasive tumor to invasive carcinoma. The invasive component arising in association with mucinous cystic neoplasms is usually the tubular/ductal type; colloid infiltration is extremely rare. Interestingly, these cases have been found to have a more indolent course than ordinary infiltrating ductal adenocarcinoma, with a degree of aggressiveness from intratumoral invasion, capsular invasion to extensive pancreatic tissue invasion.

If completely resected, the prognosis of noninvasive cases is excellent despite the level of dysplasia [15]. Staging follows the protocol for ductal adenocarcinoma [16].

The differential diagnosis includes other cystic neoplasms of the pancreas and pseudocysts. The best way to reach a diagnosis is based on combined evaluation of clinical, radiologic and pathologic data.

sometimes reaching a proper differential diagnosis with pseudocyst can be difficult (Fig. 12.19). An extensive sampling of the lesion usually leads to the identification of at least some ovarian-like stroma.

There are some features suggestive of an associated invasive carcinoma: large size with multilocular appearance; irregular thickening of the cystic wall; mural nodules. These neoplasms should be sampled extensively for microscopic examination, to look for an invasive component.

Microscopy

MCNs are characterized by tall, columnar mucin-producing cells with various degrees of atypia, associated with the presence of a distinctive subepithelial cellular

12.4.2.2 Intraductal Papillary Mucinous Neoplasms (IPMNs)

- IPMN with low or intermediate-grade dysplasia
- IPMN with high-grade dysplasia
- IPMN with an associated invasive carcinoma

IPMNs are epithelial neoplasms with ductal differentiation that characteristically grow primarily within the ductal system of the pancreas. They form intraductal masses that are radiographically and grossly detectable: an arbitrary minimal size criterion of 1cm has been suggested to define this family.

IPMNs can involve the main pancreatic duct (MD-IPMNs/main duct type) or its secondary branches (BD-IPMNs/branch duct type) in a segmental or multifocal/diffuse fashion.

The incidence of IPMNs in the general population is poorly defined because most subjects are asymptomatic. The lesions are fairly common, especially in the elderly; the incidence rate seems to increase with age.

IPMNs are estimated to account for 1-3% of all exocrine pancreatic neoplasms and almost 20% of cystic tumors. Unlike other cystic tumors they usually give symptoms (70% of the cases) that mimic those of chronic pancreatitis. However, an increasing number of IPMNs is incidentally discovered during radiologic investigations performed for other purposes.

Gross Findings

IPMNs are characterized by cystic dilatation of the pancreatic ducts with an intraductal proliferation of neoplastic mucin-producing cells usually arranged in papillary patterns, leading to diffuse or segmental main duct/secondary ducts dilatation.

Mucin production by the neoplastic cells is usually associated with intraluminal mucin which leads to cystic dilatation of the ducts, and at times, to mucin extrusion from the ampulla of Vater, a finding that is virtually diagnostic of IPMN.

Macroscopic examination of IPMNs is imperative for documenting involvement of the pancreatic ductal system and the distribution of the disease within the ductal system. Most IPMNs (70-80%) are located in the head of the pancreas (Fig. 12.20).

Branch duct type IPMN usually form a cystic mass in the uncinate process (Fig. 12.21); main duct type IPMN can involve the entire main pancreatic duct.

The intraductal growth may be either flat or papillary. The papillae may range from microscopic to large macro-

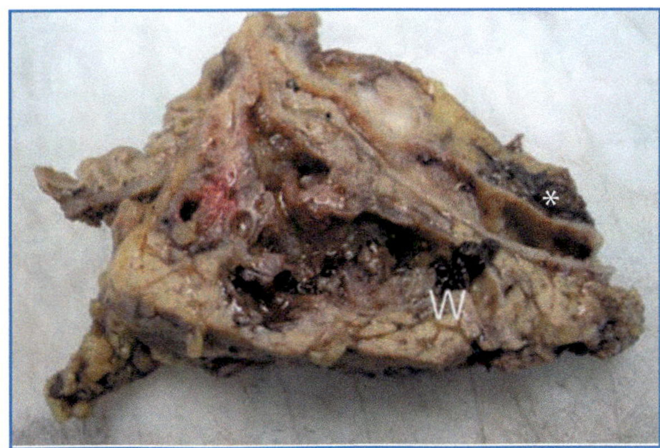

Fig. 12.20 Main duct type IPMN of the head of the pancreas: duct of Wirsung dilation (*W*) with macroscopic visible papillae (*)

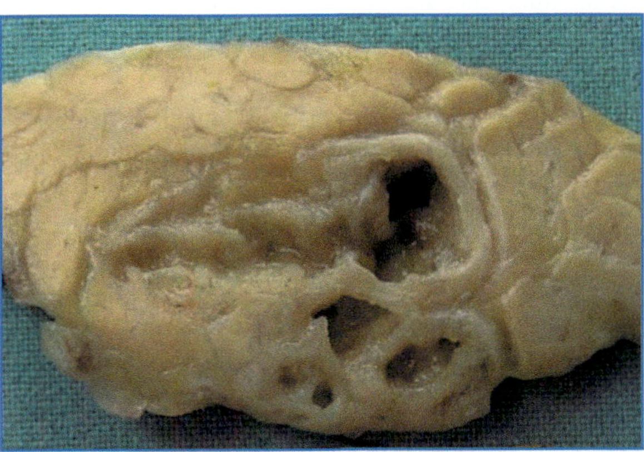

Fig. 12.21 Small "branch duct" type IPMN of uncinate process, gross section of a DCP specimen

scopically detectable proliferations. Papillary projection can be detectable at imaging as a non filled tract.

Main duct type IPMN is characterized by dilation that can involve a segment or the entire main pancreatic duct with the tortuous and irregular duct often being filled with mucin (Fig. 12.20). This type usually arises in the head of the pancreas and progresses along the main duct. The neoplastic growth leads to grossly recognizable lesions that distend the duct and compress the nearby pancreatic parenchyma finally to a peripheral rime, reflecting changes of extensive chronic obstructive pancreatitis.

The documentation of involvement of the pancreatic main duct has clinical importance because this type is associated with higher risk of high-grade dysplasia and invasive carcinoma.

Sometimes the preoperative localization of a main-

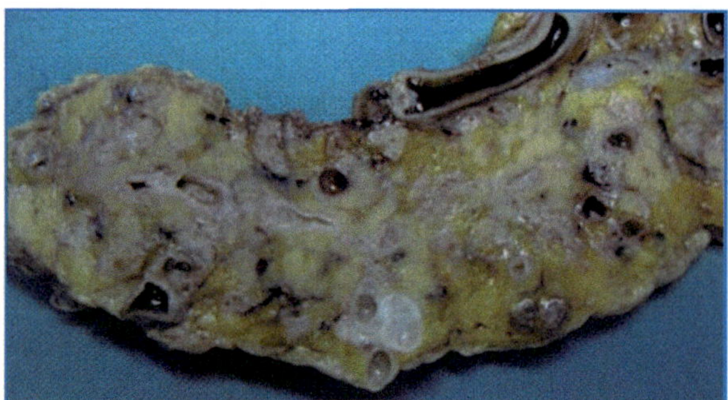

Fig. 12.22 Multifocal IPMN involving ducts all over the pancreas

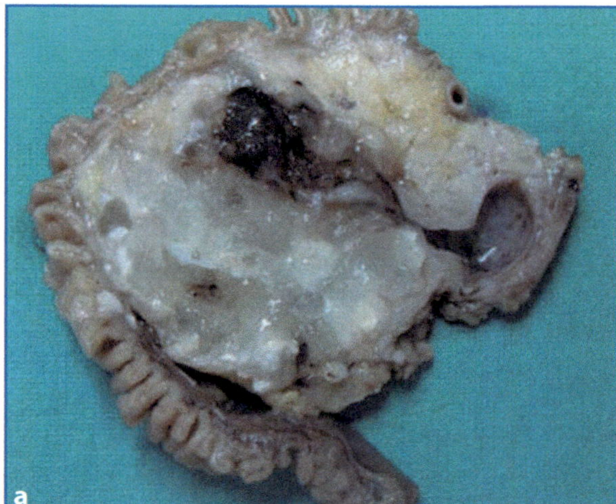

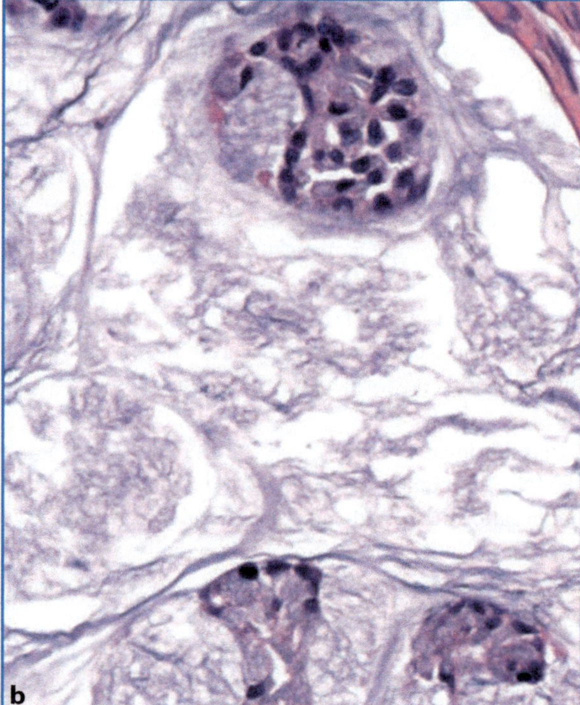

Fig. 12.23 a,b IPMN with infiltration as a colloid carcinoma: gross (**a**) and microscopic (**b**) appearance

duct IPMN may be difficult. High-resolution imaging (CT, MRI with MRCP) may show a dilated main pancreatic duct, but the dilation might also occur both proximal and distal to the IPMN because of overproduction of mucus and/or associated chronic pancreatitis.

Branch duct type IPMN primarily involves the branch ducts. This type arises most often in the uncinate process (Fig. 12.21) in the form of multicystic, grape-like structures. The adjacent pancreas is generally normal.

BD-IPMNs are associated with malignancy in about 25% of cases, and parameters associated with the presence of a malignancy are the presence of symptoms, larger lesions (>3 cm) and mural nodules.

IPMNs may be focal (localized), multifocal (multicentric) (Fig. 12.22) (in up to 40% of cases) or diffuse.

Infiltration usually has the appearance of colloid carcinoma with gelatinous stromal masses (Fig. 12.23a,b). This explains, in large advanced tumors, the frequent presence of fistula with the common bile duct and extrapapillary duodenum, or the peritoneal diffusion as pseudomyxoma peritonei.

Multifocal disease and haphazard distribution of carcinoma, which may develop both adjacent to and away from the IPMN and which may also be macroscopically undetectable, necessitates the extensive sampling of these lesions and careful histologic examination is needed to rule out invasion [17-20].

Microscopy

The cystically dilated ducts are characterized by columnar mucin-producing cells with various degrees of atypia. Architecturally the epithelium can be flat or form papillae. The papillae range from microscopic fold of epithelium to grossly evident finger-like projections.

The WHO classification classifies the noninvasive tumors on the basis of the highest degree of cytoarchitectural atypia (low-grade/intermediate-grade or high-grade dysplasia). The presence of invasive carcinoma leads to the designation IPMN with an associated invasive carcinoma.

Neoplastic epithelium may present different differentiation: gastric, intestinal, pancreatobiliary and oncocytic. IPMNs can be subclassified on the basis of the predominant cellular type [21].

Invasive adenocarcinoma, which is seen in almost 30% of cases, is usually either of the colloid or tubular (ordinary ductal) histotypes. The former has been found to have indolent behavior. Staging follows the protocol for ductal adenocarcinoma [16].

Overall 5-year survival for patients with an IPMN is 70%. This is not surprising, considering that most IPMNs are noninvasive.

The differential diagnosis for larger IPMNs includes other macrocystic/oligocystic lesions such as mucinous cystic neoplasms and macrocystic serous cystadenomas. Small IPMNs can be distinguished from microscopic lesions of the pancreatic ducts known as pancreatic intraepithelial neoplasia (PanIN) (less than 1 cm) and retention cyst. At last IPMNs must be microscopically differentiated from intraductal growth of neoplasms such as acinar cell carcinomas or neuroendocrine tumors [22].

12.4.3 Squamous-Lined Cysts

12.4.3.1 Lymphoepithelial Cysts (LECs)

Lymphoepithelial cysts are benign cystic lesions seen predominantly in males, in the fifth to sixth decade of life. Grossly they may be unilocular or multilocular. The cyst contents may vary from serous to cheesy/caseous-appearing depending on the degree of keratin formation. The cyst wall and trabeculae are usually thin. Microscopically, the cysts are lined by well-differentiated stratified squamous epithelium, without atypia which may or may not have prominent keratinization. The squamous epithelium is surrounded by a band of dense lymphoid tissue composed of mature T-lymphocytes with intervening germinal centers formed by B cells, which may be abundant in some cases. In many cases, the lymphoid tissue is immediately adjacent to the epithelium, while in others there is a band of fibrous tissue separating them. Solid lymphoepithelial islands (microscopic clusters of epithelial cells admixed with lymphocytes, similar to the so-called *epimyoepithelial islands* in salivary gland LECs) may also be present. Some of these epithelial nests form microcysts.

12.4.3.2 Epidermoid Cysts within Intrapancreatic Accessory Spleen

These are rare. They occur almost exclusively in the tail of the pancreas where accessory spleens are not too uncommon. They are seen in younger patients (2nd–3rd decades). The cysts are lined by attenuated squamous cells, usually nonstratified, surrounded by normal-appearing splenic tissue.

12.4.3.3 Dermoid Cysts

Dermoid cysts are also exceedingly rare tumors in the pancreas region. They are reported in younger patients (2nd–3rd decades) and are morphologically similar to the teratomas seen in other sites, although some examples are composed predominantly of epidermal elements, such that they are difficult to distinguish from LECs. The presence of sebaceous glands or hair follicules is more typical for dermoid cysts.

12.4.3.4 Squamoid Cyst of Pancreatic Ducts

Squamoid cyst of pancreatic ducts is a recently recognized type of cystic lesion in the pancreas in which cystically dilated ducts are lined by a squamous/transitional epithelium without keratinization. The larger and clinically manifested examples reported are unilocular. The cysts typically contain distinctive acidophilic acinar secretions that form concretions, more evident in medium-sized examples, confirming their communication with the acinar system, and suggesting a localized obstruction in their pathogenesis.

12.4.4 Cysts Lined by Acinar Cells

12.4.4.1 Acinar Cell Cystadenocarcinomas

A cystic form of acinar cell carcinoma is well documented but is extremely uncommon; only a handful of cases have been documented in the literature. True acinar cell cystadenocarcinomas are composed of neoplastic cells that form normal pancreatic acinar structure with prominent lumen formation (in contrast to ordinary acinar cell carcinomas which have a more solid growth pattern). Some show significant cystic dilatation that may measure up to several centimeters. The cysts in this neoplasm are true cysts with an epithelial lining composed of cells with acinar differentiation rather than a degenerative phenomenon. The cells often contain abundant apical, acidophilic (zymogenic) granules, and immunolabeling will reveal the presence of pancreatic exocrine enzymes. In the examples we have seen, the cysts contained enzymatic concretions admixed with crystalline material, presumably composed of enzymatic secretions. Acinar cell cystadenocarcinomas are often large. Their biology seems not to be significantly different from their solid counterparts, with liver metastases developing early in the course of the disease, although some with intraductal growth had protracted clinical courses [23].

12.4.4.2 Acinar Cell Cystadenomas

Until recently, the conventional thought was that all acinar neoplasms in the pancreas are malignant, albeit solid or cystic. In 2000, however, an entity referred to as acinar cell cystadenoma (also called cystic acinar transformation) was described. This phenomenon is uncommon, often incidental, but may on occasion produce a clinically detectable cystic mass (measuring up to several centimeters), in which the cysts are lined by cytologically bland acinar cells. Acinar cell cystadenoma is seen in young adults and children, and the consensus is that it is a benign process [24].

12.4.5 Endothelial-Lined Cysts

12.4.5.1 Lymphangiomas

Lymphangiomas may also present as pancreatic and peripancreatic cystic masses and may closely mimic LECs (especially those with denuded epithelium) because they also contain prominent lymphoid tissue. Lymphangiomas are lined by endothelial cells as demonstrated by immunohistochemical labeling for endothelial markers (CD31, CD34 or D2–40) and lack staining for epithelial markers (cytokeratins). Lymphangiomas may become very large, measuring up to 25 cm. They are benign.

12.5 Cystic Lesions – Cystic Variant of Solid Tumors

This group constitutes an estimated 10% of the pancreatic cysts [25].

12.5.1 Solid-Pseudopapillary Neoplasm [26]

These make up about 0.9-2.7% of exocrine pancreatic neoplasm and 5% of cystic pancreatic tumors and occur predominantly in young women.

Solid-pseudopapillary neoplasm is the most recent name advocated by the WHO for a distinctive tumor type in the pancreas that often presents as a cystic mass, described for the first time by Franz in 1959. The plethora of names used previously reflects the enigmatic nature of this neoplasm. It is now known that cavities present in these tumors are not *true* cysts (there is no

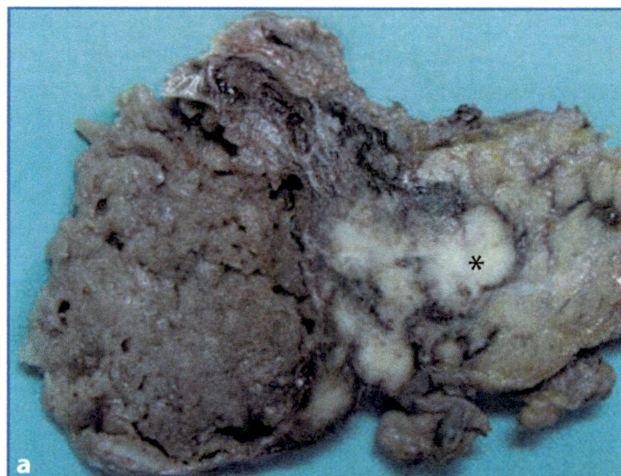

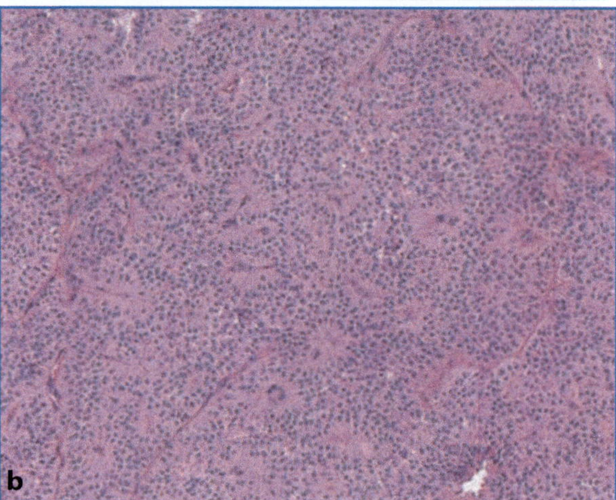

Fig. 12.24 a,b Solid-pseudopapillary tumor, with solid areas (*) and areas with fleshy pseudopapillary vegetations (**a**). Microscopic image of a solid-pseudopapillary tumor (**b**). Note the delicate vessels surrounded by neoplastic cells

epithelial lining), but they rather represent a necrotic/degenerative process. When the neoplastic cells drop away they leave aggregates of cells around a fibrovascular core, thus forming pseudo-papillae rather than real ones. The lesion does not show clear-cut pathogenetic relationship to any of the cells normally found in the pancreas; there is no evidence of ductal, acinar, or frank endocrine differentiation. Even the epithelial differentiation of this tumor type is incomplete and doubtful.

Grossly (Fig. 12.24a) it usually presents as a round well-defined mass, mainly located in the head of the pancreas, with a fibrous capsule and frequently calcified. It shows a typical alternation of solid and cystic areas without inner septations which frequently become a huge lesion with a higher proportion of degenerative necrotic-hemorrhagic events. Occasionally, the hemorrhagic-cystic changes may be extensive, mimicking a pseudocyst.

The cystic areas often contain blood, necrotic debris, and clusters of foamy macrophages. The solid component is characterized by poorly cohesive monomorphic cells with typical grooved nuclei, admixed with thin-walled blood vessels (Fig. 12.24b).

Another peculiar aspect of the tumor is its clinical behavior. The majority of cases (85-95%) are cured by surgical resection. Metastases (either to liver or peritoneum, but only seldom to lymph nodes) may be seen in a small percentage of patients, but even some patients with metastases are cured. Seldom has any death been attributed to solid-pseudopapillary neoplasm. There do not appear to be any reliable histopathologic criteria to distinguish cases that can metastasize from those that do not.

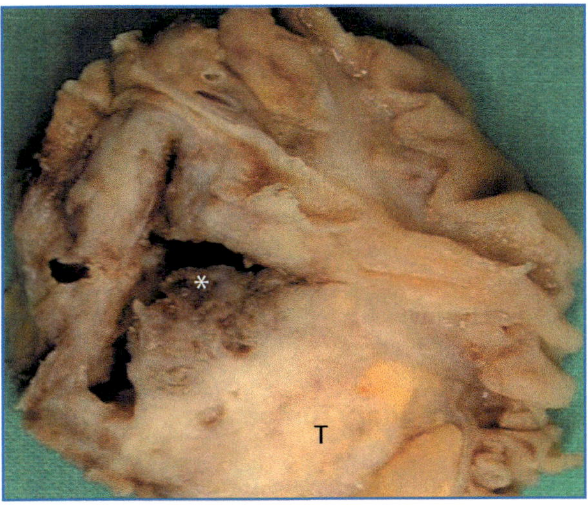

Fig. 12.25 Cystic degeneration (*) in a ductal adenocarcinoma (T)

12.5.2 Cystic Change in Ordinary Ductal Adenocarcinoma

Rarely ductal adenocarcinoma of the pancreas may undergo cystic change due to necrosis and hemorrhagic events. This occurs in less than 1% of cases. In some pancreatic cancers, a large cyst, detectable at imaging, may form because of central necrosis (Fig. 12.25). In these cases, what appears at imaging to be a cyst (a macrocyst), however, often proves microscopically to be solid, nonviable tissue surrounded by a cuff of viable carcinoma. Such cases can be misdiagnosed preoperatively as *pseudocysts*.

In other cases, ductal adenocarcinoma can obstruct the pancreatic duct and lead to cystic dilatation of the upstream duct. The dilated duct can show reactive epithelial changes, which may be indistinguishable from IPMNs or MCNs [27].

12.5.3 Cystic Pancreatic Neuroendocrine Neoplasia

Cystic pancreatic endocrine neoplasms are rare and predominantly nonfunctioning. They constitute 5-10% of pancreatic endocrine neoplasms reported in literature. In contrast to the cystic change in other solid tumors, the cyst formation in these neoplasms does not appear to be due to necrosis. Rather, the cysts are lined by a ragged cuff of well-preserved neoplastic endocrine cells, and filled with a clear fluid instead of necrotic debris. The cyst formation is usually unilocular (Fig. 12.26 a,b) and at the centre of the tumor. In some cases, however, the process is more microcystic with multiple small cysts. Some cystic pancreatic endocrine neoplasms achieve significant size, up to 25 cm. Microscopic examinations of the solid areas of the tumors

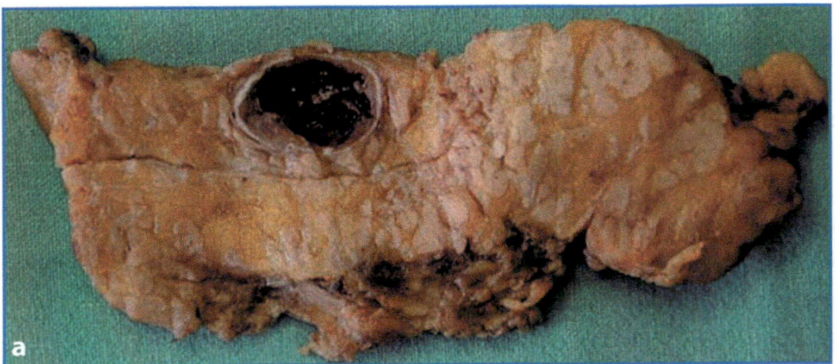
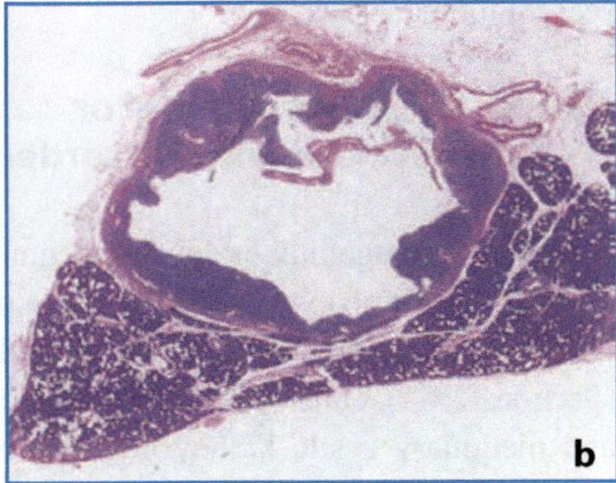

Fig. 12.26 a,b Cystic neuroendocrine tumor of the body of the pancreas (a). Macrosection image (b)

reveal characteristic features of a well-differentiated pancreatic neuroendocrine neoplasm [28].

12.5.4 Cystic Mesenchymal Neoplasms

Some mesenchymal neoplasms that occur in the pancreatic region may present as cystic lesions. Schwannomas in the pancreas especially tend to be cystic. Some sarcomas, especially GISTs, may also be cystic. Other nonepithelial tumors of this region such as paragangliomas have also been reported to present as a cyst.

12.5.5 Secondary Tumors

Rarely, metastatic neoplasms (or neoplasms that secondarily involve the pancreas) can exhibit cystic change, such as metastatic ovarian and renal cell carcinoma.

12.6　Cystic Lesions - Non Neoplastic

Other rare cystic lesions [29, 30] are cystic hamartoma, enterogenous cyst and duodenal diverticula. Cystic lesions of the common bile duct (choledochal cyst) and duodenum may also mimic pancreatic cysts.

12.6.1 Congenital Cysts

Congenital cysts of foregut derivation may also occur in the pancreas although very rarely. Essentially, these are regarded as gastrointestinal (enteric) duplications. They may have respiratory (bronchogenic) or simple ciliated epithelium.

12.6.2 Endometriotic Cyst

Endometriotic cyst with massive hemorrhage may be seen in the pancreas.

12.6.3 Cyst in Congenital or Developmental Disorders

A variety of congenital or developmental disorders may be associated with cyst formation in the pancreas, in addition to VHL-associated cystic changes discussed above (Section 12.4.1). Others include polycystic kidney disease and medullary cystic kidney. Patients with polycystic kidney disease, both adult and infantile types, may have cystic lesions in the pancreas. Rarely, patients with

medullary cystic kidneys may also have pancreatic cysts.

In patients with cystic fibrosis, the genetic defect in the cystic fibrosis transmembrane conductance regulator protein increases the viscosity of pancreatic secretions, which in turn leads to the cystic dilatation of the pancreatic ducts causing intraluminal impaction, in addition to lobular atrophy and parenchymal fibrosis. This dilatation in the ducts, however, is generally not clinically detectable. If clinically detectable it may lead to a wrong diagnosis of intraductal papillary mucinous neoplasm, but the young age should be suggestive of cystic fibrosis.

12.6.4 Cystic Lesions with no Lining – Pseudocysts

Most cavity-forming lesions of the pancreatic region are pseudocysts. The entity referred to as *pseudocyst* is a non-neoplastic complication of pancreatitis caused by alcoholic, biliary, or traumatic acute pancreatitis. It develops when a focus of peripancreatic fat necrosis is reabsorbed, producing a debris-filled space rich in pancreatic exocrine enzymes. Pseudocysts may measure up to several centimeters. The pathologic findings may vary depending on the stage of the process. The cyst contents, originally necrotic fat, transform into a mixture of necrotic cells, enzymes, scavenger cells, hematoidin pigment, cholesterol clefts, and sometimes neutrophils. There is no epithelial lining. The adjacent stroma may be hypercellular. The tissue that surrounds the necrotic material first produces granulation tissue, and eventually becomes a fibrotic pseudocapsule. Depending on the severity and duration of the pancreatitis, the pseudocyst may resolve spontaneously, or may achieve a size that

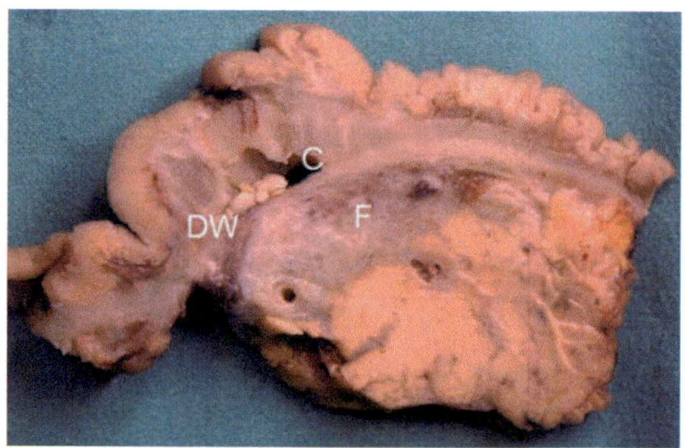

Fig. 12.27 Paraduodenal pancreatitis, cystic variant. Fibrotic area (*F*) with cyst and gallstone (*C*) in the lumen. Note the hyperplasia of the duodenal wall (*DW*)

is no longer self-absorbable, and require surgical intervention. Pseudocysts do not present a risk of malignant degeneration, and the treatment of pseudocysts differs dramatically from that of cystic neoplasms of the pancreas. Fortunately, the clinical diagnosis of a pseudocyst is usually straightforward; however, proper sampling is essential for the correct diagnosis.

12.6.5 Cyst in Paraduodenal Pancreatitis (Paraduodenal Wall Cyst/Cystic Dystrophy/Groove Pancreatitis) (Fig. 12.27)

Cysts formation is one of the complications of a subset of chronic pancreatitis that involves the second portion of the duodenum, centered on the minor papilla.

These cysts appear to occur as a consequence of chronic inflammation in the periampullary region in which one or more of the accessory ducts form a cyst on the duodenal wall. This usually occurs in the background of fibrosis and prominent proliferation of smooth muscle cells often arranged in a whorling pattern, changes that form a *pseudotumor* which frequently also involve the adjacent pancreas and the groove area (so-called groove pancreatitis). The cyst wall may be partially lined by ductal epithelium and partly by inflammation as well as granulation tissue. Total erosion of the duct epithelium may result in pseudocyst formation. Brunner's gland hyperplasia contributes to the thickening of the duodenal wall. This process may be associated with scarring of the common bile duct, mimicking pancreatic cancer [31, 32].

Other rare inflammatory cysts that can occur in the pancreas include parasitic cysts such as hydatid cyst and necrotic tuberculous infections.

References

1. Bosman FT, Carneiro F, Hruban RH et al (2010) Tumors of the pancreas. In: WHO classification of Tumors of the digestive system. IARC, Lyon, pp 279-334
2. Klimstra DS, Pitman MB, Hruban RH (2009) An algorithmic approach to the diagnosis of pancreatic neoplasms. Arch Pathol Lab Med 133:454-464
3. Capelli P, Martignoni G, Pedica F et al (2009) Endocrine neoplasm of the pancreas. Arch Pathol Lab Med 33:350-364
4. Lloyd RV, Mervak T, Schmidt K et al (1984) Immunohistochemical detection of chromogranin and neuron-specific enolase in pancreatic endocrine neoplasms. Am J Surg Pathol 8:607–614
5. Ordonez NG (2001) Pancreatic acinar cell carcinoma. Adv Anat Pathol 8:144–159
6. Klimstra DS, Heffess CS, Oertel JE et al (1992) Acinar cell carcinoma of the pancreas: a clinicopathologic study of 28 cases. Am J Surg Pathol 16:815– 837
7. Klimstra DS, Wenig BM, Adair CF et al (1995) Pancreatoblastoma: a clinicopathologic study and review of the literature. Am J Surg Pathol 19:1371–1389
8. Adsay NV, Andea A, Basturk O et al (2004) Secondary tumors of the pancreas: an analysis of a surgical and autopsy database and review of the literature. Virchows Arch 444:527–535
9. Adsay NV, Basturk O, Klimstra DS et al (2004) Pancreatic pseudotumors: non-neoplastic solid lesions of the pancreas that clinically mimic pancreas cancer. Sem Diagn Pathol 21:260-267
10. Zamboni G, Capelli P, Scarpa A et al (2009) Nonneoplastic mimickers of pancreatic neoplasms. Arch Pathol Lab Med 133:439-453
11. Zamboni G, Lüttges J, Capelli P et al (2004) Histopathological features of diagnostic and clinical relevance in autoimmune pancreatitis: a study on 53 resection specimens and 9 biopsy specimens. Virchows Arch 445:552-563
12. Kosmahl M, Pauser U, Peters K et al (2004) Cystic neoplasms of the pancreas and tumor-like lesions with cystic features: a review of 418 cases and a classification proposal. Virchows Arch 445:168–178
13. Adsay NV, Klimstra DS, Compton CC (2000) Cystic lesions of the pancreas. Introduction. Semin Diagn Pathol 17:1–6
14. Yasuhara Y, Sakaida N, Uemura Y et al (2002) Serous microcystic adenoma (glycogen-rich cystadenoma) of the pancreas: study of 11 cases showing clinicopathological and immunohistochemical correlations. Pathol Int 52:307–312
15. Zamboni G, Scarpa A, Bogina G et al (1999) Mucinous cystic tumors of the pancreas: clinicopathological features, prognosis, and relationship to other mucinous cystic tumors. Am J Surg Pathol 23:410-422
16. Edge SB, Byrd DR, Compton CC et al (2010) Exocrine and endocrine pancreas. In: AJCC Cancer Staging Manual. 7th edn. New York: Springer 24:285-296
17. Adsay NV, Longnecker DS, Klimstra DS (2000) Pancreatic tumors with cystic dilatation of the ducts: intraductal papillary mucinous neoplasms and intraductal oncocytic papillary neoplasms. Semin Diagn Pathol 17:16–30
18. Klöppel G (1998) Clinicopathologic view of intraductal papillary-mucinous tumor of the pancreas. Hepatogastroenterology 45:1981–1985
19. Crippa S, Partelli S, Falconi M (2010) Extent of surgical resections for intraductal papillary mucinous neoplasms. World J Gastrointest Surg 2:347-351
20. Zamboni G, Capelli P, Bogina G et al (2003) Pathology of intraductal cystic tumors. In: Procacci C, Megibow AJ (eds) Imaging of the pancreas. Cystic and rare tumors. Springer, Berlin Heidelberg New York, pp 85-94
21. Furukawa T, Klöppel G, Adsay NV et al (2005) Classification of types of intraductal papillary-mucinous neoplasm of the pancreas: a consensus study. Virchows Arch 447:794–799
22. Basturk O, Zamboni G, Klimstra DS et al (2007) Intraductal and papillary variants of acinar cell carcinomas: a new addition to the challenging differential diagnosis of intraductal neoplasm. Am J Surg Path 31:363-370
23. Colombo P, Arizzi C, Roncalli M (2004) Acinar cell cys-

tadenocarcinoma of the pancreas: report of rare case and review of the literature. Hum Pathol 35:1568–1571

24. Zamboni G, Terris B, Scarpa A et al (2002) Acinar cell cystadenoma of the pancreas: a new entity? Am J Surg Pathol 26: 698–704

25. Adsay NV, Klimstra DS (2000) Cystic forms of typically solid pancreatic tumors. Semin Diagn Pathol 17:66–81

26. Klimstra DS, Wenig BM, Heffess CS (2000) Solid-pseudopapillary tumor of the pancreas: a typically cystic carcinoma of low malignant potential. Semin Diagn Pathol 17:66–80

27. Lee LY, Hsu HL, Chen HM et al (2003) Ductal adenocarcinoma of the pancreas with huge cystic degeneration: a lesion to be distinguished from pseudocyst and mucinous cystadenocarcinoma. Int J Surg Pathol 11:235–239

28. Ligneau B, Lombard-Bohas C, Partensky C et al (2001) Cystic endocrine tumors of the pancreas: clinical, radiologic, and histopathologic features in 13 cases. Am J Surg Pathol 25:752–760

29. Basturk O, Coban I, Adsay NV (2009) Pancreatic cysts. Arch Pathol Lab Med 133:423-438

30. Klöppel G (2000) Pseudocysts and other non-neoplastic cysts of the pancreas. Semin Diagn Pathol 17:1–7

31. Adsay N, Zamboni G (2005) Paraduodenal pancreatitis: a clinico-pathologically distinct entity unifying 'cystic dystrophy of heterotopic pancreas', 'para-duodenal wall cyst' and 'groove pancreatitis'. Semin Diagn Pathol 21:247–254

32. Procacci C, Graziani R, Zamboni G et al (1997) Cystic dystrophy of the duodenal wall: radiologic findings. Radiology 205:741–747

Clinical and Imaging Scenarios

13

Anna Gallotti and Riccardo Manfredi

13.1 Introduction

Conventional ultrasonography (US) is the imaging modality of choice for the first-line evaluation of patients with suspected abdominal disease, to screen abdominal diseases and for the preliminary evaluation of patients with nonspecific symptoms. Conventional US is usually the first imaging method performed in symptomatic patients.

Contrast-enhanced US (CEUS) has significantly improved the accuracy of the first-line examinations, influencing the choice of second-line investigations. Contrast-enhanced multidetector computed tomography (CE-MDCT) is the criterion standard for the assessment of solid pancreatic lesions and tumor staging. Magnetic resonance imaging (MRI) with MR cholangiopancreatography (MRCP) remains the imaging modality of choice for the study of pancreatic cystic lesions and the ductal system. Other imaging modalities can be useful as third-line examinations in some cases, as subsequently described. In this chapter, the typical features of solid and cystic lesions of the pancreas according to their clinical presentation are reported. Throughout the text, a work-up algorithm is briefly proposed.

13.2 Symptomatic Solid Pancreatic Masses

1) The detection of a solid hypoechoic focal pancreatic lesion suggests the diagnosis of ductal adenocarci-

noma, which is the most common primary malignancy of the pancreas. The hypoechoic appearance and infiltrative margins, ill-defined at US, are typical US features. Most often, an upstream dilation of the main pancreatic duct is documented; if located in the pancreatic head, the *double duct sign* is often observed.

Ductal adenocarcinoma of the pancreas usually shows absence of vascular signals at Doppler study. The Doppler-study is mandatory to accurately evaluate potential vascular involvement.

The immediate administration of contrast agent (microbubbles) should be performed in the same US section. The detection of a solid hypoechoic lesion at US and hypovascular hypoenhancing lesion at CEUS should be considered a ductal adenocarcinoma until proven otherwise. A markedly hypovascular lesion is usually poorly differentiated and characterized by a worse prognosis.

The resectability or un-resectability of a lesion can be confirmed after the administration of contrast agent. The accurate evaluation of the liver during the late phase of CEUS is important to rule-out potential hepatic metastases.

2) The detection of vascular signals at Doppler study within a solid pancreatic lesion occurs in neuroendocrine tumors. However, the *Doppler silence* does not exclude this potential diagnosis. Functional endocrine pancreatic tumors are most often small in size, well marginated and related to specific clinical symptoms owing to an overproduction of pancreatic hormones. Nonfunctional endocrine pancreatic tumors usually present with mass effects, owing to their larger size; they usually present with irregular margins, sometimes with calcification and intralesional necrotic areas. The detection of a solid

A. Gallotti (✉)
Department of Radiology, IRCCS Policlinico S. Matteo
Pavia, Italy
e-mail: annagallotti@virgilio.it

hypervascular pancreatic lesion after the administration of microbubble suggests the diagnosis of a neuroendocrine tumor.

3) According to the clinical and laboratory data, a differential diagnosis between neoplastic masses and focal pancreatitis has to be considered. At US, a focal pancreatitis presents as a focal hypo-isoechoic mass; the main pancreatic duct is not infiltrated. At CEUS, it typically presents as an isoechoic mass with a parenchymal enhancement pattern.

A solid pancreatic lesion should be confirmed at CE-MDCT examination, which is useful for the staging of the disease.

In resectable lesions, surgical treatment is recommended. The endoscopic US (EUS) examination plays an important role in the T and N staging of lesions already studied by other noninvasive imaging techniques, improving the evaluation of size and shape and its relation with adjacent structures, such as pancreatic duct, bile duct and large vessels. Moreover, contrast enhancing techniques can be applied. PET/CT can be a well-established imaging method to visualize neuroendocrine pancreatic tumors, allowing a better detection of occult intrapancreatic lesions and small, unsuspected distant metastases. Especially in cases of functional neuroendocrine tumors, the intraoperative US (IOUS) can be useful for ruling out the potential coexistence of synchronous lesions hidden at preoperative imaging and to evaluate the relationship between the lesion, the main pancreatic duct and the adjacent vessels assessing the possible presence of very small liver metastases.

In cases of unresectable lesions, a fine-needle-aspiration or biopsy has to be performed before any palliative therapy (chemotherapy or radiation therapy or thermal ablation). They are almost always performed under US guidance, percutaneously or endoscopically, with better results in the presence of pathologists who can immediately evaluate the sample.

13.3   Incidental Solid Pancreatic Lesion

1) Rarely, ductal adenocarcinoma of the pancreas is incidentally discovered. As reported above, the presence of a focal solid hypoechoic hypovascular lesion of the pancreas could suggest a ductal adenocarcinoma even in asymptomatic patients. If small in size or peripherally located, in the absence of any

infiltration of nervous and vascular peripancreatic structures, they can be diagnosed in asymptomatic patients. At any rate, the upstream dilation of the main pancreatic duct can be present. The same rules described above should be applied in these cases. The Doppler study and the immediate administration of contrast agent should always be performed in the same session.

2) The incidental detection of a focal solid hypoechoic, hypervascular lesion of the pancreas should suggest the diagnosis of neuroendocrine tumor. These lesions usually consist of nonfunctioning tumor, by definition. In both cases liver metastases can be observed at the time of diagnosis even in asymptomatic patients.

A solid pancreatic lesion should be confirmed at CE-MDCT examination, which is particularly useful for the staging of the disease.

In cases of resectable lesions the surgical resection is recommended, being the treatment of choice if possible. In some cases, it could be helpful to complete the imaging staging performing a PET/CT or an EUS examination. In cases of unresectable lesions, a fine-needle-aspiration or biopsy has to be performed before any treatment is undertaken.

13.4   Symptomatic Cystic Pancreatic Lesion

1) In symptomatic patients with a history of acute or chronic pancreatitis, the pancreatic cystic lesion most frequently detected consists of pseudocysts (PSC). These appear as well marginated, rarely calcified, irregular in shape and most often unilocular anechoic lesions at conventional US. A heterogeneous content can be observed owing to the presence of debris or hemorrhagic content. After the administration of microbubbles, the complete lack of enhancement of these inclusions is mandatory to confirm the diagnosis. Moreover, this leads to making a differential diagnosis with pancreatic cystic tumors. The main pancreatic duct can be irregularly dilated in chronic pancreatitis. A pseudocyst may be suspect after at least 4-5 weeks from the acute clinical symptoms. It can become complicated by developing into a pseudoaneurysm. This is the reason why the detection of an anechoic lesion at US needs Doppler-evaluation to avoid vascular damage.

2) In young females, the detection of a large solitary lesion, grossly rounded and most often located in the pancreatic tail, characterized by a solid and cystic appearance should suggest the diagnosis of solid pseudopapillary tumor (SPT). Peripheral or central calcifications may be present. It usually shows heterogeneous content owing to the hemorrhagic degeneration and hypervascularity of the solid portion is documented. Owing to their typical location, the main pancreatic duct is usually normal in caliber. They can present with abdominal pain, most often due to recent hemorrhage.

3) In elderly males, the detection of multifocal or unifocal cystic lesions of the pancreas communicating with the main pancreatic duct should suggest the diagnosis of an intraductal papillary mucinous neoplasm (IPMN). This can be hard to detect at conventional US, as the evaluation of the communication is often too thin. Therefore, MRI with MRCP still remains the imaging modality of choice to detect an IPMN. However, CEUS plays an important role in defining the vascularity of potential inclusions, with the high spatial and contrast resolution together with the real-time evaluation of the enhancement. The symptomatic secondary-branch IPMN is usually located in the uncinate process and is usually larger than 30 mm in size, presenting with recurrent acute pancreatitis. The presence of mural nodules, thick septa and a duct of Wirsung diameter greater than 10 mm are highly suggestive for malignancy.

On the other hand, IPMN of the main duct can sometimes present with atypical symptoms, mainly related to pancreatic exocrine insufficiency. As is well known, they require a different treatment strategy compared to other forms of IPMNs, but they do need an MRI with MRCP as the criterion standard.

A cystic pancreatic lesion should be confirmed at MRI with MRCP, which is better able to define the pancreatic ductal system. The functional evaluation after secretin administration can sometimes be performed to better evaluate the exocrine pancreatic reserve.

Symptomatic pseudocysts undergo percutaneous or surgical drainage, depending on their content, which is best evaluated at MRI. PST requires surgical resection owing to its high risk of hemorrhage and potential local invasion and hepatic or peritoneum spread, even though rare. In patients with symptomatic side-branch IPMNs, a surgical resection could be recommended to avoid recurrent pancreatitis. Main type IPMNs require a multidisciplinary judgment to choose the best treatment in each patient.

As reported in the literature, PET/CT is not recommended in cystic pancreatic lesions owing to the poor FDG uptake of cystic lesions. In some cases, EUS can be helpful to better evaluate the smallest cystic lesions and their potential connection with the main pancreatic duct. Moreover, rarely, a fine-needle-aspiration of the cystic fluid can be obtained under EUS-guidance to add complementary information to the diagnosis.

13.5 Incidental Cystic Pancreatic Lesion

1) The detection of a single grossly rounded cystic lesion, usually located in the tail of the pancreas, with heterogeneous content, irregular thick wall and sometimes peripheral calcifications should be considered a mucinous cystadenoma (MCA) until proven otherwise. It is a potentially malignant tumor usually presenting as a poorly-locular round lesion, without communication with the main pancreatic duct. MCA is most frequently diagnosed in asymptomatic patients. The immediate administration of contrast agent allows its differentiation with a pseudocyst, often similar at conventional US. As reported above, the detection of vascular inclusions (irregular thick septa or mural nodules), enhancing at CEUS, rules out the diagnosis of a pseudocyst and should suggest the diagnosis of an MCA.

2) Serous cystadenoma (SCA) is a benign tumor, almost always incidentally observed in asymptomatic patients, appearing as a multiloculated lesion at conventional US, with internal thin septa oriented towards the center. The main pancreatic duct is usually normal in caliber and the lesion does not communicate with the ductal system. In some extremely microcystic types, SCA can resemble a pancreatic solid lesion.

3) In some asymptomatic patients, IPMNs and PSTs can also be detected. They show the same features reported above. Some small PSTs appear solid at diagnosis.

An incidental pancreatic cystic lesion also should be confirmed at MRI completed by MRCP, to better define the pancreatic ductal system. The functional evaluation after the administration of secretin can sometimes be performed to better evaluate the exocrine pancreatic reserve.

MCA is a premalignant lesion and thus requires surgical resection. As reported above, PST should be resected owing to its high risk of hemorrhage and its albeit low risk of local or hepatic spread. In patients with asymptomatic side-branch IPMNs imaging follow-up is recommended.

13.6   Jaundice and Double Duct Sign

In patients with jaundice, conventional US still remains the first imaging modality of choice to screen abdominal disease. The *double duct sign* consists of both the dilation of the main pancreatic duct and the common bile duct. Since ductal adenocarcinoma of the pancreas is the most frequently encountered malignant tumor and 80% of adenocarcinomas are located in the pancreatic head leading to ductal obstruction, the double duct sign should suggest the presence of pancreatic cancer until proven otherwise.

13.7   Main Pancreatic Duct Dilation

The dilation of the main pancreatic duct can be both an incidental finding at conventional US or can present as an imaging feature suggestive of specific diseases, even in symptomatic patients.

1) Considering that 80% of ductal adenocarcinoma are located in the pancreatic head and lead to duct obstruction, the detection of an irregular and marked dilation of the pancreatic duct should suggest the presence of pancreatic cancer. The ductal system usually shows an abrupt cut-off at the level of the pancreatic lesion: it is markedly dilated upstream, with pancreatic atrophy, describing the so-called *obstructive pancreatitis.*

2) IPMN of the main pancreatic duct consists of a focal or diffuse dilation of the ductal system, with a grossly tubular shape, usually reaching the papilla of Vater. Mural nodules may sometimes be detected.

3) Unlike the pattern described above, in severe chronic pancreatitis a *pearl-like duct* is often observed, characterized by an alternation between stenosis and dilations, sometimes associated with parenchymal or ductal calcifications. The main duct can be followed from the tail of the gland to the papilla without any abrupt cut-off.

As reported, the imaging modality of choice to most effectively study the pancreatic ductal system remains MRI with MRCP. However, the high spatial resolution of MDCT provides multiplanar images with higher resolution, similar to those obtained at MRI.

Flowcharts in Pancreatic Diseases

Elisabetta Buscarini

The main indications for imaging investigations of the pancreas are:

1. Jaundice
2. Midline upper abdominal pain, acute or chronic/ Upper abdominal mass/Idiopathic acute pancreatitis
3. Evaluation of acute pancreatitis: etiology?
4. Evaluation of acute pancreatitis: complications?
5. Solid pancreatic masses
6. Cystic pancreatic masses

E. Buscarini (✉)
Department of Gastroenterology,
Maggiore Hospital, Crema, Italy
e-mail: ebuscarini@rim.it

M. D'Onofrio (ed.), *Ultrasonography of the Pancreas*, © Springer-Verlag Italia 2012

14.1 Jaundice

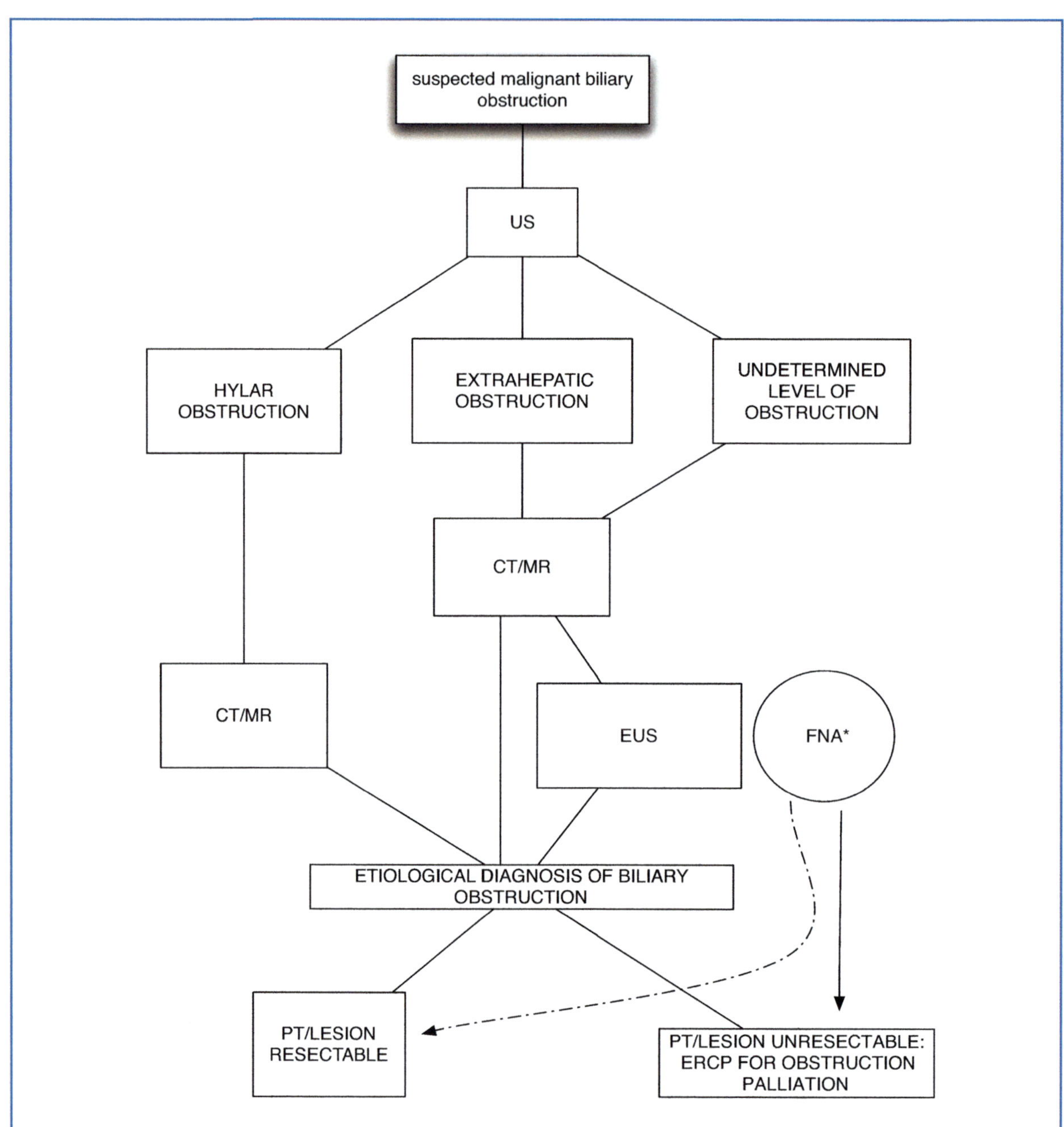

PT, patient.

Note: the use of FNA in resectable pancreatic lesions is still debated. The decision to biopsy a resectable pancreatic lesion is made on a case-by-case basis, according to the clinical, imaging and biochemical data.

*either EUS-guided or percutaneous US (CT)-guided.

14.2 Midline Upper Abdominal Pain, Acute or Chronic/Upper Abdominal Mass/Idiopathic Acute Pancreatitis

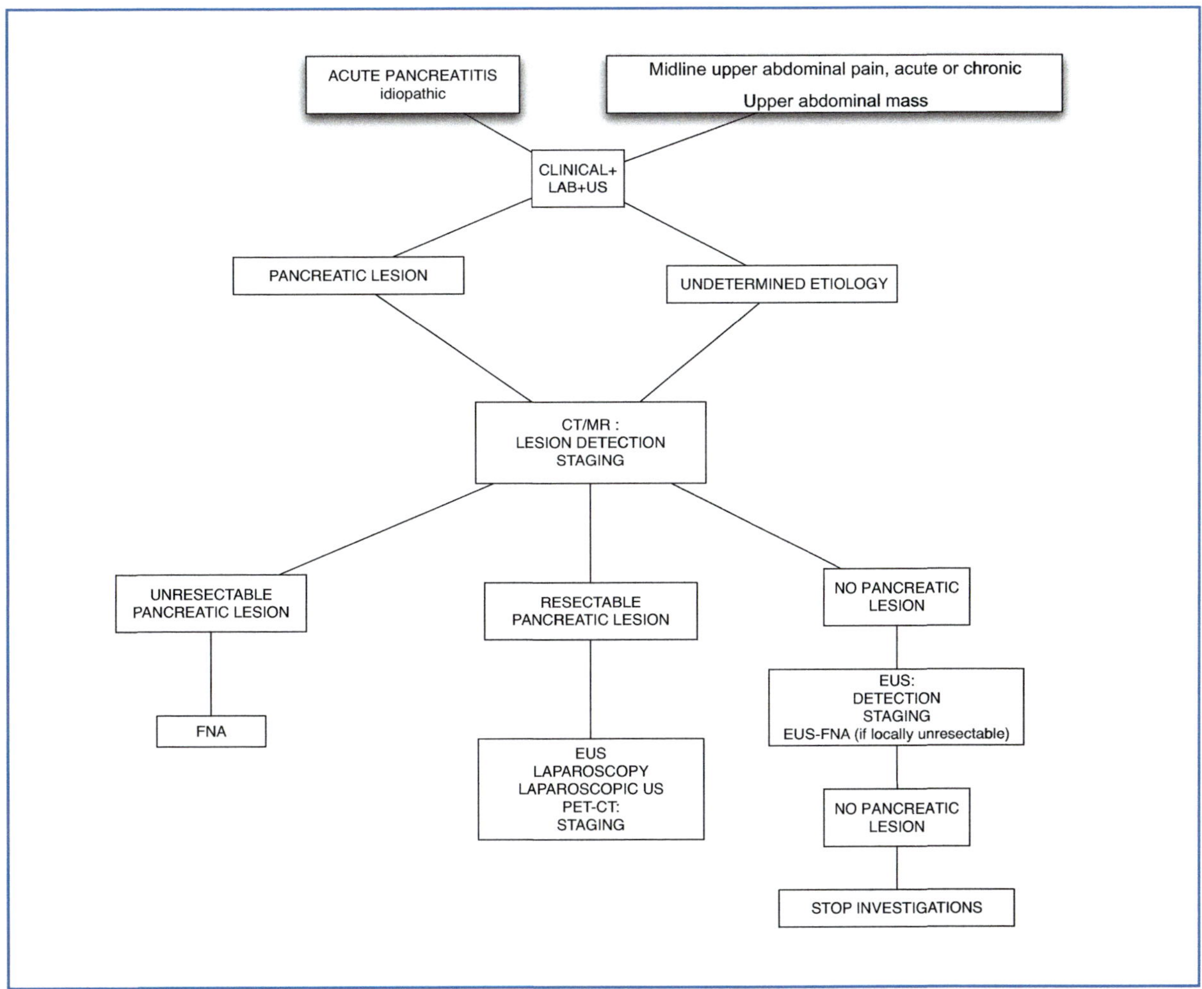

14.3 Evaluation of Acute Pancreatitis: Etiology?

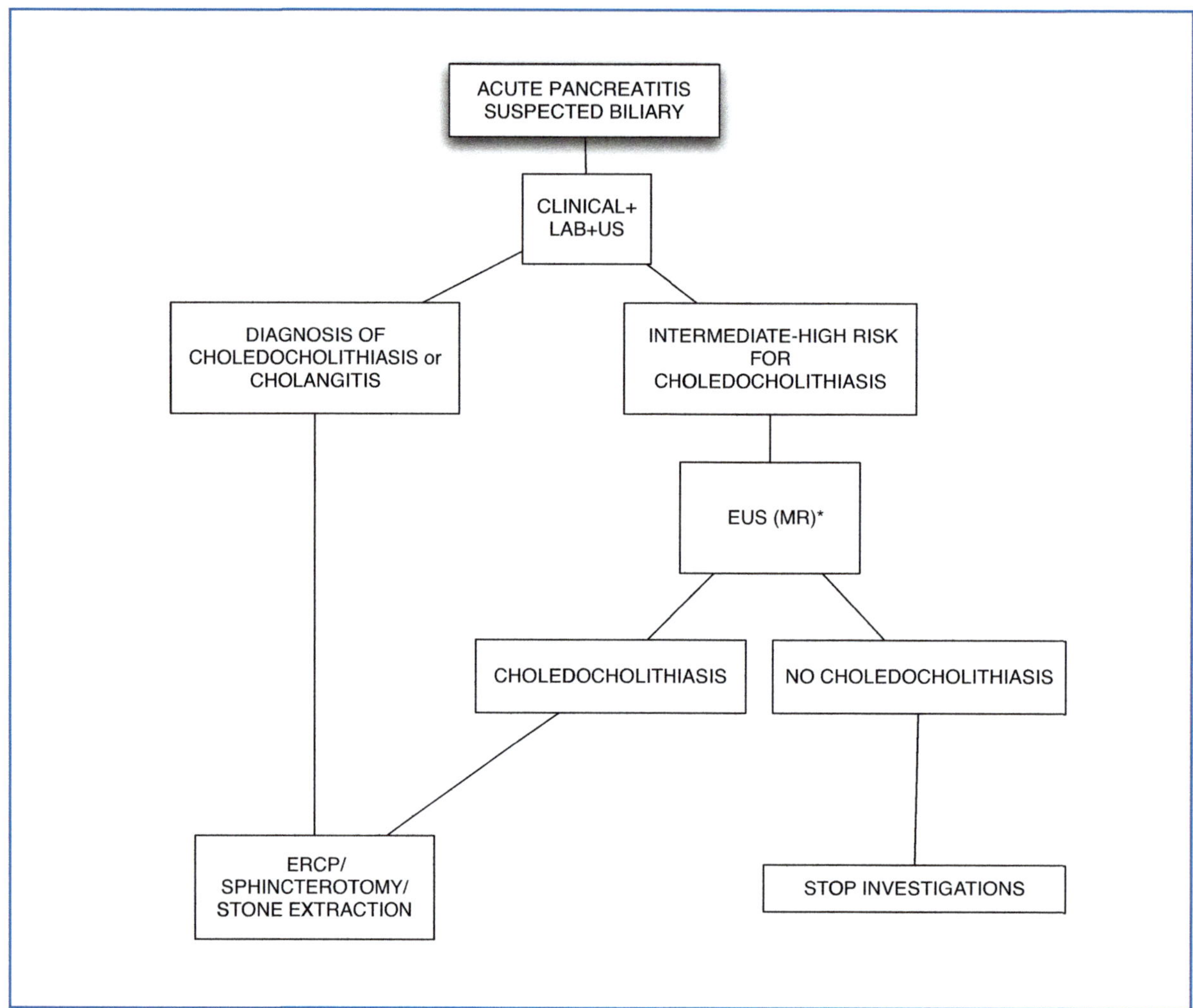

*In centers where EUS is not available, or in patients where EUS can not be performed, MR is proposed for choledocholithiasis detection.

14.4 Evaluation of Acute Pancreatitis: Complications?

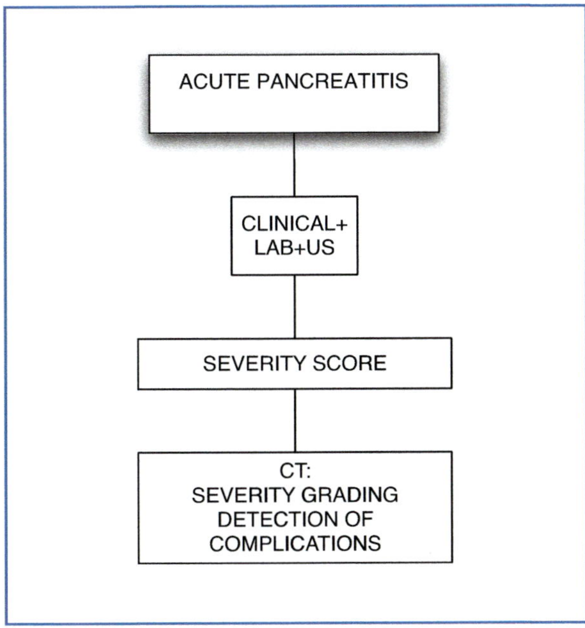

14.5   Solid Pancreatic Masses

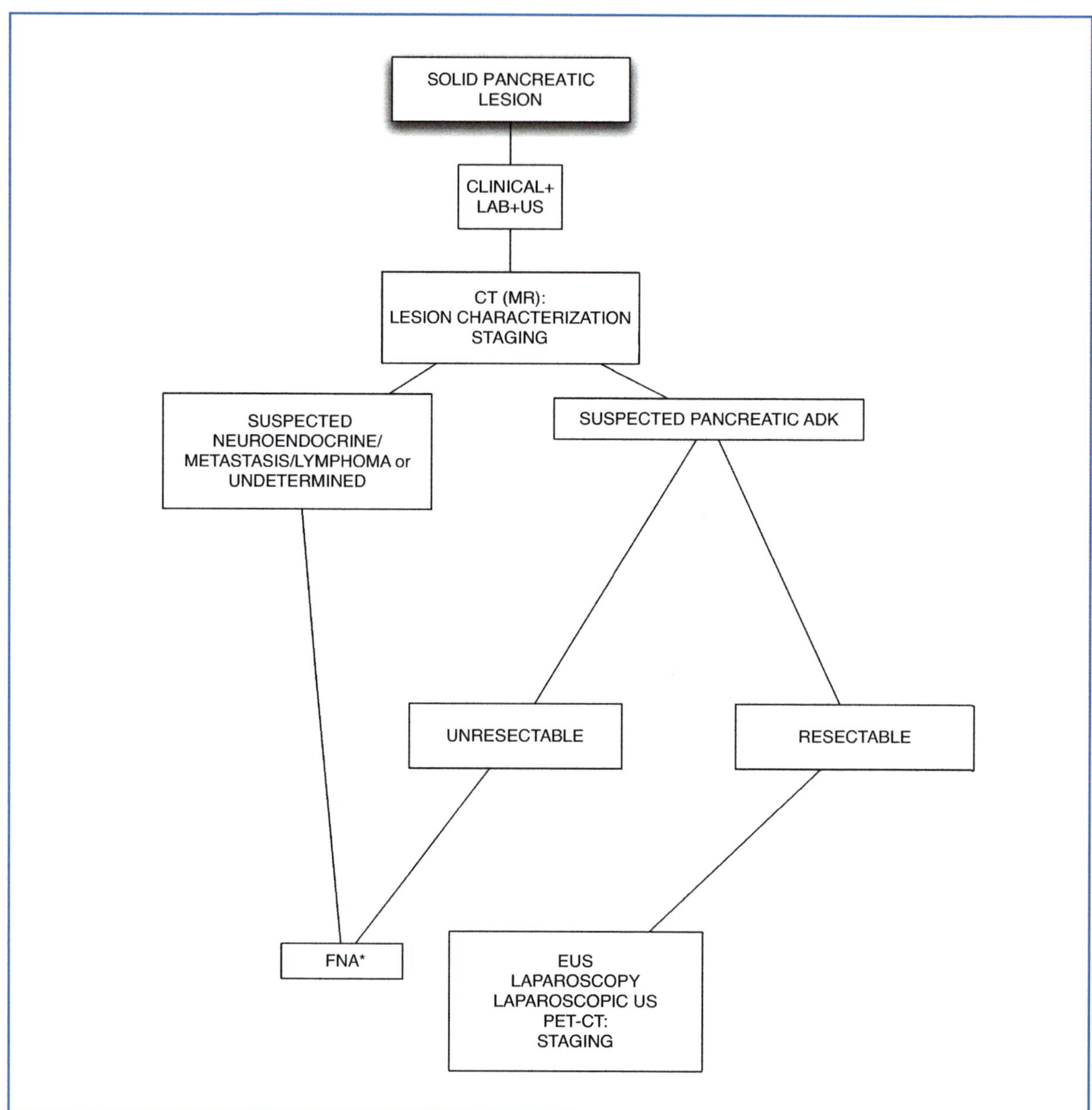

*either EUS-guided or percutaneous US (CT)-guided.

14.6   Cystic Pancreatic Masses

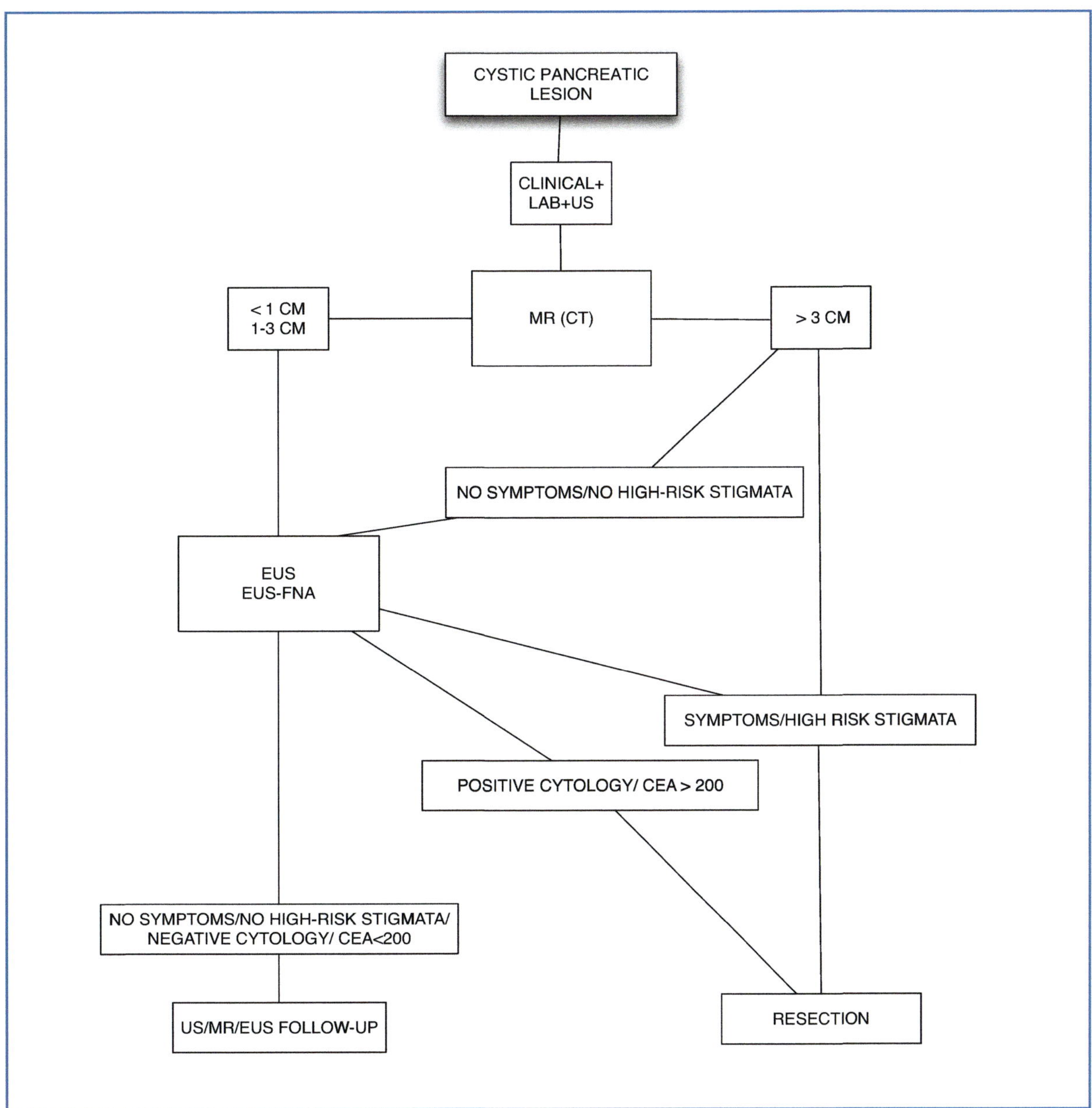

Subject Index

A

Acinar cell carcinoma 137, 166, 171, 181
Acoustic Radiation Force Impulse (ARFI) 1, 9-12, 97-98, 114-115, 121, 123-124, 127
Acute pancreatitis 19-21, 25, 34, 39-40, 65, 71, 83-86, 90, 141, 160-161, 184, 189, 191, 193-195
Adenocarcinoma 11, 14, 23, 25, 27, 33-35, 38-40, 42, 59, 88-89, 93-101, 103-107, 111, 120-122, 124-126, 128-129, 135, 137, 140-142, 148-151, 153-157, 160-161, 165-175, 178, 181, 183, 187-188, 190
Adenosquamous 168-169
Ampullary carcinoma 168
Ampullary tumor 38
Anaplastic 129, 169
Autoimmune disease 173
Autoimmune pancreatitis 22-23, 40-41, 88-89, 107, 154-155, 161, 166, 172-173, 175

B

Biopsy 9, 11, 18, 24, 31, 47-52, 55, 88, 112, 140-142, 153, 157, 174, 188, 192
Bleeding 32, 34, 52, 78, 90, 129, 140, 159
B-Mode 2-4, 9, 11, 13, 83, 85, 87, 101, 105
Branch duct type 27, 36, 125, 179

C

Calcification 3-4, 21-22, 25, 27, 33, 36, 41, 63, 72, 87-88, 103, 115, 119, 127, 129, 136-138, 141, 148, 151, 154-155, 157-160, 177, 188-190
Catheter 12, 42, 47, 50-51
CA 19-9 50, 112, 137, 140
Capsule 65, 85, 129, 135-137, 142, 158-159, 177, 182
CBD stones 19
CD 34 120, 142
CEA 36, 50, 112, 117, 122, 137, 140, 197
Central necrosis 129, 183
CEUS *see* Contrast-enhanced Ultrasound
Choledocholithiasis 40, 84, 194
Chronic pancreatitis 7, 19-23, 27, 34-36, 40-42, 58, 63-64, 74, 78, 86-89, 106-107, 111, 148, 151, 157, 161-162, 166, 168, 173-174, 179-180, 185, 188, 190
Coarse needle 47
Collateral vessel 34, 86
Colloid 107, 178, 180-181
Color-power study 7

Common bile duct 3, 17-19, 23-25, 32-33, 38-39, 41, 75, 78-79, 89, 96, 103, 166-167, 173, 180, 184-185, 190
Compounding 4
Congenital cyst 141, 184
Contrast agent 152
Contrast resolution 3-5, 10, 13, 27, 55, 71, 73-74, 88, 93, 103, 111, 150, 189
Contrast-enhanced EUS (CE-EUS) 31, 33-35, 38-40, 98-99, 104, 106
Contrast-enhanced Ultrasound (CEUS) 1, 11, 13-14, 24, 31, 39, 56-57, 73 83, 85-86, 88-89, 94-100, 102-106, 111, 113, 115-122, 125-130, 136-137, 139, 142, 147, 149-154, 156-157, 159-160, 187-189
Conventional US 1-7, 9-14, 85, 96-97, 100, 104, 114, 148-149, 152-153, 187-190
Cyst hemorrhage 151
Cystic change 25, 103, 111, 129, 137, 166, 183-184
Cystic dystrophy of the duodenal wall 28, 90
Cystic lesion 1, 3, 7, 11, 13, 26-27, 32, 36-37, 50, 86, 104, 111-125, 127-130, 142, 147, 149-152, 157-159, 161, 166, 174-175, 177, 181-182, 184, 187-189
Cystic neoplasm 4-5, 12, 25-27, 36, 112, 122, 130, 136-137, 142, 166, 175-178, 181, 185
Cystic pancreatic lesion 4, 25, 111-113, 120, 122, 124, 130, 151, 188-189, 197
Cystic pancreatic mass 5, 125-126, 191, 197

D

Detection 4, 8, 10, 19, 23, 25, 31, 35, 37-38, 40, 55-57, 60, 84-86, 93-96, 98, 102-104, 111-112, 121, 125, 128-129, 147, 149, 151, 160, 165, 168, 176-177, 187-190, 193, 195
Diagnostic procedures 47, 49-51, 112
Dilation of the main pancreatic duct 3, 27, 97, 125, 187-188, 190
Doppler 5-9, 11-12, 21-23, 26, 31, 39-40, 42, 48, 52, 56, 59, 70, 73, 83, 86-87, 90, 98, 100-104, 106-107, 111-112, 115-116, 149-150, 187-189
Doppler imaging 1, 5-6, 13, 57, 59, 122, 124
Double duct sign 23, 96-97, 153, 187, 190
Drainage of fluid 47, 84
Drainage of pseudocysts 41
Ductal adenocarcinoma 11, 23, 34, 88-89, 93-94, 96, 98-100, 103-105, 107, 111, 128, 140-142, 148-150, 153, 155-157, 161, 165-175, 178, 181, 183, 187-188, 190
Ductal obstruction 190

Duplex Doppler imaging 6
Dynamic evaluation 13, 120, 125, 150, 156

E
Elasticity modulus 10
Elastography 1, 9, 28, 35, 39-41, 86, 97-98, 104, 106, 114, 122, 160
Embryogenesis 177
Endocrine cystic tumor 129
Endocrine differentiation 169, 182
Endocrine tumor 23, 25, 38-39, 56-57, 98, 103-105, 115, 129, 137, 139, 142, 150, 154-155, 160, 169-171, 174
Endoscopic Retrograde Cholangiopancreatography (ERCP) 40, 71, 74, 78-79, 84, 86, 125, 192, 194
Endoscopic Ultrasonography 31, 49, 84
Endoscopic Ultrasound (EUS) 95, 111
Enucleation 57, 142
ERCP 40, 71, 74, 78-79, 84, 86, 125, 192, 194
Ethanol ablation 43
EUS Color Doppler 31, 39, 42
EUS criteria 33-34, 36, 40
EUS elastography 35, 39-41
EUS-guided therapy 42

F
Fat 1, 18-21, 31, 57, 63, 65-66, 71, 75, 137, 141-142, 148, 151, 156, 174, 184
Fibrotic pseudocapsule 170, 184
Fibrus content, contrast-enhancement 150
Fine-needle aspiration (FNA) 56
Fistula 90, 177, 180
Flat-T probe 55-56
Fluid collection 3, 19-21, 47, 50-52, 83-86, 89
Fluid-solid differentiation 3-4
FNA 31-32, 34-37, 39-40, 47-48, 50, 56, 88, 112, 117, 122, 128, 130, 192
Follow-up 13, 27, 36, 43, 51, 84, 86, 117, 130, 190, 197
Functioning endocrine tumor 139, 142

G
Gallbladder 19, 24, 65, 67-69, 71, 76-78, 80-81, 84, 168
Gastrinoma 23, 25, 102-103, 138-139
Gauge 31, 42, 47, 50, 75, 112
Groove pancreatitis 28, 75, 90, 173, 185

H
Hemorrhagic 129, 136-137, 151, 158-159, 170, 175, 177, 182-183, 188-189
Histologic sampling 47
Hypervascular pancreatic lesion 188
Hypovascular hypoenhancing lesion 187

I
IgG4 173
Image fusion 3
Image quality 3-4, 9, 56, 93, 125, 149, 151, 159
Incidentaloma 170
Incidental pancreatic cyst 129-130, 189
Infiltrative 74, 97, 153, 166, 170, 187
Insulinoma 23, 25, 38, 56-57, 102-103, 138, 169-170

International normalized ratio 49
Interstitial edema 19, 84
Interventional procedure 3, 19, 31, 47, 55, 58, 71, 84, 160
Intraductal calculi 22-23
Intraductal papillary mucinous neoplasm (IPMN) 56, 76, 107, 113, 114, 125, 128, 149-151, 153, 159, 161, 166, 177, 179-181, 183, 189-190
Intraductal papillary mucinous tumor (IPMT) 27, 36-37
Intraductal ultrasonography (IDUS) 31, 33, 36-37
Intraoperative ultrasonography (IOUS) 55
Intraperitoneal space 64, 66, 76, 80
IOUS-guidance 55-59
I-shaped transducer 55

J
Jaundice 23, 137-138, 140, 165-166, 169, 171, 174, 176, 190-192

K
K-ras 128
Ki67 104, 169

L
Laparoscopic 1, 55-56, 58-60, 193, 196
Lesion conspicuity 4, 149
Linear scanning 31-32
Liver staging 56-57, 99-100
Lymph nodes 9, 25, 27, 34, 39, 41, 121, 124, 128, 129, 135, 138-139, 168, 171, 173, 175, 183
Lymphangioma 141, 166, 182
Lymphoid tissue 175, 181-182
Lymphoma 24-25, 40, 49, 137-138, 140-141, 166, 172, 175, 196

M
Macrocystic 117, 118, 157-159, 176, 181
Magnetic Resonance Colangiopancreatography (MRCP) 111, 114
Magnetic Resonance Imaging (MRI) 1, 31, 56, 63, 86, 95, 111, 136, 147, 187
Main duct type 26-27, 37, 125, 179
Main pancreatic duct 3, 22, 26-27, 31, 33, 36, 38, 40, 41, 56-57, 63, 73-74, 88, 90, 96-97, 113-115, 117, 118, 125-130, 148, 151-153, 155, 170, 173, 179-180, 187-190
MDCT 104, 111, 127, 136-138, 141-142, 147-161, 187-188, 190
Mean vascular density (MVD) 99, 105
Menghini needle 49
Mesenteric vein 8, 17-19, 21, 23, 31, 34, 58, 67-70, 75-76, 79-80, 96, 100-101, 161, 167
Mesenteric vessel's bed 167
Metastasis 34-35, 39, 49, 58, 60, 102, 135, 137, 139, 165-166, 168, 172, 196
Microbubbles 11-14, 56, 86, 104, 120, 128, 149-152, 154, 187-188
Microcystic 26, 39, 113-117, 137, 153, 157-158, 176, 183, 189
Microcystic cystadenoma 26, 176
Midazolam 32
Misdiagnosed 140, 173-174, 183
MRI 1, 13, 31, 35-36, 38, 56-57, 63, 65-66, 69, 71-75, 86, 89,

95, 104, 111, 113, 115-118, 120-125, 127, 129-130, 136-142, 147-161, 180, 187, 189-190
Mucinous cystadenocarcinoma 121, 123, 125, 126
Mucinous cystadenoma (MCA) 117, 119-121, 124, 157, 189
Mucinous cystic neoplasm 4-5, 12, 27, 122, 129, 137, 166, 177-178, 181
Mucinous noncystic carcinoma 169
Multidetector Computed Tomography (MDCT) 104, 111, 147
Multifrequency transducers 2
Multiplanar reconstruction 5
Mural nodule 27, 36-37, 111, 121, 124, 127, 128, 150, 153, 159, 178, 180, 189-190
MVD 13, 99, 105

N
Necrosis 13, 19-21, 23, 25, 33, 35, 42-43, 83-86, 89, 93, 97, 99, 103, 107, 129, 137, 160, 166, 169, 171, 183-184
Necrotizing pancreatitis 20, 85
Needle 11, 31, 37, 41-42, 47-52, 56, 58-59, 88, 107, 112, 141, 153, 188-189
Neuroendocrine carcinoma 24, 169
Neuroendocrine tumor 25, 32, 35, 38-40, 49, 67, 102-104, 106, 111, 128, 138, 140, 153-154, 166, 169, 177, 181, 183, 187-188
Neurolysis of the celiac plexus 41, 42
Nodule 9, 25, 27, 36, 40, 57, 58, 94, 98, 102, 103, 111, 112, 115, 119-122, 124-129, 137, 150-153, 159, 175, 178, 180, 189, 190
Nonfunctioning endocrine tumor 142
Nonfunctioning islet cell tumors (NFETs) 103

O
Obstructive chronic pancreatitis 166, 168
Obstructive pancreatitis 139, 167, 179, 190
Oligocystic serous cystadenoma 26
Onsite cytology 52
Ovarian-like stroma 178

P
Pancreatic
    abscess 21, 86
    adenocarcinoma 14, 33-35, 39-40, 42, 59, 88, 94-101, 105-107, 135, 137, 148-149, 151, 153, 156, 160, 167
    cancer 4, 23, 31, 33-35, 40, 42, 49, 51, 59, 77, 88, 93, 96, 101, 106, 140-141, 156-157, 165, 172, 174, 183, 185, 190
    cystic lesion 11, 32, 111-112, 114-115, 121, 123, 125, 129, 151, 187-189
    embryology 76
    endocrine component 66
    exocrine component 65, 68
    fluid collection 3, 50-51, 85
    lymphoma 24-25, 137, 140-141
    metastases 25, 142, 172
    microscopy 65, 137, 168, 170, 178, 180
    portion 167, 173
    pseudocyst 20, 86, 89-90, 137, 141
    pseudolesion 80
    uncinate process 139
    volume 21, 80, 86
Pancreatic anatomic variants
    annular pancreas 75, 78, 79, 175

ectopic pancreas 78, 80
    pancreas divisum 19, 76-88
    pancreatic agenesis 76, 79, 80
Pancreatic anatomy
    axial planes 67, 68, 70, 72
    coronal planes 72
    sagittal planes 67-69, 72
    calcification 22, 88, 148, 160
Pancreatic duct
    dilatation 20-21, 23, 26, 33, 36, 40
    accessory 71, 75, 77-79, 185
    anatomic variant 66, 71, 76, 78-80
    Santorini 66, 71, 74-79, 173
    second order 66, 76
Pancreatitis, focal 19, 23, 49, 84, 88, 157, 188
Pancreatoblastoma 137-138, 166, 171
PanIN 107, 181
Papillary projection 27, 177, 179
Pararenal space
    compartment anterior 18, 20, 64, 84
    compartment posterior 64
Parenchymal enhancement pattern 188
Pearl-like duct 190
Perfusion 14, 20, 85, 93, 105-106, 120, 124, 129, 136, 155
PET/CT 95, 188-189
Platelet count 32, 49
Posterior lamina 166-167
Progression 40, 107, 178
Prothrombin 49
Pseudocyst 20-21, 25, 36-37, 41-42, 50-52, 83, 86, 89-90, 111-113, 120, 122, 129, 137, 141, 150-152, 157, 159-161, 166, 175, 177-178, 183-185, 188-189
Pseudolymphoma 166, 175
Pseudomyxoma peritonei 180
Pseudo-papillae 182
Pseudopapillary and solid tumor 158, 159
Pseudotumor 23, 40, 154-155, 161, 166, 172-175, 185

R
Radial scanning 31-32
Radiofrequency ablation (RFA) 56, 71
Real-time evaluation 1, 13, 35, 42, 105, 111, 128, 152, 154, 189
Resectability 8, 13, 34-35, 56-57, 100, 187
Resectable lesions 100, 188
Resectable/unresectable pancreatic tumor 50, 56, 59
Retroperitoneal margin 167
RFA 56, 59, 71
Risk factor 32, 104, 129

S
Salt-and pepper 171
Seldinger technique 50
Septa 4, 27, 36, 39, 41, 111, 113, 115-122, 125, 127, 129, 136, 138, 141-142, 150-153, 156-159, 176-177, 189
Serous cystadenoma (SCA) 113, 153, 189
Shear wave 10-12
Solid pancreatic lesion 31, 104, 151, 187-188, 196
Solid pancreatic mass 35, 93, 187, 191, 196
Solid-pseudopapillary tumor (SPT) 129, 135-137, 166, 189

Somatostatin 66-67, 139-140, 170
Sonoelasticity 1, 9
Spatial resolution 2, 4, 8-9, 71, 94, 102, 122, 128, 149, 160, 190
Splenic vein 3, 5, 17-22, 24, 26, 31, 33, 38, 64, 66-70, 75, 137
Staging of pancreatic cancer 34-35
Superior mesenteric artery 8, 17-18, 23-24, 33-34, 48, 64, 66-70, 75-76, 79-80, 100, 161, 167
Superior mesenteric vein 8, 17-19, 21, 23, 31, 34, 58, 67-70, 75-76, 79-80, 96, 100-101, 161
Symptomatic 27, 41, 50, 78, 112, 117, 121, 128-130, 139, 168, 170, 174, 179, 187-190

T
Temporal resolution 8, 12, 150
Therapeutic procedure 47, 50-51, 57, 71
Tissue characterization 11, 150-151
Tissue harmonic imaging (THI) 1-4, 10, 86, 149
Tissue stiffness 9-11, 35, 96
TNM 34, 169
Transabdominal conventional ultrasonography (US) 17
Trocar technique 50-51
Tru-cut needle 49

Tumor seeding 51

U
Unresectable adenocarcinoma 148
Unresectable lesion 188
Upper abdominal mass 191, 193
US examination 2, 5, 11, 14, 17, 21, 27-28, 72, 94, 136, 147
US flow imaging modalities 9
Us-guided fine-needle biopsy (FNB) 49

V
Vascular
    complications 21, 84, 86
    invasion 7, 34, 36, 57, 100, 138, 166, 168
    structures 3, 5-7, 9, 52, 56-57, 72, 85, 100, 149
Vessel 5-7, 9-10, 13, 17-18, 21, 23, 26, 31, 33-34, 41-42, 48, 55, 57-58, 63-64, 70, 72, 74, 86, 90, 97-103, 106-107, 112, 115-116, 120, 138, 142, 167-168, 170-171, 182-183, 188
Volumetric image acquisition 4
Von-Hippel Lindau 113

W
Wirsung 19, 22-24, 26, 32-33, 37, 39, 41, 66-68, 70-71, 73-79, 128, 166-167, 170,

9788847023789